Qualitative Research
in Nursing and Healthcare

Qualitative Research
in Nursing and Healthcare

Immy Holloway
Stephanie Wheeler

Third Edition

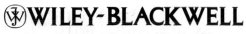

A John Wiley & Sons, Ltd., Publication

This edition first published 2010
Second edition published 2002
First edition published 1996
This edition © 2010 by Immy Holloway and Stephanie Wheeler
First and second editions © 1996, 2002 by Blackwell Publishing Ltd

Blackwell Publishing was acquired by John Wiley & Sons in February 2007. Blackwell's publishing programme has been merged with Wiley's global Scientific, Technical, and Medical business to form Wiley-Blackwell.

Registered office
John Wiley & Sons Ltd, The Atrium, Southern Gate, Chichester, West Sussex, PO19 8SQ, United Kingdom

Editorial offices
9600 Garsington Road, Oxford, OX4 2DQ, United Kingdom
2121 State Avenue, Ames, Iowa 50014-8300, USA

For details of our global editorial offices, for customer services and for information about how to apply for permission to reuse the copyright material in this book please see our website at www.wiley.com/wiley-blackwell.

The right of the author to be identified as the author of this work has been asserted in accordance with the Copyright, Designs and Patents Act 1988.

Wiley also publishes its books in a variety of electronic formats. Some content that appears in print may not be available in electronic books.

Designations used by companies to distinguish their products are often claimed as trademarks. All brand names and product names used in this book are trade names, service marks, trademarks or registered trademarks of their respective owners. The publisher is not associated with any product or vendor mentioned in this book. This publication is designed to provide accurate and authoritative information in regard to the subject matter covered. It is sold on the understanding that the publisher is not engaged in rendering professional services. If professional advice or other expert assistance is required, the services of a competent professional should be sought.

Library of Congress Cataloging-in-Publication Data

Holloway, Immy.
  Qualitative research in nursing and healthcare / Immy Holloway, Stephanie Wheeler. – 3rd ed.
    p. ; cm.
  Rev. ed. of: Qualitative research in nursing / Immy Holloway, Stephanie Wheeler. 2nd ed. 2002.
  Includes bibliographical references and index.
  ISBN 978-1-4051-6122-0 (pbk. : alk. paper) 1. Nursing – Research – Methodology. 2. Qualitative research.
I. Wheeler, Stephanie. II. Holloway, Immy. Qualitative research in nursing. III. Title.
  [DNLM: 1. Nursing Research – methods. 2. Health Services Research – methods. WY 20.5 H745q 2010]
  RT81.5.H656 2010
  610.73072 – dc22

                                                                                    2009019840

A catalogue record for this book is available from the British Library.

Typeset in 10/13 Sabon by Laserwords Private Limited, Chennai, India
Printed and bound in Malaysia by KHL Printing Co Sdn Bhd

1   2010

Contents

Preface

In this, the third edition of our book, we consider some of the changes that have taken place since the last edition. All chapters, and most of the examples within them, have been updated. In the light of developments in qualitative health research, a mixed methods research chapter was added.

The reference lists at the end of each chapter are still long and include significant and foundational texts as well as less important references. We aimed to give qualitative health researchers a variety of articles and books which they can follow up themselves depending on their choice of approach. The references provide guidance for further and more detailed reading.

The book addresses a somewhat wider readership than before. Nurses, midwives and health visitors are still the main professions which will use the text; however, it could also be helpful for other health researchers such as doctors and professions allied to medicine, for instance physio- and occupational therapists. The groups for whom this book is intended are thus

1. professionals in the healthcare field who wish to carry out qualitative research in clinical or educational settings;
2. undergraduates, especially mature students who already have some research experience;
3. pre-registration students with an appreciation of research who wish to learn about qualitative perspectives;
4. postgraduates who undertake a qualitative research project and want to revise qualitative research strategies and procedures before proceeding to more sophisticated texts.

We have attempted to provide researchers with theoretical understanding and practical knowledge. Novice researchers might find some of the issues rather complex, and we tried to make abstract ideas more understandable and explained practical procedures in some detail but, we hope, without too much simplification.

How to read this book

Researchers need not read this book from start to finish, although it would help them understand the nature of qualitative research. In particular, they can be selective about part three, depending on the approach they choose.

Acknowledgements

We are grateful to our editor Katrina Hulme-Cross for her patience and support. Thanks are also due, as always, to our friend Dr. Jan Walker for her advice, and to a variety of colleagues who reviewed individual chapters.

PART ONE

Introduction to Qualitative Research: Initial Stages

CHAPTER 1

The Nature and Utility of Qualitative Research

What is qualitative research?

Qualitative research is a form of social inquiry that focuses on the way people make sense of their experiences and the world in which they live. A number of different approaches exist within the wider framework of this type of research, and many of these share the same aim – to understand, describe and interpret social phenomena as perceived by individuals, groups and cultures. Researchers use qualitative approaches to explore the behaviour, feelings and experiences of people and what lies at the core of their lives. For example, ethnographers focus on culture and customs; grounded theorists investigate social processes and interaction, while phenomenologists consider and illuminate a phenomenon and describe the 'life world' or *Lebenswelt*. Qualitative approaches are useful in the exploration of change or conflict. The basis of qualitative research lies in the interpretive approach to social reality and in the description of the lived experience of human beings.

The main features of qualitative research

Different types of qualitative research share common characteristics and use similar procedures though differences in data collection and analysis do exist.
The following elements are part of most qualitative approaches:

- The data have primacy (priority); the theoretical framework is not predetermined but derives directly from the data.
- Qualitative research is context-bound and researchers must be context sensitive.
- Researchers immerse themselves in the natural setting of the people whose behaviour and thoughts they wish to explore.
- Qualitative researchers focus on the 'emic' perspective, the views of the people involved in the research and their perceptions, meanings and interpretations.

- Qualitative researchers use 'thick description': they describe, analyse and interpret but also go beyond the constructions of the participants.
- The relationship between the researcher and the researched is close and based on a position of equality as human beings.
- Reflexivity in the research makes explicit the stance of the researcher, who is the main research tool.

The primacy of data

Researchers usually approach people with the aim of finding out about their concerns; they go to the participants to collect the rich and in-depth data that can then become the basis for theorising. The interaction between the researcher and the participants leads to an understanding of experience and the generation of concepts. The data themselves have primacy, generate new theoretical ideas, and they help modify already existing theories or uncover the essence of phenomena. It means that the research design cannot be predefined before the start of the research. In other types of research, assumptions and ideas lead to hypotheses which are tested (though this is not true for all quantitative research); sampling frames are imposed; in qualitative research, however, the data have priority. The theoretical framework of the research project is not predetermined but based on the incoming data. Although the researchers do have knowledge of some of the theories involved, the incoming data might confirm or contradict existing assumptions and theory.

This approach to social science is, initially at least, inductive. Researchers move from the specific to the general, from the data to theory or analytic description. They do not impose ideas or follow up assumptions but give accounts of reality as seen by the participants. Researchers must be open-minded – though they cannot help having some 'hunches' about what they may find, especially if they are familiar with the setting and some of the literature on the topic.

While some qualitative inquiry is concerned with the generation of theory such as grounded theory, many researchers do not achieve this; others, such as phenomenologists, focus on a particular phenomenon to illuminate it. All approaches usually provide descriptions or interpretation of participants' experiences and the phenomenon to be studied but go to a more abstract and theoretical level in their written work, especially when they carry out postgraduate research. Qualitative inquiry is not static but developmental and dynamic in character; the focus is on process as well as outcomes.

Contextualisation

Researchers must be sensitive to the context of the research and immerse themselves in the setting and situation. Both personal and social context is important. The context of participants' lives or work affects their behaviour, and therefore researchers have to realise that the participants are grounded in their history and temporality. Researchers take into account the total context of people's lives and the broader political and social framework of the culture in which it takes place. The conditions in which they gather the data, the locality, time and history are all involved. Events and actions are studied as they occur in everyday 'real life settings'. Koro-Ljungberg (2008) states that participants not only have personal values and beliefs but are also connected with their environment, and this influences their interactions with the researcher. It is important to respect the context and culture in which the study takes place. If researchers understand the context, they can locate the actions and perceptions of individuals and grasp the meanings that they communicate. The interest in context and contextualisation goes beyond that which influences the research; it also affects its outcomes and applications in the clinical situation. Scott *et al.* (2008) add that organisational context, group membership and other factors are also important in the applications and use of the research in healthcare settings.

Immersion in the setting

Qualitative researchers use the strategies of observing, questioning and listening, immersing themselves in the 'real' world of the participants. Observing, listening and asking questions will lead to rich data. Involvement in the setting also assists in focusing on the interactions between people and the way they construct or change rules and situations. Qualitative inquiry can trace progress and development over time, as perceived by the participants.

For the understanding of participants' experiences, it is necessary to become familiar with their world. When professionals do research, they are often part of the setting they investigate and know it intimately. This might mean that they could miss important issues or considerations. To better be able to examine the world of the participant, researchers must not take this world for granted but should question their own assumptions and act like strangers to the setting or as 'naïve' observers. They 'make the familiar strange' (Delamont and Atkinson (1995) called their book *Fighting Familiarity*). Immersion might mean attending meetings with or about informants, becoming familiar with other similar situations, reading documents or observing interaction in the setting. This can even start before the formal data collection phase.

Most qualitative inquiry investigates patterns of interaction, seeks knowledge about a group or a culture or explores the life world of individuals. In clinical, social care or educational settings, this may be interaction between professionals and clients or relatives, or interaction with colleagues. It also means listening to people and attempting to see the world from their point of view. The research can be a macro- or micro-study – for instance, it may take place in a hospital ward, a classroom, a residential home, a reception area or indeed the community.

Immersion in the culture of a hospital or hospital ward, for instance, does not just mean getting to know the physical environment but also the particular ideologies, values and ways of thinking of its members. Researchers need sensitivity to describe or interpret what they observe and hear. Human beings are influenced by their experiences therefore qualitative methods encompass processes and changes over time in the culture or subculture under study.

The 'emic' perspective

Qualitative approaches are linked to the subjective nature of social reality; they provide insights from the perspective of participants, enabling researchers to see events as their informants do; they explore 'the insiders' view'. Anthropologists and linguists call this the *emic perspective* (Harris, 1976). The term was initially coined by the linguist Pike in 1954. It means that researchers attempt to examine the experiences, feelings and perceptions of the people they study, rather than immediately imposing a framework of their own that might distort the ideas of the participants. They 'uncover' the meaning people give to their experiences and the way in which they interpret them, although meanings should not be reduced to purely subjective accounts of the participants as researchers search for patterns in process and interaction, or the invariant constituents of the phenomenon they study.

Qualitative research is based on the premise that individuals are best placed to describe situations and feelings in their own words. Of course, these meanings may be unclear or ambiguous and they are not fixed; the social world is not frozen in a particular moment or situation but dynamic and changing. By observing people and listening to their accounts, researchers seek to understand the process by which participants make sense of their own behaviour and the rules that govern their actions. Taking into account their informants' intentions and motives researchers gain access to their social reality. Of course, the report individuals give are *their* explanations of an event or action, but as the researcher wishes to find people's own definition of reality, these reports are valid data. Researchers cannot always rely on the participants' accounts but are able to take their words and actions as reflections of underlying meanings. The qualitative approach requires 'empathetic understanding', that is, the investigators must try to examine the situations, events and actions from the participants' – the social actors' – point of view and not impose their own perspective. The meanings of participants are interpreted or a phenomenon identified and described. Researchers have access to the participants' world through experience and observation. This type of research is thought to empower participants, because they do not merely react to the questions of the researchers but have a voice and guide the study. For this reason, the people studied are generally called *participants* or *informants* rather than subjects. It is necessary that the relationship between researcher and informant is one of trust; this close relationship and the researcher's in-depth knowledge of the informant's situation make deceit unlikely (though not impossible).

Of course, researchers theorise or infer from observed behaviour or participants' words. The researcher's view, the analytical and more abstract interpretation and description, is the *etic perspective* – the outsider's view (Harris, 1976). Researchers move back and forth between the emic perspective of the participants and their own etic view. These ideas correspond directly to those of Denzin (1989) who speaks of first- and second-order constructs. First-order constructs are those used in the common-sense perspective on everyday life, while second-order constructs are more abstract and imposed by the researcher. For instance, individuals often mention the term 'learning the job' which could be called a first-order concept recognised by people in everyday life. A social scientist would call the same concept 'occupational socialisation', a second-order concept. The two terms show the difference between 'lay language' and 'academic language'. It must be kept in mind, however, that the emic view cannot be simply translated into an etic perspective but demands analysis and reflection from the researcher.

Thick description

Immersion in the setting will help researchers use *thick description* (Geertz, 1973; first used by the philosopher Gilbert Ryle). It involves detailed portrayals of the participants' experiences, going beyond a report of surface phenomena to their interpretations, uncovering feelings and the meanings of their actions. This also means that researchers create and produce another layer constructed from that of the participants. Thick description develops from the data and the context. The task involves describing the location and the people within it, giving visual pictures of setting, events and situations as well as verbatim narratives of individuals' accounts of their perceptions and ideas in context.

The description of the situation or discussion should be thorough; this means that writers describe everything in vivid detail. Indeed Denzin (1989: 83) defines thick description as: 'deep, dense, detailed accounts of problematic experiences... It presents detail, context, emotion and the webs of social relationship that join persons to one another.' Thick description is not merely factual, but includes theoretical and analytic description.

Thick description helps readers of a research study to develop an active role in the research because the researchers share their knowledge of the participants' perspective with the readers of the study. Through clear description of the culture, the context and the process of the research, the reader can follow the path of the researcher and share some understanding of the phenomenon or the culture under study. Thick description not only shows readers of the story what they themselves would experience were they in the same situation as the participants, but it also generates theoretical and abstract ideas which the researcher has developed.

Ponterotto (2006) develops the concept of 'thick description', traces its evolution and stresses the importance of context. He states that the discussion of a qualitative research report 'successfully merges the participants' lived experiences with the interpretations of these experiences...' (p. 547)

The importance of the research relationship

In order to gain access to the true thoughts and feelings of the participants, researchers adopt a non-judgemental stance towards the thoughts and words of the participants. The relationship should be built on mutual trust. This is particularly important in interviews and observations. The listener becomes the learner in this situation, while the informant is the teacher who is also encouraged to be reflective. Rapport does not automatically imply an intimate relationship or deep friendship (Spradley, 1979), but it does lead to negotiation and sharing of ideas though each relationship is unique in the context of time and place. Rapport and trust make the research more interesting for the participants because they feel able to ask questions. Negotiation is not a once and for all event but a continuous process, indeed Boulton (2007: 2191) speaks of social science relationships as 'more enduring, negotiated and equal'. In qualitative inquiry the participants have more power because they can guide the researcher to issues that are of concern for them. Miller and Boulton (2007: 2200) state that the relationship between participants is one of continuously shifting boundaries between the professional and the personal.

The researcher should answer questions about the nature of the project as honestly and openly as possible without creating bias in the study.

Reflexivity

Reflexivity is critical reflection on what has been thought and done in a qualitative research project. It locates the researcher in the research project. Finlay (2002a: 531) names reflexivity as the process 'where researchers engage in explicit, self-aware analysis of their own role'. It is a conscious attempt by researchers to acknowledge their own involvement in the study – a form of self-monitoring in relation to the research that is being carried out. It also includes awareness of the interaction between the researcher, the participants and the research itself and it takes into account how the process of the research affects findings and eventual outcomes.

'Critical subjectivity', as Etherington (2004) calls it, means adopting a critical stance to oneself as researcher. Personal response and thoughts about the research and research participants is taken into account, and researchers are aware and take stock of their own social location and how this affects the study. This is of major importance in health research where researchers often have been socialised into professional ways of thinking. Although they do not take centre stage in the research, they have a significant place in its process during collection and interpretation of data as well as in the relationship they have to participants and to the readers of their research. The researchers' own standpoint and values shape the research, and this needs to be made explicit in qualitative inquiry. Researchers should be aware of and present their own preconceptions and assumptions while attempting to understand the effect they have on the data and be conscious of both structural and subjective elements in their research. The researcher is part of the research but also the conditions and problems which are encountered and the context in which it occurs; all these become a focus for reflexivity. In other words, reflexivity is not only critical reflection on the researcher's place in the inquiry but also on the process of knowledge generation and the factors which have influenced it (Guillemin and Gillam, 2004). Thus the concept of reflexivity is concerned with the awareness of socially located and constituted knowledge.

Finlay (2002b) discusses five types of reflexivity:

1. *Introspection:* This is an exploration of one's own experience and meaning to further insights and interpretations in the research.
2. *Intersubjective reflection:* This type of reflexivity focuses on the relationship between the researcher and the participants. The researcher has to be aware of the way in which the relationship affects the research.
3. *Mutual collaboration:* The participants are part of the research and their own reflection on it influences the context of the relationships, and this in turn affects the process of the research. The account is an outcome of collaboration between the partners, the researcher and the participant. Researchers must be aware of this.
4. *Social critique:* Reflexivity as social critique is linked to the power relationship and the social position of researcher and participant which have an impact on the research and which the researcher must acknowledge.
5. *Discursive deconstruction:* This type of reflexivity is linked to language and the variety of meanings inherent in it. Researchers concede in their writing that the findings can have multiple meanings and focus on the construction of the text.

There are dangers inherent in reflexivity even on the simplest level: the researchers might take self-reference too far, and some qualitative writers are prone to this. The voice of the participants and the illumination of the phenomenon under study should have priority. Nevertheless, **the researcher is the main research instrument;** he or she decides what constitutes data and where the focus should be located; researchers analyse the data and determine how to illuminate the phenomenon under study. They also write the research report and choose what to include and exclude.

Some of the differences between qualitative and quantitative inquiry are listed in Table 1.1.

Table 1.1   Some differences between qualitative and quantitative research

	Qualitative	Quantitative
Aim	Exploration, understanding and description of participants' experiences and life world	Search for causal explanations
	Generation of theory from data	Testing hypothesis, prediction, control
Approach	Initially broadly focused	
	Process oriented	Narrow focus
	Context-bound, mostly natural setting	Product oriented
	Getting close to the data	Context free, often in laboratory settings
Sampling	Participants, informants	
	Sampling units such as place, time, concepts	Respondents, participants (the term 'subjects' is now discouraged in the social sciences)
	Purposive and theoretical sampling	Randomised sampling
	Flexible sampling that can develop during the research	Sample frame fixed before the research starts
Data Collection	In-depth non-standardised interviews	Questionnaire, standardised interviews
	Participant observation/fieldwork	Tightly structured observation
	Documents, diaries, photographs, videos	Documents
		Randomised controlled trials
Analysis	Thematic or constant comparative analysis, latent content analysis ethnographic, narrative analysis, etc.	Statistical analysis
Outcome	A story, ethnography, a theory	Measurable and testable results
Relationships	Direct involvement of researcher	Limited involvement of researcher with participant
	Researcher relationship: close	Researcher relationship: distant
Rigour	Trustworthiness, authenticity	Internal/external validity, reliability
	Typicality and transferability	Generalisability
	Validity	

These differences are not absolute; they are mainly at the end of a continuum. For instance, some approaches seek causal factors or explanations such as grounded theory. The term validity is used often in qualitative research – although it has an alternative meaning; quantitative research is not always context free, nor completely objective. The researcher can have a relationship with participants in quantitative research, and qualitative inquiry might seek generalisability (these aspects are discussed later in the book).

The place of theory in qualitative research

What place has theory in qualitative research? Theory is a framework or set of statements about concepts that are related to each other and useful for understanding the phenomena under study. Silverman (2006:14) states that theory provides a 'framework for critically understanding phenomena'. Novice researchers sometimes believe that they do not need theories in the beginning of their research because qualitative inquiry is inductive, that is, it goes from the specific and unique cases to the general and hence develops theory or theories. Indeed many qualitative approaches explicitly develop theory, such as grounded theory, and theorising prior to the study is not encouraged. However, the inductive nature and the lack of a hypothesis in the beginning of research do not mean that no existing theories are needed or used in the research. For instance, a colleague might research ethnic differences in professional education. Her or his data from interviews have primacy. This means that the theories of culture, ethnicity and social interaction are part of the framework of the research, regardless of the data obtained and the theory developed. In chronic illness, theories of identity or gender might be important. Existing theory illuminates the findings (Reeves et al., 2008) and might even be modified through these. Researchers also need some knowledge about the related literature on major theoretical concepts which could be important for the research. Health researchers sometimes present a-theoretical studies though the empirical content is useful and valuable. In a piece of research for practical purpose this might be acceptable but not in an academic project.

Creswell (2009) ascribes a place to theory and calls it a general 'orientating lens' through which the research can be seen. It helps researchers to formulate the research question and – eventually – locate their own research inside or outside an existing framework. As well as the theories mentioned above, there are many pre-existing social theories, such as feminist theory, critical theory, symbolic interactionism etc, and any of these might explain the standpoint of the researcher. Too much theory in the beginning of the research, however, might generate preconceptions and assumptions rather than leaving the researchers with an open mind and free to develop their own theoretical ideas.

The usefulness of qualitative research in healthcare

Qualitative researchers adopt a person-centred and holistic perspective. The approach helps develop an understanding of human experiences, which is important for health professionals who focus on caring, communication and interaction. Through this perspective, nurses and other health researchers gain knowledge and insight about human beings – be they patients, colleagues or other professionals. Researchers generate in-depth accounts that present a lively picture of the participants' reality. They focus on human beings within their social and cultural context, not just on specific clinical conditions or professional and educational tasks. Qualitative health research is in tune with the nature of the phenomena examined; emotions, perceptions and actions are qualitative experiences.

The essence of work in the health professions contains elements of commitment and patience, understanding and trust, give and take, flexibility and openness (Paterson and Zderad, 1988). These traits mirror those of qualitative inquiry. Indeed, flexibility and openness are as essential in qualitative study as they are in the tasks of the health worker. In the clinical arena too, health professionals often have to backtrack as they do in research, return to the situation and try something new, because the situation is constantly evolving.

Health professionals, in particular midwives and nurses, have long recognised that individuals are more than diagnostic cases (Leininger, 1985) and therefore research must focus on the whole person rather than merely on physical parts. The researcher, taking a holistic view, observes people in their natural environment, and the researcher–informant relationship is based on trust and openness. Both professional caring and qualitative research depend on knowledge of the social context. The settings in which individuals live or stay for a time, the social support they have and the people with whom they interact, have a powerful effect on their lives as well as on health and illness.

Built-in ethical issues exist in both caring and qualitative research. Health researchers are ethically bound to act in the interest of clients or participants in the setting and to empower them to make autonomous decisions. This does not mean that conventional forms of inquiry have no ethical basis; however, the closer relationships forged in qualitative research enable researchers to be more focused on ethical values and achieve empathy with the participants in the research. These relationships also help health researchers to be more aware that their clients are human beings and not just body parts.

In their assessment, health professionals use inductive thinking but also make deductions before coming to conclusions, piecing together the full picture of the patient's or client's condition from specific observations and individual pieces of information. Listening carefully and asking relevant questions without being judgemental enables them to gain insights into problems and a deeper understanding of the people with whom they interact. Qualitative research too, proceeds from collecting specific data to more general conclusions.

There are many uses and applications of qualitative inquiry for health researchers and there are reasons why it might be helpful in the clinical or educational setting. In the social and political arena, it can reveal the perspectives of the policy makers in health services and organisations as well as examine strategies for development. More importantly however, qualitative research can explore the cultural, social and uniquely personal aspects of living with illness, pain and disability. While studying how people make sense of their experience

and suffering, nurses and other health researchers also gain th
care and treatment and are able to evaluate management an
of illness and health from both the professional and client ¡
fessional education too, qualitative inquiry can be a usefu
thoughts and ideas of both teachers and students.

In uncovering motivations, values and expectations, the health researcher
translates the findings of the research to clinical practice. Kuper *et al.* (2008)
argue that this research helps health professionals in the understanding of
clinical issues; for instance, reasons for adhering to or abandoning medical
commendations can be elicited.

There are many more cases when qualitative inquiry can be of use. Sandelowski
(2004: 1368) summarises the topics and utilisation of qualitative research which
can be helpful to examine the following:

- The social constructions of illness, prevention, treatment and risk
- Experiencing and managing the effects of disease and its treatment
- Decisionmaking around the areas of birth, dying and potential technological
  interventions
- Factors affecting the quality of care either positively or negatively, linked to
  access to care, promotion of good health and prevention of disease and the
  reduction of inequalities

Indeed she suggests that other researchers too now use some of the language
which started in qualitative inquiry. Evidence-based practice, which is meant to
include the best evidence on which to develop patient care, has generally meant
the evaluation and utilisation of evidence from the field of randomised controlled
trials. However, it has recently been recognised that qualitative research too
can contribute to the evidence base (Newman *et al.*, 2006) and indeed add
to practical knowledge which is valued highly because of its applicability to
the clinical setting. Sandelowski confirms the recent return to emphasis on the
'primacy of the practical' over pure knowledge, and the latter could be translated
into utilisation in professional practice.

Choosing an approach for health research

Adopting approaches because researchers find them easy or interesting is not an
appropriate way of doing research. Methodology and procedures depend on

- the nature and type of the research question or problem;
- the epistemological stance of the researcher;
- the capabilities and knowledge of the researcher;
- skills and training of the researcher;
- the resources available for the research project.

> In the main, the research approach should depend on the intentions of the researcher and the aims of the inquiry.

Researchers do have to think of the practicalities of the research such as their own competence and interest, the scope and time of the research and available funds and resources, all factors that influence the undertaking of a project. A qualitative methodology is generally applied in healthcare settings when the focus is on feelings, experience and thoughts, change and conflict.

Researchers do have a variety of choices on the approach to adopt. Holloway and Todres (2003: 355) advise health researchers to consider carefully the research question, including the phenomenon to be studied, and the type of knowledge which they seek. Once they have chosen their approach, they need to study it with care and get to know it in detail, even though they might eventually diverge from some of its more rigid elements.

If researchers wish to study a specific phenomenon or the life world of the participants they might take a *phenomenological approach*, usually through interviewing participants. For instance, a researcher might interview new fathers or mothers about the phenomenon of becoming a parent.

A *grounded theory* method would generate theory directly from the data; although it can be used in any field of qualitative health research, it often focuses on interaction and has interviewing and/or participant observation as its main data collection procedures; a researcher might observe the interaction between hospital consultants and patients or doctors and nurses. After observation, the researcher might interview the people who were observed about these interactions.

In *narrative analysis*, for instance, the researcher will ask for a first-hand account of insiders who are asked for their experiences; for instance they might narrate the story about living with multiple sclerosis or chronic pain. *Ethnographers* study the culture or subculture of a particular group in which they have an interest. The culture of midwifery teachers or that of orthopaedic nursing might be explored through observation and interviews. Of course, the preceding are not the only approaches, but each has a distinct focus and theoretical base or framework.

These are only some examples that could be investigated (many will have been carried out already).

Problematic issues in qualitative research

There are problematic issues in all research, and qualitative research is no exception. However, some concerns are specific to qualitative inquiry. Researchers also make mistakes which range from attempting to study a topic which is too complex to making the research too broad-based or too narrow. Some problems are set out below.

Lack of methodological knowledge

Some researchers see no need to study the methodology and methods before starting the research. Not knowing about the complexities of qualitative inquiry, many researchers are so eager to start that they neglect to gain this knowledge. Without it, however, the research can go wrong. For instance, researchers need to have information about interview procedures – such as having an interview guide rather than a structured questionnaire. Another example would be within grounded theory: for example, researchers need to know about the interaction of data collection and analysis as well as theoretical sampling before starting a study. The data are not all collected and then analysed together, rather the analysis process is ongoing through the data collection. Most approaches have their own way of collecting and analysing data and reporting on the findings.

Drowning in data and the need for time

Qualitative researchers often produce great amounts of data and lack the time for analysis and reflection. Each interview produces many tapes and pages of text which researchers need to reduce and collapse without losing the core ideas; hence, knowledge of procedures is essential. Richards (2005) advises new researchers to have plans for reduction in place. They are sometimes overambitious and want to include everything related to the topic. Qualitative research takes time, and poor preparation puts the study in jeopardy. Unlike quantitative research where a clear framework has been established from the beginning, the tentative and flexible character of qualitative research hinders early completion of research, although funding bodies sometimes believe that it can be done quickly. As Silverman (2006) advises the amount of data and the available time must be reconciled.

Methodolatry

The research methodology and the methods inherent in it are not the only consideration for researchers though. 'Methodolatry', about which Janesick (2000: 390) warns us, is a danger in any research. Methodolatry means an obsession with method without reflection, an overemphasis on method rather than substance in the research. This can lead to distancing from participants by valuing method over their thoughts and ideas.

Romanticism and 'emotionalism'

Because researchers get close to the participants while also describing a phenomenon from the inside, qualitative research is sometimes romanticised especially in health research, where participants are often vulnerable and lack power in the clinical setting.

Most texts advise researchers to listen to the voice of the people with whom they carry out their research or explore their 'life world'. However, researchers cannot put themselves 'into other people's shoes' and see the world from exactly the same perspective or the authentic view of the participant even though they inhabit the same world. Indeed many novice researchers wish to study experiences that they themselves have had (we remember students with epilepsy and chronic pain, for instance) because they empathise or feel that their own experience gives them special insight into the condition. Although this research is feasible and one's own experience can be a valuable source of knowledge, researchers, in particular neophytes, need be aware that they might have preconceptions which could influence their interviews and observations.

With Silverman (2006: 123–5) one might call this empathic and feeling-centred research 'emotionalism'. He maintains that this position is seductive, particularly in interview research. Indeed, the researcher might never hear the true voice of the participant; researchers, after all, translate, describe and interpret the voice of the participants and go to a level of abstraction to do this.

Method slurring

Qualitative research includes a variety of diverse approaches for the collection or analysis of data, based on different philosophical positions and rooted in various disciplines. Some are in fact philosophies rather than methods of data collection and/or analysis – for instance phenomenology – others present approaches to data collection, analysis and theorising such as grounded theory and ethnography. Yet others are textual analyses like discourse and conversation analysis. Even within a single method, different schools compete with each other and their followers sometimes take a strong position.

Students cannot always differentiate between methods, and some expert researchers strongly argue against 'slurring' or 'muddling' them (Boyle *et al.*, 1991; Baker *et al.*, 1992). These writers point out that each approach in qualitative research has its own assumptions, procedures and unique features. Holloway and Todres (2003) warn against interchanging these as this might lead to inconsistency and harm the integrity of the chosen approach. They explore the tensions between *flexibility* – seeing what can be mixed and used in any approach – and *coherence* – clarity and constancy within a single approach.

A researcher using one of the methods should make sure that language, philosophical underpinnings and procedures are appropriate to that which has been chosen. Commonalities do exist, of course. Most of these ways of researching focus on the experiences of human beings and the perspectives of the participants, interpreted by the researcher. They uncover meanings that people give to their experiences. Most of these types of research result ultimately in a coherent story with a strong storyline (the problem with generalisability in Chapter 18).

These are not the only issues in qualitative research that might be problematic. Throughout this text, we attempt to show how these problems can be overcome.

Conclusion

Nurses and other health researchers do not use qualitative approaches without reflection and evaluation. To be of value to healthcare, a critical and rigorous stance is necessary. We repeat in this book the tenets of Atkinson *et al.* (2001: 5)

> 'As qualitative research methods achieve ever-wider currency...we need to apply a critical and reflexive gaze. We cannot afford to let qualitative research become a set of taken for granted precepts and procedures. Equally, we should not be so seduced by our collective success or radical chic of new strategies of social research as to neglect the need for methodological rigour.'

Summary

- Qualitative research is an exploration of the perspectives and life world of human beings and the meanings they give to their experiences. It is used for a variety of reasons.
- In this type of inquiry, the data collected by the researcher have priority over hypotheses and theories, and the research is initially inductive.
- Context and contextualisation are of major importance.
- Researchers have continual and prolonged engagement.
- Some of the main features are thick or exhaustive description and reflexivity.
- The power relationships of researcher and participants are based on equality as persons.
- The approach chosen should 'fit' the research question and the epistemological stance of the researcher.

Those who wish to be acquainted with the paradigm debate would be advised to read the next chapter.

References

Atkinson, P., Coffey, A. & Delamont, S. (2001) A debate about our canon. *Qualitative Research*, **1** (1), 5–21.

Baker, C., Wuest, J. & Stern, P.N. (1992) Method slurring: the grounded theory/phenomenology example. *Journal of Advanced Nursing*, **17** (11), 1355–60.

Boulton, M. (2007) Informed consent in a changing environment. *Social Science and Medicine*, **65** (11), 2187–98.

Boyle, J.S., Morse, J.M., May, K.M. & Hutchinson, S.A. (1991) Dialogue. On muddling methods. In *Qualitative Nursing Research: A Contemporary Dialogue* (ed. J.M. Morse), p. 257. Newbury Park, CA, Sage.

Creswell, J.W. (2009) *Research Design: Qualitative, Quantitative and Mixed Methods Approaches*. Los Angeles, CA, Sage.

Delamont, S. & Atkinson, P. (1995) *Fighting Familiarity: Essays on Education and Ethnography*. Cresskill, NJ, Hampton Press.

Denzin, N.K. (1989) *Interpretive Interactionism*. Newbury Park, CA, Sage.

Etherington, K. (2004) *Becoming a Reflexive Researcher: Using Our Selves in Research*. London, Jessica Kingley.

Finlay, L. (2002a) Outing the researcher: the provenance, process and practice of reflection. *Qualitative Health Research*, **12** (4), 531–45.

Finlay, L. (2002b) Negotiating the swamp: the opportunity and challenge in research practice. *Qualitative Research*, **2** (2), 209–30.

Geertz, C. (1973) *The Interpretation of Cultures*. New York, NY, Basic Books.

Guillemin, M. & Gillam, L. (2004) Ethics, reflexivity and 'ethically important moments' in research. *Qualitative Inquiry*, **10** (2), 261–80.

Harris, M. (1976) History and significance of the emic/etic distinction. *Annual Review of Anthropology*, **5**, 329–50.

Holloway, I. & Todres, L. (2003) The status of method: flexibility, consistency and coherence. *Qualitative Research*, **3** (3), 345–7.

Janesick, V.A. (2000) The choreography of qualitative research design. In *Handbook of Qualitative Research*. (eds N.A. Denzin & Y.S. Lincoln), 2nd edn, pp. 379–99. Thousand Oaks, CA, Sage.

Koro-Ljungberg, M. (2008) Validity and validation in the context of qualitative research. *Qualitative Health Research*, **18** (7), 983–89.

Kuper, A., Reeves, S. & Levinson, W. (2008) An introduction to reading and appraising qualitative research. *British Medical Journal*, **337**, a288.

Leininger, M. (1985) *Qualitative Research Methods in Nursing*. Orlando, Grune and Stratton.

Miller, T. & Boulton, M. (2007) Changing constructions of informed consent: qualitative research and complex social worlds. *Social Science and Medicine*, **65** (11), 2199–211.

Newman, M., Thompson, C. & Roberts, A.P. (2006) Helping practitioners to understand the contribution of qualitative research to evidence-based practice. *Human Behaviour*. Glendale, CA, Summer Institute of Linguistics (later editions of this book have been published).

Paterson, J.G. & Zderad, L.T. (1988) *Humanistic Nursing*. New edn. New York, NY, National League for Nursing.

Ponterotto, J.G. (2006) Brief note on the origins, evolution and meaning of the qualitative research concept 'thick description'. *The Qualitative Report*, **11** (3), 538–49. Retrieved August 2008 from http://www.nova.edu/ssss/QR/QR11-3/ponterotto.pdf.

Reeves, S., Albert, M., Kuper, A. & Hodges, B.D. (2008) Why use theories in qualitative research? *British Medical Journal*, **337**, a949.

Richards, L. (2005) *Handling Qualitative Data: A Practical Guide*. London, Sage.

Sandelowski, M. (2004) Using qualitative research. *Qualitative Health Research*, **14** (10), 1366–86.

Scott, S.D., Estabrooks, M.A. & Pollock, C. (2008) A context of uncertainty: how context shapes nurses' utilization behaviors. *Qualitative Health Research*, **18** (3), 347–57.

Silverman, D. (2006) *Interpreting Qualitative Data*, 3rd edn. London, Sage.

Spradley, J.P. (1979) *The Ethnographic Interview*. Fort Worth, TX, Harcourt Brace Johanovich College Publishers.

Further reading

Finlay, L. & Gough, B. (eds.) (2003) *Reflexivity: A Practical Guide for Researchers in Health and Social Sciences*. Oxford, Blackwell.

May, T. (2007) *Reflexivity*. London, Sage.

CHAPTER 2

The Paradigm Debate: The Place of Qualitative Research

There are many books which trace the background and theoretical framework of qualitative research. They focus mainly on epistemological and methodological issues, and most experienced qualitative health researchers are acquainted with the debates surrounding it. For novice qualitative researchers it might be useful to rehearse these arguments and give an (admittedly simple) overview of the debates, as was done in previous editions. Although many writers maintain that the dispute about 'research paradigms' has been settled and the 'paradigm wars' are over, new researchers need to know about early discussions on these issues.

Theoretical frameworks and ontological position

Social inquiry can be approached in several different ways, and researchers will have to select between varieties of approaches. Whilst often making a choice on practical grounds, they must also understand the theoretical and philosophical ideas on which the research is based.

Approaches to social inquiry consist not only of the procedures of sampling, data collection and analysis, but they are rooted in particular ideas about the world and the nature of knowledge which sometimes reflect conflicting and competing views about social reality. Some of these positions towards the social world are concerned with the very nature of reality and existence (*ontology*). From this, basic assumptions about knowledge arise: *epistemology* is the theory of knowledge and is concerned with the question of what counts as valid knowledge. *Methodology* refers to the principles and ideas on which researchers base their procedures and strategies (*methods*). To assist in understanding the background to the interpretive/descriptive approach to research, the following section will describe epistemological and methodological ideas about the rise and development of qualitative research. (See the discussion in the book by Willis (2007), Chapters 1 and 2 in particular.)

Conflict and tension between different schools of social science have been in existence for a long time. Several sets of assumptions underlie social research;

in their most basic form they describe the dichotomy between the *positivist* and the *interpretivist* (interpretive) paradigms (Bryman, 2008).

In the early days of positivism, the focus was on the methods of natural science that became a model for the social sciences such as psychology and sociology. Interpretivists stressed that human beings differ from the material world and the distinction between humans and matter should be reflected in the methods of investigation. Much social research developed from these ideas. Qualitative research was critical of the natural science model and a reaction against the tenets of this model. Researchers held a 'separatist' position and believed the world views of qualitative and quantitative researchers to be incompatible. They initially rejected a mix of the two (Murphy and Dingwall, 2001).

Social scientists continue to raise the paradigm debate but stress that simplistic polarisation between positivist and qualitative inquiry will not do. Atkinson (1995), in particular, criticised the use of the concept of the term *paradigm* and the 'paradigm mentality'. Health researchers, too, accused their professions of unwarranted 'paradigmatic thinking' and maintain that it restricts rather than extends knowledge (Thorne *et al.*, 1999). Nevertheless, qualitative researchers are still defensive of their methodology and tend to develop arguments against other approaches. Indeed, they sometimes do that of which they accuse quantitative researchers and seem to be absolutist in their statements and uncritical of their own approach.

The natural science model: positivism, objectivism and value neutrality

From the nineteenth century onwards, the traditional and favoured approaches to social and behavioural research were quantitative. Quantitative research has its root in the positivist and early natural science model that has influenced social science throughout the nineteenth and the first half of the twentieth century. The description that follows here is core to the debate.

Positivism was an approach to science based on a belief in universal laws and attempts to present an objective picture of the world. Positivists followed the natural science approach by testing theories and hypotheses. The methods of natural – in particular physical – science stem from the seventeenth, eighteenth and nineteenth centuries. Comte (1798–1857), the French philosopher who created the terms 'positivism' and 'sociology', suggested that the emerging social sciences must proceed in the same way as natural science by adopting natural science research methods.

One of the traits of this type of research is the quest for objectivity and distance between researcher and those studied so that biases can be avoided. Investigators searched for patterns and regularities and believed that universal laws and rules, or law-like generalities, exist for human action. Behaviour could be predicted, so they believed, on the basis of these laws. Researchers thought that findings would and should be generalisable to all similar situations and settings. Even today many researchers think that numerical measurement, statistical analysis and the search for cause and effect lie at the heart of much research, and of course, that is so. Not many researchers now feel that detachment and objectivity are possible, and that only numerical measurement results in objective knowledge. In the positivist approach, researchers control the theoretical framework, sampling frames and the structure of the research. This type of research seeks causal relationships and focuses on prediction and control.

Popper (1959) claimed falsifiability as the main criterion of science. The researcher formulates a hypothesis – an expected outcome – and tests it. Scientists refute or falsify hypotheses. When a deviant case is found the hypothesis is falsified. Knowledge is always provisional because new incoming data may refute it. (There has been criticism of Popper's ideas but the debate cannot be developed here. It is discussed in philosophy of science texts.)

The positivist approach develops from a theoretical perspective, and a hypothesis is often, though not always, established before the research begins. The model of science adopted is hypothetico-deductive; it moves from the general to the specific, and its main aim is to test theory. The danger of this approach is that researchers sometimes treat perceptions of the social world as objective or absolute and neglect everyday subjective interpretations and the context of the research.

Nineteenth-century positivists believed that scientific knowledge can be proven and is discovered by rigorous methods of observation and experiments, and derived through the senses. However, this is a simplistic view of science and there has been major change. Even natural scientists – for instance biologists and physicists – do not necessarily agree on what science is and adopt a variety of different scientific approaches and inductive methods as well as deduction. Social scientists too, use a number of approaches and differ in their understandings about the nature of science. Scientific knowledge is difficult to prove.

The search for objectivity may be futile for all scientists. They can strive for it, but their own biases and experiences intrude. Science, whether natural or social science, cannot be 'value free', that is, it cannot be fully objective as the values and background of the researchers affect the research.

The paradigm debate

In the 1960s the traditional view of science was criticised for its aims and methods by both natural and social scientists. The new and different evolutionary stance taken within disciplines such as biology and psychology had gone beyond the simplistic positivist approach. Qualitative researchers go further still. Lincoln and Guba (1990), for instance, argue that a 'paradigm shift' occurred – in line with the ideas of Kuhn (1962, 1970).

Kuhn's thinking has had great impact on the paradigm debate. 'Normal science', with its community of scholars, he asserts, proceeds through a series of crises that hinder its development. Earlier methods of science are questioned and new ways adopted; certain theoretical and philosophical presuppositions are replaced by another set of assumptions taking precedence over the model from the past. Eventually, one scientific view of the world is replaced by another. Although Kuhn wrote about the physical sciences and was a natural scientist, later writers have used his work to draw analogies with the shift in the ideas of social science. Kuhn's (1962: 162) definition of paradigm is 'entire constellation of beliefs, values, techniques, and so on, shared by the members of a given community'.

Thus a paradigm consists of theoretical ideas and technical procedures that a group of scientists adopt and which are rooted in a particular world view with its own language and terminology. Kuhn's ideas have been extensively criticised (Fuller, 2000), but the critique cannot be developed here.

Qualitative social researchers often claim that a 'paradigm shift' in social science has occurred – in the same way in which Kuhn discussed it – that a whole world view is linked to the new paradigm. They attack the positivist stance for its emphasis on social reality as being 'out there', separate from the individual, and maintain that an objective reality independent of the people they study is difficult to grasp.

Quantitative research, in all its variations, is useful and valuable, but it is sometimes seen as limited by qualitative researchers, because it neglects the participants' perspectives within the context of their lives. Lather (2004) reminds researchers, that the shift to qualitative approaches in the 1970s was partly due to the difficulties of measurement and the 'limits of causal models'. (Although she speaks of education in particular, her ideas can also be applied to health research.)

The controlled conditions of traditional approaches sometimes limit practical applications. This type of research does not always or easily answer complex questions about the nature of the human condition. Researchers using these approaches are not inherently concerned about human interaction or feelings, thoughts and perceptions of people in their research but with facts, measurable behaviour and cause and effect; of course both types of research are necessary.

> Both qualitative and quantitative methodologies in research are important, but researchers ask different questions suitable to each approach and generate different answers.

It must not be forgotten that natural scientists, too, have criticised the often mechanistic natural science view of the world which in the view of many researchers, including many natural scientists, is at least to some extent socially constructed and defined. Indeed one could argue that there has not been a 'scientific revolution' with a new paradigm. A decade ago many, such as Atkinson (1995) and Thorne *et al.* (1999), challenged the notion of paradigm shift and suggested that the debate is an oversimplification of complex issues.

The interpretive/descriptive approach

The interpretive or interpretivist model and descriptive research (descriptive phenomenologists would not call their approach interpretive) have their roots in philosophy and the human sciences, particularly in history, philosophy and anthropology. The methodology centres on the way in which human beings make sense of their subjective reality and attach meaning to it. Social scientists view people not as individual entities who exist in a vacuum but explore their world within the whole of their life context. Researchers with this world view believe that understanding human experiences is as important as focusing on explanation, prediction and control. The interpretive/descriptive model has a long history, from its roots in the nineteenth century and Dilthey's philosophy, Max Weber's sociology and George Herbert Mead's social psychology.

The interpretivist view can be linked to Weber's *Verstehen* approach. Philosophers and historians such as Dilthey (1833–1911) considered that the social sciences need not imitate the natural sciences; they should instead emphasise empathetic understanding. Understanding in the social sciences is inherently different from explanation in the natural sciences. Weber was well aware of the two approaches that existed in the nineteenth century. The concept of *Verstehen* – understanding something in its context – has elements of empathy, not in the psychological sense as intuitive and non-conscious feeling, but as reflective reconstruction and interpretation of the action of others. Weber believed that social scientists should be concerned with the interpretive understanding of human beings. He claimed that meaning could be found in the intentions and goals of the individual.

Weber argued that *understanding* in the social sciences is inherently different from *explanation* in the natural sciences, and he differentiates between the nomothetic, rule-governed methods of the latter and idiographic methods that are not related to general laws and rules but to the actions of human beings. This was linked to the *Methodenstreit* – the conflict between methods – which historians and philosophers such as Dilthey (1833–1911) and Windelband (1848–1915) had discussed in the nineteenth century. Weber believed that numerically measured probability is quantitative only, and he wanted to stress that social science concerns itself with the qualitative. We should treat the people we study, he advised, 'as if they were human beings' and try to gain access to their experiences and perceptions by listening to them and observing them. Weber did not have a direct impact on early qualitative researchers (Platt, 1985), nor did he discuss qualitative inquiry as we now understand it, but he influenced sociologists in particular, and his ideas have helped shape the qualitative perspective. Sociologists developed further the interpretive perspective that initially stemmed from the writings of Mead, Weber, Schütz and others in the early twentieth century; grounded theory as well as some other approaches acknowledge these influences.

Phenomenology as a qualitative research approach is based on philosophy in the nineteenth and early twentieth centuries too, starting with Dilthey, but in particular on the ideas of the mathematician and philosopher Husserl (1859–1938), and the philosopher Heidegger (1889–1976) who focused on ontological questions of meaning and lived experience. The theoretical framework has developed through time and includes the work of other philosophers. In practical terms it has benefited from the work of psychologists and sociologists. Qualitative researchers claim that the experiences of people and other phenomena are essentially context-bound, that is, they cannot be free from time and location or the mind of the human actor. Researchers are urged to grasp the socially constructed nature of the world and realise that values and interests become part of the research process. Complete objectivity and neutrality are impossible to achieve; the values of all participants become an integral part of the research. Researchers are not divorced from the phenomenon under study (Mantzoukas, 2004). This means reflexivity on their part; they must take into account their own position in the setting and situation, as the researcher is the main research tool. Language itself is context-bound and depends on the researchers' and informants' values as well as their social location (see also Chapter 1). Detailed replication or duplication of a piece of research is impossible because the research relationship, history and location of participants differ from study to study.

Qualitative methodology is not completely precise, because human beings do not always act logically or predictably. Indeed many writers argue that those who cannot bear ambiguity should not attempt this type of research. Investigators using a qualitative lens turn to the human participants for guidance, control and direction throughout the research. Structure and order are, of course, important for the research to be scientific. The social world, however, is not orderly or systematic; therefore it is all the more important that the researcher proceeds in a well structured and systematic way.

Recent focus on postmodernism and social constructionism

Latterly, qualitative researchers have stressed two related influences on qualitative research, those of postmodernism and social constructionism. Postmodernism is not a unitary concept but a set of ideas rooted in philosophy and sociology and also permeating recent literature, music and visual arts, and in particular, architecture. Postmodernists are critical of the traditionalist values of society and stress the plurality of beliefs. Questioning the existence of objectivity and neutrality in research, they believe that much depends on the presenter's and audience's standpoint and stance and suggest that much that people consider as facts is relative and subjective. Research is bound to the local context and is valid only in relation to our own time and community (Cahoone, 2003).

Postmodernism challenges traditional knowledge, and in qualitative research it stresses the multiplicity of perspectives and lack of a unitary view of truth. Postmodernist researchers are antifoundationalist, that means they believe that there is no absolute and universal knowledge and truth; indeed knowledge is provisional and uncertain (Willis, 2007) and there are often a variety of alternative explanations for a phenomenon.

Postmodernism and social constructionism (or similarly constructivism) are closely related. Social constructionists argue that so-called social reality is a product of social processes; it is tied and relative to context, time and culture; human beings construct it themselves (see Holstein and Gubrium, 2008). It is believed that the participants, the researcher and the reader together construct the research; in this way research is produced by social interaction. Holstein and Gubrium, however, refute in the introduction to their book that constructionism and qualitative research are synonymous, and not all this type of inquiry can be labelled social constructionist.

Critical theory is another basis of some qualitative research approaches such as critical ethnography and critical discourse analysis. The critical approach takes account of power and inequalities in society and has its roots in Marxist and neo-Marxist thought. Proponents are Habermas (b. 1929) and the members of the 'Frankfurt School' (desiring social change after the Second World War) who point to oppressive relationships in society. Researchers who base their inquiry on critical theory take account of these unequal relationships and aim their research at empowerment of those whose voices cannot be heard (Willis, 2007). Critical theorists want to change existing inequalities through their research.

Conflicting or complementary perspectives?

Some social scientists believe that qualitative and quantitative approaches are merely different methods of research to be used pragmatically, dependent on the research question (Bryman, 2008). Others decide that they are incompatible and mutually exclusive on the basis of their different epistemologies (Lincoln and Guba, 1985; Leininger, 1992; Denzin and Lincoln, 2005). Researchers sometimes carry out one or the other, depending on their own epistemological stance, or they use both. Silverman (2006) and many others argue that neither school is better or more valid than the other, and that an emphasis on the polarities does not result in a useful debate as both are valid approaches.

Many sociologists, psychologists and health professionals work in the quantitative tradition. In much of health, education and social work, however, the qualitative perspective has been in the ascendant for some decades, in particular in nursing. One might suggest that qualitative research is a coherent way of researching human thought, perception and behaviour (not new or uni-linear but developed to answer different questions from those of traditional approaches).

The positivist and the interpretive/descriptive model of social research have their roots in different assumptions about social reality. While early positivism is based on the belief that reality has existence outside and is independent of individuals, those who adopt new approaches to research claim that *social* reality is constructed and is not independent from the people creating it, although they usually do acknowledge that there is a reality 'out there'. Not only qualitative researchers hold this view, but many quantitative researchers also believe this.

Oakley (2000) claims that qualitative researchers sometimes use the term 'positivism' as a form of abuse. She criticises this and those researchers who neglect experimental and other forms of quantitative research. She asserts that both qualitative and quantitative approaches have a place. In any case, the terms are not absolute, as numbers are often used in qualitative research, and quantitative inquiry includes elements of quality. Also, research, whether quantitative or qualitative, can be presented in a positivist or non-positivist frame, aim or direction. Crotty (1998: 41) suggests '... it is a matter of positivism vs. non-positivism, not a matter of qualitative vs. quantitative'. Methodological debates often suffer from oversimplification.

Bryman (2008) argues that qualitative research became popular initially because of dissatisfaction with quantitative research. The latter could not, in the view of many researchers, answer the important questions in which they were interested. In qualitative health research, the 'voices' of patients and clients are heard, and feelings and experiences can be grasped. Although there are distinct differences between the major methodological approaches, many argue against their polarisation. Ercikan and Roth (2006) reiterate the view of these and claim that the dichotomy between qualitative and quantitative research is meaningless: phenomena under investigation have both qualitative and quantitative features. Qualitative research is often seen as subjective and quantitative as objective and neutral. In research, however, subjectivity and objectivity are at the end of a continuum – qualitative inquiry is at the more subjective end, while quantitative research has some subjective features but attempts to be more objective. There is neither total objectivity nor complete subjectivity in either approach.

The two approaches should not be seen as dichotomous although of course they are different (see Table 1.1).

Final comment

To add to the confusion and ambiguity of the paradigm debate, many researchers see other types of research such as those based on critical theory or mixed methods research as separate 'paradigms'. The term 'paradigm' though overused, is still seen as a valid concept in methodology (Morgan, 2007). There are many philosophical and epistemological directions which have had an impact on qualitative research; there is no space for all these in this text. Qualitative researchers choose a variety of approaches and procedures to achieve their aims. These include ethnography, grounded theory, phenomenology, narrative research, conversation analysis, discourse analysis and others. Some forms of social inquiry such as action research, ethnography and feminist approaches often use qualitative methods and techniques but sometimes include quantitative strategies.

Regardless of the epistemological stance or perspective of the researchers who carry out this type of inquiry, however, they must at least appreciate some of the important issues which might affect qualitative research. This includes knowledge of the paradigm dialogue and the philosophical and theoretical ideas which have had an influence on qualitative research.

References

Atkinson, P. (1995) Some perils of paradigms. *Qualitative Health Research*, 5 (1), 117–24.

Bryman, A. (2008) *Social Research Methods*, 3rd edn. Oxford, Oxford University Press.

Cahoone, L. (ed.) (2003) *From Modernism to Postmodernism: An Anthology*. Malden, MA, Blackwell.

Crotty, M. (1998) *The Foundations of Social Research: Meaning and Perspective in the Research Process*. London, Sage.

Denzin, N.K. & Lincoln, Y.S. (eds) (2005) *Handbook of Qualitative Research*, 3rd edn. Thousand Oaks, CA, Sage.

Ercikan, K. & Roth, W.M. (2006) What good is polarisation between qualitative and quantitative research? *Educational Researcher*, 35 (5), 13–23.

Fuller, S. (2000) *Thomas Kuhn: A Philosophical History for our Times*. Chicago, IL, University of Chicago Press.

Holstein, J.A. & Gubrium, J.F. (eds) (2008) *Handbook of Constructionist Research*. New York, NY, Guilford Publications.

Kuhn, T.S. (1962; 2nd edn 1970) *The Structure of Scientific Revolutions*. Chicago, IL, University of Chicago Press.

Lather, P. (2004) This is your father's paradigm: Government intrusion and the case of qualitative research. *Qualitative Inquiry*, 10 (1), 15–34.

Leininger, M. (1992) Current issues, problems, and trends to advance qualitative paradigmatic research methods for the future. *Qualitative Health Research*, 2, 392–415.

Lincoln, Y.S. & Guba, E.G. (1985) *Naturalistic Inquiry*. Beverly Hills, CA, Sage.

Lincoln, Y.S. & Guba, E.G. (eds) (1990) *The Paradigm Dialogue*. Newbury Park, CA, Sage.

Mantzoukas, S. (2004) Issues of representation within qualitative inquiry. *Qualitative Health Research*, 14 (7), 924–1007.

Morgan, D. (2007) Paradigms lost and pragmatism regained: methodological implications of combining qualitative and quantitative methods. *Journal of Mixed Methods Research*, **1** (1), 48–76.

Murphy, E. & Dingwall, R. (2001) Qualitative methods in health technology assessment. In *The Advanced Handbook of Methods in Evidence Based Healthcare* (eds A. Stevens, K. Abrams, J. Brazier, R. Fitzpatrick, & R. Lilford), pp. 166–78. London, Sage.

Oakley, A. (2000) *Experiments in Knowing: Gender and Method in the Social Sciences*. Cambridge, Polity Press.

Platt, J. (1985) Weber's *Verstehen* and the history of qualitative research: the missing link. *British Journal of Sociology*, **36**, 448–66.

Popper, K. (1959) *The Logic of Scientific Discovery*. London, Routledge & Kegan Paul.

Silverman, D. (2006) *Interpreting Qualitative Data*, 3rd edn. London, Sage.

Thorne, S.E., Kirkham, S.R. & Henderson, A. (1999) Ideological implications of the paradigm discourse. *Nursing Inquiry*, **4**, 1–2.

Willis, J.W. (2007) *Foundations of Qualitative Research*. Thousand Oaks, CA, Sage.

Further reading

Most textbooks on qualitative research contain chapters on these issues. A very clear article discussing the paradigm debate for a nursing readership is the following:

Mead, G.H. (1934) *Mind, Self and Society*. Chicago, IL, University of Chicago Press.

Weaver, K. & Olsen, J. (2006) Understanding paradigms used for nursing research. *Journal of Advanced Nursing*, **53** (4), 459–69.

CHAPTER 3

Initial Steps in the Research Process

At the beginning of their study, researchers go through the process of selecting the research topic and defining the research question. They must make sure of a sound design, and that this design fits the chosen topic. Although the initial steps in different types of research are similar, qualitative researchers use a distinct terminology and adopt different principles, and this is reflected in the way they design their project. The initial phase is important as it sets the scene for the progress of the research. Qualitative inquiry suits studies where little is known about the specific research topic, as researchers should not start with assumptions or preconceived ideas.

Selecting and formulating the research question

The first step in the process is the selection of the research area, topic and question. Although the terms are often used interchangeably, Punch (2006) believes that they are a hierarchy of concepts with different levels of abstraction. The research area and topic are more general than the research question. A research question or problem is a question about an issue that researchers examine to gain new information. It differs from data collection questions that are at the lowest level of abstraction. The latter are the steps to gather data in order to answer the research question. The conclusions of any study are intended to answer the research question. The question should be explicit as well as meaningful and coherent (Mantzoukas, 2008).

Examples

An *area* of research may be 'the experience of chronic pain', or 'living with diabetes'. A *topic* would be a more specific aspect of the area, for instance, 'old people's experience of chronic pain and their coping strategies' or 'chronic back pain and changes in identity'. The *research question* or problem might be phrased: 'How do old people experience and cope with pain?' or 'The relationship between chronic illness and self perception.'

A *data collection question* is much more specific, such as 'How did you feel when you had that asthma attack?' or 'Tell me how you coped with your pain?' These are not research questions but interview questions.

Nurses and other health researchers often notice problems in their work setting which they feel need investigation so that solutions or remedies for unsatisfactory situations or behaviour may be found. Sometimes the topic emerges from the literature linked to a particular area of professional work where gaps in knowledge can be identified. Nursing/midwifery and other health research studies contribute to existing knowledge and enhance understanding of the area under investigation. Knowledge and understanding of an issue are not always enough, however; health professionals also seek solutions to problems in the clinical setting.

Personal observation and experience, as well as discussion with others, guide individuals towards the topic for research. Events and interactions often provide an interest or a puzzle and generate the wish to know more. The research question is a statement about what they want to find out and stems directly from a problem experienced in the clinical area or in their personal and professional lives. Holliday (2007) argues that research questions develop during the process of the research; they vary on a continuum from the broader and more general to the very specific and might be changed. Many health researchers have a question from the beginning of the study based on their clinical work.

It is important that the problem is related to professional work; for instance if nurses are working in the field of paediatrics it would be inappropriate (though not wrong) for them to undertake a project with old people, however much it might arouse their interest. A nurse on a ward for confused elderly people who had worried about accidents and falls might explore nurses' perspectives on the care of old people and the problems involved in their care. A midwife who notices the reluctance of some women to breastfeed might use this as an area of investigation.

Certain criteria should be considered when identifying a research problem:

- The question must be researchable.
- The topic must be relevant and appropriate.
- The work must be feasible within the allocated time span and resources.
- The research should be of interest to the researcher.

The question must be researchable

Health researchers are often confronted with an important ethical or philosophical dilemma that cannot be solved through research. A moral or philosophical question is not researchable; for instance, the question of whether nurses or doctors should become involved in euthanasia is answerable only in philosophical but not in research terms.

Although the research problem need not be a practical one, it must nevertheless result in findings and outcomes. Research could not answer the question whether health professionals 'should' use euthanasia, but the topic of nurses' perceptions of euthanasia would be researchable. 'Do' and 'should' questions are difficult to answer. 'Do new mothers have feelings of inadequacy?' would become 'What are the feelings of new mothers about coping with their babies?' to transform it into a research question.

Examples of researchable questions and topics

Fathers' perspectives on the chronic illness of their children.
Nurse practitioners' interactions with general practitioners.
How do people experience and cope with chronic pain?
The experience of a Caesarian section for first-time mothers.
(These questions would be more specific in the design of a study.)

The topic should be relevant and appropriate

Relevance means that the research is linked to clinical practice or professional issues. The question might also be important for patients or clients, the health professions or for society in general, and the answer will advance theoretical nursing and healthcare knowledge. The results should be applicable to practice, education or management, legitimising existing practices or leading the way towards change.

The work must be feasible

Health professionals are sometimes overambitious, especially if they are new to research. Rather than reflecting on the time the study may take and some of the detailed procedures and the complexity of analysis, they want to start the study straight away, before they have a thorough knowledge of methodology. Learning about methodology should be one of the first steps in research.

Time can become a problem in qualitative research because it is eaten up by transcribing, coding and categorising data. A simple small-scale study using a well-documented research strategy is far less time consuming than a complex piece of triangulation.

The research should be feasible in terms of resources and accessibility of participants, and researchers should identify whose resources will be used. The topic might be inappropriate because of major ethical and access problems which cannot be overcome, such as superiors not giving permission to do the research, or patients' vulnerability. The research should also be feasible in terms of participant numbers or availability. Last but not least, it must be within the researcher's knowledge and capability and the time frame available.

The research should be of interest to the researcher

If the topic is interesting, it can stimulate and motivate rather than generate boredom during the course of the study, and it can be sustained only if the researcher is fully involved. The storyline of the project is not merely controlled by the participants but it reflects the interest of the researcher.

The selection of the focus takes time, reflection and discussion with others who have knowledge in the field of study. Students in particular should discuss the focus of their work with their tutors and supervisors. All too often, new researchers in qualitative research choose a question that is designed to deal with factual issues and needs a survey rather than a qualitative approach.

Example

A nurse decides to research the availability of counselling services in the area. He or she decides to ask questions from patients and nurses in the community about access to these services. A qualitative study would not be useful, as a questionnaire is more appropriate to elicit this detailed information about facts. If however the experience of the counselling services by patients is the topic of the research, a qualitative study would be useful.

Quantitative researchers focus on a very specific area and plan every detail before the start of the study, while qualitative researchers initially formulate the question in more general terms and develop and focus it during the research process. Qualitative researchers generally begin with a broad question and become more specific in the process of the research, responding to what they hear and find in the setting (progressive focusing). The research design is evolutionary rather than strictly pre-defined. This needs flexibility on the part of researchers.

Example

A community nurse might be interested in the perspectives of diabetic patients on their condition. As many of her clients are elderly patients with diabetes, she decides that the focus of the study should be their experience. However, on searching the literature on this topic, she might find that a large number of studies exist on the perspectives of older people with diabetes, but nobody might yet have examined children's experiences or those of their parents. The final aim of the project then could be 'to explore the experience and management of diabetes by children and their parents' (or similar).

Practical issues

Beginners, such as pre-registration students, might undertake a simple study suitable to show that they understand the research process and can produce a valid and useful project. We advise novice researchers not to carry out research involving patients except in exceptional circumstances, for instance if they have long nursing experience, special expertise in their field and expert supervision. For inexperienced researchers it is particularly important to be clear and straightforward. The clearer the question, the clearer is the outcome of the study.

The research design and choice of approach

The research design needs to be appropriate for the chosen topic and research question. The design of the study depends entirely on the topic to be studied and on the developing research question. There is of course no reason why researchers may not choose to develop a qualitative research project but the method must fit the problem or question.

The literature review

After identifying the research question, investigators review the important literature consisting of the information published and closely related to the area of the project, including both *primary* and *secondary* sources. Primary sources are produced by researchers who developed original work on a subject or researched this topic. For the researcher this means searching for the topic area in research and academic journals and books. Secondary information consists of reports, summaries or references to original work originating from a person other than the researcher. Library catalogues and on-line data bases are useful locations for research in the general area of the researcher's topic; Hansen (2006) adds government reports and conferences to the list of places for finding relevant literature. The literature reviewed before the start of the inquiry and during the process would include foundational early texts and up-to-date references. The literature search involves searching data bases and journals which are of relevance for the topic area.

Researchers review the literature for the following reasons at the beginning:

- To find out what is already known about the subject and acknowledge those who have worked in this area
- To identify gaps in knowledge
- To describe how the study contributes to existing knowledge of a topic area
- To avoid duplicating other people's work
- To assist in defining the research question
- To place their research in the context of other studies
- To show that they have reflected on the research question

Punch (2006) points out the specific importance of certain aspects:

1. The identification of the literature relevant to the topic
2. The relationship of the literature to the proposed study
3. The way the researcher uses the literature in the research

Through reading reports (articles and books) researchers can identify what knowledge about the subject of their study already exists, the way in which it was generated, and the methods that were adopted. They may find a large number of studies on the particular topic and decide to avoid it, not wishing to focus on issues that others have thoroughly examined at an earlier stage. There is little justification for researchers to keep to their original research question if the topic has already been addressed exhaustively and adequately elsewhere. However, the literature sometimes points to problems within the subject area that have not yet been investigated.

Examples

A Scottish nurse researcher wishes to examine the topic of interprofessional mentorship and finds that several research studies have been carried out in the United States. He did however not find studies in Scotland and proceeds to investigate this.

A physiotherapist seeks to gain perspectives on a specific chronic illness condition. Many professionals have written about this condition, but there is no study about the perceptions and experience of patients themselves. Although much literature exists in the field, the researcher is justified in carrying out a study with patient participants if this is new and has not been done before.

A simple detailed description of the literature is not enough. It must be critically reviewed and evaluated, even in the initial literature review; researchers appraise others' work within the context of what they themselves intend to do.

The use of literature in qualitative research

Although the literature review is not extensive in a qualitative proposal, researchers need to know from the beginning how other writers' work is used in a piece of qualitative research; they also must be aware that the initial literature review is not exhaustive as it should not direct the study since researchers initially take an inductive approach.

There is a debate about the place of the literature in qualitative research. We know that in quantitative studies researchers read the literature about a topic area and give a detailed evaluative report in the literature review before they start the fieldwork. In the early days of qualitative investigations, researchers were encouraged to start without a literature review so that they would not be directed in their research, as it was believed that a detailed review would invalidate the qualitative research study; indeed Glaser (2004) and earlier writings strongly advise against any type of literature review on the specific topic in the beginning of the study, and advocate instead a wider view which includes the areas around a study rather than specifically addressing the particular topic area. However, some sort of trawl and search for literature should be carried out, because an answer to the question may already exist in the public domain. In any case, researchers' minds are not a *tabula rasa*, a blank sheet, especially not when they are already experienced professionals. Although it is inappropriate to start with a fully developed theoretical model and an in-depth literature review, it is dangerous to start without any prior ideas of what has already been done in the field. The introductory literature review (or overview) should not be seen to direct the research. However, as Haverkamp and Young (2007) point out, the literature review for a research project is not about the knowledge researchers already possess but how they make use of what they know while carrying out a study.

Researchers do not start the study with a rigid framework, hypotheses or fully developed theories for their research. In qualitative research a flexible conceptual framework is necessary, as the study is linked to other research and ideas about the topic. For instance, one of our students researched a specific topic in which gender and class were important aspects. His theoretical position on gender and class were developed from the beginning and formed a framework within which his study proceeded.

An overview of the literature often takes place prior to the study, but the literature search and review proceeds throughout. The literature might even become another source for data in the main body of the study, where it is guided by the findings and emerging themes of the researcher. The researchers compare or contrast their own findings with those of other studies and engage in an active debate and dialogue with results reported in the literature. This happens throughout the study. Metcalfe (2003) advises researchers that previous authors should be treated as 'experts' or authorities in the field in much the same way that witnesses are called to court to give evidence. The researcher must make a case for calling on the work of these authors and show that they have credibility. Hence it is not necessary to quote each single piece of research that has ever been done; it suffices if credible experts have been consulted in each major area of the research. Their studies and writing is to confirm or disconfirm (challenge) the findings and the argument that the researcher has established, indeed, they form 'building blocks' for the argument. The publications chosen, however, must demonstrate that the researcher does not show only one single point of view but has presented a balanced choice.

Often, a category or construct that researchers discover and develop is reflected in other disciplines or areas of knowledge. Ideas about the emerging concepts can then be followed up in the literature. A look at the nursing or health literature does not always suffice; psychological, educational or sociological literature might also be useful.

Example

An investigator finds that 'returning to normal' is a major issue for people who have had a myocardial infarction (MI). He or she then follows up the idea of 'becoming normal, being normal, normalisation' etc. in other fields of study. Research accounts about people with a disability or an illness condition, and how they try to achieve normality, can then become part of the dialogue between findings and literature in the study of MI patients.

The literature will become integrated at a later stage. As data collection and analysis proceed at the same time in many qualitative approaches, there is an ongoing process of searching the literature that is linked to the findings in the data. Qualitative researchers have an ongoing dialogue with the literature related to their themes, categories or constructs.

Practicalities

Hart (1998) identifies the steps to be taken by researchers in a literature review:

- Collect background information.
- Start mapping the topic.
- Focus the topic.
- Search the sources of literature.
- Build up early bibliographies.
- Search for critical evaluations of the literature.

Many researchers summarise research studies from the literature and the major concepts involved on cards that they file alphabetically from the beginning of their research. This way they can access the ideas and topic areas more quickly when they want them at a later stage.

Novice researchers often take an uncritical stance to the literature, but it is important to evaluate critically rather than merely describe. If factual claims are made in the introduction or literature review (for instance: 'Recent research has shown ...' or: 'Midwife researchers suggest ...') they must be substantiated with names and dates; evidence should be given. Sometimes older foundational texts are used; reasons for the inclusion of this work must, however, be given otherwise the review does not seem up-to-date for the reader.

There are a variety of search and retrieve strategies for qualitative research, some of which are described by Barroso *et al.* (2003) and Shaw *et al.* (2004).

Writing a research proposal

In an academic situation the term research proposal is used, but in professional settings it is sometimes called the research protocol. Before starting the project, researchers write a proposal – a summary of what they will be examining, why they adopt the particular research focus, and how they will proceed. It also includes information about where and when the research will be carried out. It is useful to add intended outcomes and the potential benefits for patients and service. Researchers also describe the design of the study.

The proposal justifies and clarifies the proposed study for submission to ethics committees, funding agencies, official gatekeepers such as managers and, for student work, to supervisors. The proposal is a detailed plan of action to convince the reader that the researcher knows enough to undertake the project and can show that the completed study will contribute to knowledge in the field.

Structure of a proposal

The proposal consists of the following main elements:

1. Working title
2. Abstract
3. Introduction
   - Problem statement and rationale of the study (justification; demonstration of importance for the profession and clinical practice)
   - Context and setting
   - The aim of the research
4. Brief discussion of the relevant literature
   - A discussion of other researchers' work demonstrating the need for this particular study

5. Design and methodology
   - Theoretical basis and justification of the methodology (including references on the chosen approach)
   - Delimitations and limitations of the study
   - Sample selection and sampling procedure
   - Data collection and analysis
   - Ethical and entry issues
   - Bibliography and references
6. Timetable and costing
7. Potential dissemination

Researchers generally proceed in this order, though reviewers (supervisors, ethics committees or funding bodies) might have their own format for the proposal. There may be change and reformulation at a later stage during the process. Although the research design is not rigid, we advise inexperienced researchers to follow clearly structured, conventional guidelines.

Working title

The working title can be changed as the research evolves, although permission for change might have to be sought from supervisors, research committees or funding bodies. (Discussion of titles in Chapter 19.)

Abstract of proposal

The abstract in the research proposal is a brief summary of the aim, methods, potential outcomes and usefulness.

Introduction

This section sets the scene for the research and must be clear and precise. Readers can only understand the proposal in context. In the introduction researchers demonstrate quality and feasibility of the study and the reasons for it.

The problem statement and rationale

This briefly describes the research focus, the way in which researchers became aware of the problem, and why they want to find out about it. They describe the context in which it takes place. It is important that the research problem is not trivial but has significance for healthcare. The potential usefulness of the project for the profession and clinical setting might be explained. Researchers can address a new problem that occurred in the setting or adopt a new approach to a familiar problem. They demonstrate the significance of the work by explaining why the research is important, and/or how it could possibly help in improving healthcare practice. Research funded by the National Health Service or related funding agencies must identify potential benefits to the National Health Service.

The rationale gives the reasons for the research that might have emerged through observation of a problem in a particular situation or were stimulated by reading about an event, a crisis or question in the clinical or community setting. At this stage researchers can mention some of the claims and suggestions that other writers make about the topic or area of study. The investigation of the problem should fill a gap in professional knowledge, however small that gap may be. The proposal is a starting point for the writing-up stage; indeed, some sections can be taken over directly into the research report and then extended or modified appropriately.

Context and setting

The context includes the environment and the conditions in which the study takes place as well as the culture of the participants and location. The setting is the physical location of the research, for instance a ward in a hospital, a clinic or the community.

The aim of the research

The aim of the study – a statement of the researcher's intentions and purpose – is made explicit. A statement of the aim is sufficient; objectives might constrict the study by directing it from the outset rather than following the guidance from the ideas of participants. Specific steps to reach the aim will develop as the research proceeds. The overarching purpose of the study reflected in the stated aim is usually concerned with an understanding of participants' feelings, experiences and perceptions as they have developed in the setting and context. Some researchers fail to distinguish the aim from the outcome of the research – the aim is always the specific research aim. For instance, 'the aim of the study is to develop a model of...' is not a research aim but an outcome of the inquiry. Instead the sentence should read something like ' the aim of the study is to explore... in order to develop a model...'

Examples of aims

The aim of this study is to explore the interactions of surgical patients and their consultants.

The purpose of my study is to describe the perspectives of nurse practitioners on their role and role relationships.

The study aims to examine people's perceptions of their visits to alternative practitioners and on the treatment they receive from them.

Creswell (2009) advises qualitative researchers to keep the aim non-directional, not to describe cause and effect but to give a general sense of the main idea using terms such as 'discover', 'develop', or 'describe' or 'explore'. Generally the statement of the study's aim should be crisp and not too long, otherwise it becomes unmanageable and unclear.

The literature

This is sometimes called the 'initial literature review' or 'overview of the literature'in qualitative research as it is not an exhaustive description and evaluation of all the major literature or research studies in the field of the research project. At this stage, the literature in a qualitative account broadly demonstrates the amount and level of knowledge that exists in the area of study. On the basis of an initial scan of relevant studies done by others, the researcher can decide whether to proceed with the work. It is important to mention foundational, classic studies on the subject – those which Hart (1998) calls 'landmark studies' – but also to include the most recent writing.

In a qualitative literature overview the discussion of the literature tends to be more limited than in other types of research. As the data have primacy, qualitative researchers avoid taking too much direction from the literature, and in consequence they only discuss a few major research studies.

Resources

Researchers specify the use of resources and other costs to demonstrate that the research can be adequately funded. Resourcing and costs are of major importance in proposals for grant-giving bodies and must be detailed. These include clerical costs, paper, computer, letters and mailing, as well as the researcher's time.

The research design and methodology

The research design is the overall plan and includes strategies and procedures. Researchers must also show how the conceptual framework will be developed during the research process. As stated before, methodology is concerned with the ideas and principles on which procedures are based. Methods consist of the procedures and strategies rooted in a methodology. Students must identify, describe and justify the methodology they adopt and the strategies and procedures involved. It is, of course, important that the methods fit the research question. It must be remembered that some of the details of a qualitative research project cannot be pre-specified as they arise during the research process.

Limitations of the study

Researchers should list the constraints and limitations of the study, and how they would overcome them. Locke et al. (2007) see limitations as weaknesses which constrain the research while delimitations are the boundaries around the research. By stating these, researchers show their careful preparation for the study. For example, one of the limitations of qualitative research that must be acknowledged is the lack of generalisability of findings. When stating the limitations, researchers can sometimes suggest ways to overcome them. It may be explained, for instance, how the lack of generalisability need not be a problem by describing attempts to achieve typicality or specificity, or how theoretical ideas might be generalisable.

> **Example**
>
> A midwife might plan a study researching women's experience of labour and childbirth in water. She intends to do this in her workplace through in-depth interviewing of women. She then realises that the outcome of the study would only be related to her own setting and cannot be generalised (quite apart from the ethical issues involved). To achieve typicality, she studies three other settings in different areas of the country. Important similarities in the different settings might be found. When this study is finished, it might well show that the results show typicality, meaning that they are typical not only for one, but across similar settings.

Sample selection and procedure

The access to participants and the initial sample size must be explained as well as other sampling procedures. An explanation of purposive and theoretical sampling is required, depending on the type of study.

Data collection and analysis

This section describes the way in which the data will be collected and analysed. These may include interviews, observations, diaries or other forms of data collection. The specifics of data analysis will also have to be discussed – for instance, constant comparative or thematic data analysis.

Ethical and entry issues

Researchers will give an indication as to how they will deal with these issues, where and how will they recruit their sample, for instance. They will also demonstrate how they will protect the participants from risk and safeguard them from disclosure of identity and lack of confidentiality. A statement about ethics committee approval should also be included. There is further discussion of ethical issues later in this chapter and in chapter 3.

References

The referencing must be exact, consistent and, in case of research students, compatible with the advice given by the university in which the student is registered. It is advisable to up-date the referencing towards the end of the study so that the latest edition of a book is consulted and referenced. A piece of research for a higher degree should contain the original source of an idea as far as it is known.

Timetable and costing

Reviewers wish to see a timetable for the research to become convinced of its feasibility. Therefore qualitative researchers submit a projected work schedule for the research even though they cannot always predict how long exactly each step is going to take. Each step is recorded on the time line. This time line can be written or drawn as a diagram. It must be remembered that the analysis of data in qualitative research takes a long time. The literature has to be searched after the identification of major categories and built into the findings and discussion. The write-up is revised until a storyline is clearly discernible. All this takes time.

Dissemination

Researchers identify the readership for which they write and explain the usefulness of the study for the particular group they address. They can state how they will disseminate the results of the study, be it through journals, books or other media such as conferences, video and audiotapes.

Example of time frame for an undergraduate student project
(This could be presented in diagrammatic form)

June/July

- Initial literature review/formulation of research question
- Gaining approval from gatekeepers, ethics committee and participants
- Writing proposal

August/September

- Data collection (for instance, interviewing and participant observation)
- Start of analysis (coding and categorising)

September–January

- Further data collection and analysis
- Literature review related to emerging categories
- Final decision on categories and major themes

January–March

- Writing up

Useful reading about evaluating proposals can be found in Morse (2003). It is a good idea to look at one's own proposal in the light of an evaluation checklist. We have added an example below.

Example evaluation of a qualitative research proposal

1. *The focus*
   Is the focus of the study clearly described?

2. *The aim*
   Is the aim linked to the discovery of feelings, perceptions and concepts rather than facts?
   Is the aim clearly and precisely stated?

3. *Methodology and methods*
   Is the methodology justified?
   Does the researcher show an understanding of qualitative inquiry?
   Are the methods, techniques and strategies clearly described in detail (this includes the data collection and analysis)?
   Are the methods appropriate for the problem or topic under study?

4. *The sample*
   Do the researchers state how they will gain access to the sample?
   Is there an explanation of purposive and/or theoretical sampling?
   Does the researcher describe the essential features of the sample?

5. *The literature*
   Has a gap in knowledge been identified through an initial literature review?
   Does the researcher state that the literature will be integrated into the discussion and become part of the study?

6. *Ethical and legal aspects*
   Are the relevant ethical interests of the participants respected and any conflict of interests from the researcher identified?
   Does the research study conform to the standards set out in the Research Governance Framework for Health and Social Care?
   Has permission been sought from the participants and the relevant gatekeepers including local research ethics committees?
   Will the researcher guarantee anonymity to the participants and the right to withdraw at any time?

7. *Practical issues*
   Is the topic area researchable and feasible?
   Does the researcher have enough time to undertake the study?
   Are the resources sufficient for the proposed project?

8. *Application to professional practice*
   Are there any implications for clinical practice, education or management? Will the outcome of the study have potential benefits for the participants or future participants?

9. *Trustworthiness or validity*
   Has the researcher demonstrated the trustworthiness or validity of the research?

Frisch *et al.* (2006) list the weaknesses that are present in many qualitative research proposals, of which researchers should be aware.

- The method is not appropriate for the research question.
- The researcher does not use the language of qualitative research.
- Not enough detail on data collection and analysis is given.
- The researcher does not reflect on the trustworthiness (validity) of the potential findings.

Access and entry to the setting

Health researchers, be they experienced professionals or students, must ask permission for entry to the setting and access to the participants. Gaining access means that they can observe the situation, talk to the individuals involved, read the necessary documents and interview potential participants. Formal permission is important in any research and protects both researchers and participants. Access is sought in various ways. Some health professionals put up a notice on a public board in the hospital in which they work; others ask permission from a self-help group, such as a group of carers, to talk to the members and find out whether they wish to participate. There are a number of ways to access potential informants, but voluntary participation must be ensured.

There are steps in the process of access and entry:

1. Gaining access to the participants (sometimes with the help of gatekeepers) and asking for permission to carry out the research
2. Explaining the aim and scope of the research
3. Thinking of ethical issues, particularly in their sampling decisions
4. Taking account of organisational or institutional issues
5. Counteracting the effects of reactivity

First then, researchers need to make contact with people in the setting who can give permission for access and speak to those whom they wish to observe and interview.

Second, the researcher explains early and clearly the type of project and its scope and aims. The explanation cannot be too detailed however, as the research might be prejudiced if everything is explained at this early stage, and participants would be guided towards specific issues rather than give their own ideas and perceptions to the researcher. (At the end of interviews and observation, more detail of the research must be given.)

Third, sensitive areas for research and vulnerable people must be treated with thoughtfulness and care.

Fourth, the researcher must be aware of the hierarchy in the system and know that conflicts between the interests of those at the top and those at the bottom of the hierarchy may exist. All individual participants involved should, of course be asked for permission to undertake the study.

Fifth, the researcher might have an effect on the setting. This may not only be threatening to the people involved but could also skew the research. The threat can be diminished if researchers get to know the people in the setting and establish a relationship of trust.

The choice of setting

Researchers search for an appropriate setting. The location where the research takes place must be suitable. For this the researcher has to know the setting intimately. There is, of course, a very important difference between general knowledge of, say, a paediatric oncology setting and researching it on the particular unit in which the professional has previously worked. Some settings are inappropriate or too complex for the particular research question to be answered. There is no point in planning an ambitious study if access to the setting proves impossible or difficult.

It is not advisable that health researchers carry out research in their own settings both for ethical and practical reasons (this is debated in Chapter 3). Qualitative researchers do not always choose a single setting but in an attempt to demonstrate the typicality of their findings, carry out the research in several settings. The answer to the research question needs to contribute to nursing knowledge and the existing literature (Morse, 2003).

Access to gatekeepers

Researchers negotiate with the 'gatekeepers' – the people who have the power to grant or withhold access to the setting. There may be a number of these at different places in the hierarchy of the organisation. Researchers should not just ask the person directly in charge but also others who hold power to start and stop the research. This includes managers, clinicians, consultants, nurses, general practitioners or other personnel, whose patients or clients might be observed or interviewed. For instance, if nurses wish to observe interaction on a ward, they must not only ask the consent of the manager of the NHS Trust and the local research ethics committee (LREC) but also that of the ward manager, the people working on the ward and, most importantly, the patients involved. All gatekeepers have power and control of access, but those at the top of the hierarchy are most powerful and should be asked first because they can restrict access even if everybody else agrees. If they cooperate, the path of the research can be smoothed, and their recommendations might make others more willing to collaborate, though their power might influence participants to take part, and the researcher has to ascertain that participation is entirely voluntary.

There can be problems with gatekeepers. They may make demands that the researchers cannot fulfil, trying to guide them in a particular direction or denying access to some individuals. Often their knowledge of research is based on familiarity with randomised controlled trials or surveys; hence, the nature of qualitative research and the aims and objectives of the study must be explained. The topic might have to be negotiated to fit in with the social organisation, physical environment or timetable of the setting. Although researchers cannot start without permission and must take the wishes of the gatekeepers into account, it is important that participants do not see researchers as a tool of management because this would affect the data.

Usually gatekeepers do not interfere in the research process, though ethics committees can and do. In research carried out with financial and social support from superiors, there is sometimes a danger that gatekeepers have their own expectations and attempt to manipulate the research, intentionally or unintentionally. This can affect the researchers' direction or report of the work, and they might find that they are influenced by these expectations. As gatekeepers are in a position of power, resistance might be difficult.

Example

An experienced hospital nurse wished to interview patients with a serious condition about their need for counselling. His immediate superior not only encouraged the research but she also saw it as important because of the support that might be given to future patients with the same condition. The ethics committee had given its approval. However, one of the consultants on the ward disagreed with the form of the proposed research and refused permission for interviews of the patients in his care.

A series of complications and difficulties followed. On the one hand the research was seen as important by the researcher and his colleagues. On the other, to go ahead meant directly contravening the consultant's wishes and generating conflict between him and the researcher's superiors. Endless debates and discussions would waste precious time, and in the end the researcher decided to explore the perceptions of the nurses who cared for the patients instead of interviewing the patients themselves. Although the piece of research did not directly explore the feelings of patients, it produced results that helped in their care and avoided conflict on the ward. Of course, the study became completely different from that originally planned – and possibly less useful (this example is adapted from a real case).

The above example shows that powerful people within the setting can generate difficulties for the researcher who often has to compromise. Contract arrangements might lead to more constraints on researchers as institutional objectives might take precedence over individual research interest because of the prioritising of resources. Staff time costs money.

Researchers are denied access for a variety of reasons:

- The gatekeeper sees the researcher as unsuitable.
- It is feared that an observer might disturb the setting.
- There is suspicion and fear of criticism.
- Sensitive issues are being investigated.
- Potential participants in the research may be embarrassed or fearful.

Powerful gatekeepers might see researchers as unsuitable because of gender, age or lack of trustworthiness. They must be convinced that the researcher is both able to cope with the study and trustworthy. Friends and acquaintances who are already involved in the chosen location can sometimes persuade those in power of the ability and trustworthiness of the researcher. If researchers are very young, the gatekeepers might feel that they lack credibility; some female researchers suggest that they have problems with male colleagues in positions of power.

Managers might deny access if they feel that the setting will be disturbed by the presence of researchers. A ward climate might change because everybody feels that the researchers are watching every task and movement that occurs; therefore it is important that observers and interviewers immerse themselves in the setting until they become part of it and do not create an 'observer effect'.

Researchers ask potential participants for permission to interview or observe, stating clearly the right of refusal or withdrawal and assuring confidentiality. When the main steps have been taken, the research can begin, always taking into account appropriate timing, site and situation.

Summary

Here is a brief summary of the research process:

- The first step in the process is selection of the research topic.
- After an overview of previous research the researchers identify the gaps in knowledge and define their own research focus.

- The specific topic area and the appropriate approach are selected.
- Following ethical guidelines, the researcher writes a research proposal and seeks access to gatekeepers and participants.
- It is essential that research in the healthcare arena is vetted by the relevant ethics committee.
- The researcher must obtain consent from participants, if possible in writing.
- The study must be of importance for the people or setting under investigation.

References

Barroso, J., Gollop, C.J., Sandelowski, M. *et al.* (2003) The challenges of searching for and retrieving qualitative studies. *Western Journal of Nursing Research*, **25** (2), 153–76.

Creswell, J.W. (2009) *Research Design: Qualitative and Quantitative and Mixed Methods Approaches*, 3rd edn. Los Angeles, CA, Sage.

Frisch, N.C., Rew, L. & Hagedorn, M.E. (2006) Guidelines for preparing research proposals. *The American Holistic Nurses Association* **25**(5), 2022. /ahna.org/public/Research_Guidelines.pdf

Glaser, B.G. (with the assistance of Judith Holton) (2004) Remodeling grounded theory [80 paragraphs]. *Forum Qualitative Sozialforschung (Forum: Qualitative Social Research)*, **5**(2), Art. 4. [On-line Journal]. Available at: http://www.qualitative-research.net/fqs-texte/2-04/2-04glaser-e.htm accessed December 2007

Hansen, E.C. (2006) *Successful Qualitative Health Research: A Practical Introduction.* Maidenhead, Open University Press.

Hart, C. (1998) *Doing a Literature Review: Releasing the Social Science Research Imagination.* London, Sage.

Haverkamp, B.E. & Young, R.A. (2007) Paradigms, purpose and the role of the literature: formulating a rationale for qualitative investigations. *The Counseling Psychologist*, **35** (2), 265–94.

Holliday, A. (2007) *Doing and Writing Qualitative Research*, 2nd edn. London, Sage.

Locke, L., Spirduso, W.W. & Silverman, S.J. (2007) *Proposals that Work: A Guide for Planning Dissertations and Grant Proposals*, 5th edn. Thousand Oaks, CA, Sage.

Mantzoukas, S. (2008) Facilitating research students formulating qualitative research questions. *Nurse Education Today*, **28** (3), 371–77.

Metcalfe, M. (2003) Author(ity): The literature review as expert witnesses [45 paragraphs]. *Forum Qualitative Sozialforschung (Forum: Qualitative Social Research)* 4(1). [On-line Journal], accessed February 2008. Available at: http://www.qualitative-research.net/fqs-texte/1-03/1-03metcalfee.htm

Morse, J.M. (2003) A review committee's guide for evaluating qualitative proposals. *Qualitative Health Research*, **13** (6), 833–51.

Punch, K.F. (2006) *Developing Effective Research Proposals*, 2nd edn. London, Sage.

Shaw, R.L., Booth, A., Sutton, A.J. *et al.* (2004) Finding qualitative research: an evaluation of search strategies. *BMC Medical Research Methodology* 4 (5). Available at: http://www.biomedcentral.com/1471-2288/4/5, accessed February 2008

Further reading

Marshall, K. & Rossman, G. (2006) *Designing Qualitative Research*, 4th edn. Thousand Oaks, CA, Sage (chapters 2 and 3).

CHAPTER 4

Ethical Considerations

Ethical issues must be considered in all research, be it quantitative or qualitative. Health researchers apply the principles that protect participants in the research from harm or risk and follow professional rules laid down in codes of conduct and research guidelines. The *Research Governance Framework for Health and Social Care* of the Department of Health (DH, 2005: section 2) sets out standards for all those involved in the conduct of research and is not restricted to any one professional group. The standards are organised into the following domains:

- *Ethics:* the dignity, right, safety and well-being of participants
- *Science:* the quality and appropriateness of research
- *Information:* the requirements for free access to research information
- *Health, safety and employment:* taking account of the safety of participants and of researchers and other staff
- *Finance and intellectual property:* financial probity and compliance with the law for research activity
- *Quality research culture:* application of principles and standards in an open and visible form, and promotion of expert management and leadership

(DH, 2005)

These elements are linked together and form part of the ethical framework.

The basic ethical framework for research

Historically, attempts at establishing international rules for ethical research stem from the time after the Second World War, as a result of the criminal trials in Germany. The Nuremberg Code contained guidelines for consent or discontinuation of studies and advised on the balance between risks and benefits. Most of these rules were, however, concerned with experimental research. The World Medical Association's Declaration of Helsinki (2008) lists the basic principles for all medical research (the first version appeared in 1964 and has been amended several times). Although the terminology concerns mainly medical research and human 'subjects' (*sic* – see Chapter 8), the declaration contains guidance for all research investigators and research participants. The latest revision (2008) strengthens, in particular, the aspects of informed consent.

Ethics in research has its basis in certain philosophical assumptions (which cannot be discussed here). The term originates in the Greek word 'ethos' which, according to Aristotle, means character and refers to the credibility of a speaker or writer. It is a branch of philosophy concerning value – and there are two approaches in ethics: the *normative* approach (what we should do) and the *descriptive* approach (what we actually do).

Ethics for health professionals/researchers is concerned with guiding professionals to protect and safeguard the interest of clients (for instance, see NMC, 2008). The researcher needs to draw on ethical principles and rules and balance these in the research process. Key ethicists in this field are Beauchamp and Childress (2008) in their work *Principles of Biomedical Ethics*. They view ethics as a generic concept for both understanding and examining moral life. Although the book considers bio-medical ethics in particular, it is useful for all health professionals. The authors emphasise a framework of moral norms that encompass principles, rules, rights, virtues and moral ideals and outline four basic principles as pivotal to this framework. Although this 'principlism' has found critics – in particular social scientists – it emphasises some essential human rights important for all health and social care researchers:

1. The principle of *respect for autonomy* (respecting the decision-making capacities of autonomous persons)
2. The principle of *nonmaleficence* (avoiding the causation of harm)
3. The principle of *beneficence* (providing benefits and balancing benefits against risks and costs)
4. The principle of *justice* (distributing benefits, risks and costs fairly)

Respect for autonomy (from the Greek *autos*, self; *nomos*, law) means that the participants in the research must be allowed to make a free, independent and informed choice without coercion. The counterpart in law of this principle is the right of self determination, and it underpins the notion of informed consent and refusal. The concept of respect for autonomy includes advice to the researcher to consider the social nature of individuals, the impact of their choices and actions on others and the emotions involved in the process of research (Butler, 2003).

As research is conducted for the benefit of individuals, patients/users, care professionals and the public in general (DH, 2005) these are pertinent features. The Department of Health (p. 15) makes clear that the primary consideration in any research study is to protect the dignity, rights, safety and well-being of participants. As informed consent is at the centre of all research, studies must have appropriate arrangements for obtaining informed consent (see later in this chapter).

The principles of *beneficence* and *nonmaleficence* (do good, do no harm) demand that benefits outweigh the risks for the individual and the wider society. The principles set up by the World Medical Association (WMA) add that risks must be carefully assessed and weighed against benefits not only for the population as a whole but also for the individual; these risks should be kept to a minimum.

The principle of *justice* implies that the research strategies and procedures are fair and just. In a multicultural society this includes proper representation in research samples (DH, 2005) and respect for diversity (age, gender, disability and sexual orientation). In their ethical framework, Beauchamp and Childress (2008) also discuss ethical rules, and there is a loose distinction between rules and principles in the operation of these rules. They argue that rules are more specific, giving more precise guides to action. These are related to research as set out below:

- Veracity (truth-telling)
- Privacy
- Confidentiality
- Fidelity

Veracity in healthcare involves an accurate flow of information that is comprehensive and takes account of the participant's understanding. These features are important for gaining informed consent for participation in research. The rule of 'truth-telling' links to the principle of respect for autonomy. Dishonesty would not respect the autonomy of the individual and impede the decision-making process. Similarly considerations of veracity are necessary in terms of disclosure and nondisclosure of information. An individual cannot make a fully informed decision about participation in research if some information is withheld. Giving full initial information, however, can be problematic with respect to the flexibility of qualitative research methods as shown later.

Privacy is also part of the principle of respect for autonomy. Researchers must respect privacy of the research participants which is closely linked to confidentiality. The Declaration of Helsinki (WMA, 2008: 3) states that 'every precaution must be taken to protect the privacy of research subjects (*sic*) and the confidentiality of their personal information and to minimize the impact of the study on their physical, mental and social integrity'.

Confidentiality in healthcare generally is recognised as underpinning the patient–practitioner–researcher relationship. Without such confidentiality there would be no basis for trust in these encounters. Information can only be given to a third party with the consent of the research participant. All those involved in research need be aware of their ethical and legal duties and ensure that systems are in place to protect confidentiality (DH, 2005).

Finally the ethical rule of *fidelity* concerns notions of faithfulness or loyalty. Beauchamp and Childress (2008) argue that traditionally professional loyalty concerns giving priority to the participant's interests but third-party interests such as institutional interests and the changing health professions also need consideration, and conflict might occur between these differing priorities. Beauchamp and Childress specifically examine aspects of conflicts of fidelity and stress that fidelity conflicts can occur in both therapeutic and non-therapeutic research. The Declaration of Helsinki (WMA, 2008: 3) states that research participants must be informed of any institutional affiliations or potential conflicts of interest of the researcher. The *Research Governance Framework for Health and Social Care* (DH, 2005: ii), makes clear that it is the researcher's duty 'to protect the dignity, rights, safety and well-being of participants'.

All health and social care researchers have to justify the research not only to research ethics committees (RECs) but also to participants, superiors and gatekeepers. They must recognise the right of informants to refuse participation in the project or to withdraw from it if they wish. In Britain, the National Research Ethics Service (NRES), under whose aegis RECs operate, helps to safeguard patient rights. It is an ethics service within the National Patient Safety Agency for the National Health Service. It also guides and advises research applicants, be they students or other researchers. Its purpose and functions can be found on the web and include all application forms and guidance notes. The equivalent of the NRES in the United States is the National Institute of Health (NIH) which has an ethics manual and provides training.

Ethics in qualitative research

Many aspects of the sections below would apply to all types of research, but for practical reasons they are integrated with issues particularly concerning qualitative research.

Introduction

Van den Hoonaard (2008) states that ethical guidelines for bio-medical research have – problematically in his opinion – shaped the ethical guidelines for social research, an area which encompasses qualitative health research. He suggests that the traditional medical view of the human 'subject' is inadequate in social research when compared to the holistic understanding of the World Health Organization (WHO). For qualitative researchers a holistic view of 'participant' as an active and interactive human being is of major importance, and researchers need to be aware of the social and cultural context. These issues must be considered especially in qualitative research, as it is context bound and usually interactive. The following section is a discussion of research with patients which includes the particular concerns of qualitative researchers.

Ethics in research with patients

Patients are in a particularly endangered position for two main reasons: the perceived imbalance of power in their relationship with health professionals and the special vulnerability of being ill. Participants are in a situation in which they have limited power, and they feel a lack of control. They are not always aware of their rights to refuse participation in the research, particularly if it lasts over a long period of time, and when unexpected issues arise. The researcher must understand the feeling of obligation that participants might have. Often they feel powerless to deny the researchers access to their world. While official documents focus on the rights of patients, research in healthcare often deals with people who have little real power in their situation. The power balance is perhaps more equal in the client's own setting than in the hospital situation.

Timing is an important issue in qualitative research (Cowles, 1988). Bad timing can inhibit informants, especially when they have recently had a traumatic experience. They might feel threatened at this particular time and too emotionally involved to make rational decisions about taking part or continuing the research. This leads to the problems of interviewing patients.

Interviews and observations

Interviews, in particular, may deeply affect participants who do not just reveal their experiences and deep thoughts to the researcher but also might become aware of hidden feelings for the first time. Interviews might provoke distressing memories and strong emotions (Butler, 2003), and the researcher should be prepared to allow the participant to work through these. Interviewers also might find these conversations distressing and stressful, and they too might need peer support or even counselling.

Towards the end of the research project another problem may arise: the continuous, intimate nature of the interviewer–informant relationship generates trust and sometimes friendship; therefore, it is difficult for both researcher and participants to extricate from it. A sensitive researcher does not leave the patient anxious or worried. The 'debriefing' of informants and the provision of emotional support, if needed, is important. If health researchers find strong distress in patients, there is need for debriefing and a mechanism for following up the participants.

Example

Consider a nurse who wishes to interview patients with a serious illness about their feelings and the support they receive. The study will almost certainly help in the future because of extended knowledge and information that nurses have gained. Patients, however, may well feel distressed and disturbed by the nurse's probing into private thoughts and feelings at a time when they experience pain, distress and anxiety about their future.

Mander (1988) claims that patients are particularly vulnerable because they are 'a captive population'. Patients are vulnerable especially when they are very young or very old. Interviews must take into account the difficulty they might have in sustaining long in-depth interviews; the researcher might consider several short interviews instead. Children, people with learning difficulties and those who have a mental or terminal illness need particular protection. For the children and some people with learning difficulties, researchers are obliged not only to gain permission from the participants but also from parents or legal guardians as ethical issues are particularly complex in this case. Even experienced health professionals should undertake research with these groups only after careful consideration. (NRES has specific guidance documents for research with those who cannot give consent for themselves.)

There are particular issues to be considered when carrying out research with frail older people (Harris and Dyson, 2001) as much qualitative research now focuses on this group. It is difficult for some, though by no means all, members of this group to give fully informed consent as they might be prevented from doing so by ill health, chronic disease or fatigue. Even factors such as size of writing in the information sheet or consent form or the clarity of the researcher's voice are important, as is the potential participant's ability to understand the information and to concentrate on it. Older people are sometimes loath to commit themselves to being interviewed for research purposes and must therefore be recruited with care and diplomacy.

Harris and Dyson (2001) add among other suggestions:

- Researchers should not underestimate difficulties in recruiting vulnerable older people.
- Researchers need to develop skills in recruiting members of this group while also protecting their rights to refuse to take part.
- Researchers should attempt to obtain genuine consent in a study (See Further reading).

Very similar issues are taken into account in research with children. Researchers also need special consideration of 'giving voice' to minority groups as there is often a tension between using people as sources of data and respecting the rights of individuals to be heard. Researchers must give reasons for focusing on or excluding minority groups.

Ethical questions arise in *observation*, too. Covert observation is problematic and its ethics debatable. Researchers in the field of healthcare usually disclose their presence as observers and reveal the purpose of the observation. This may generate the observer effect – the change that observers may bring about in the setting through their presence. Patton (2002) suggests that the effect can be overestimated, as participants are immersed in the setting and get used to their presence. In any case, clients and colleagues generally trust the health professional to behave ethically.

Permission for observation must always be obtained. Rogers (2008) gives the example of midwifery research where a researcher might wish to observe the empathising skills of midwives during the labour process. This means that clients and others in the setting have to be asked for permission and not only midwives.

Informed consent and voluntary participation

Informed, voluntary consent means that research participants are fully informed about the research and give their voluntary agreement to take part in it. There should be neither implicit or explicit pressure from researchers nor any inducement. The Royal College of Nursing (2005) gives guidance about informed consent in health and social care research and states: 'Informed consent is an ongoing agreement by a person to receive treatment, undergo procedures or participate in research, after risks, benefits and alternatives have been adequately explained to them' (RCN, 2005: 3).

The nature of qualitative research is its flexibility, the use of unexpected ideas arising during data collection (serendipity) and the prompts that are allowed during interviews. Qualitative research focuses on the meanings and interpretation of the participants. The developing concepts are grounded in the data rather than in a previously established framework; hence qualitative researchers have inherent problems with informed consent. When the research begins, they have no specific objectives for the research, though they have a general aim and focus. Shaw (2008) discusses this problem: the participants cannot always have full and detailed information about the project as the ideas of the researcher might change during its process. This is a dilemma of which participants must be informed. Researchers must often make difficult decisions after balancing advantages and disadvantages of giving full information from the beginning of the research. The initial lack of complete information is only justifiable because it produces data without harming the participants. By the end of the research participants need full disclosure of details, so they can make an informed decision on the use of their data; consent given before the interview cannot be taken for granted and must be confirmed throughout without putting pressure on the participants.

Consent in qualitative research is an ongoing process. Whilst consent may be implied in one phase of the research, it cannot be assumed at another stage when the researcher's ideas change on the basis of the information provided, or indeed, when participants change their minds. Thus consent is not a once and forever agreement by participants but requires ongoing consent.

The process of informed consent is located within the principle of respect for autonomy. This principle demands that participation is voluntary and that informants are aware not only of the potential benefits of the research for the population but also of the personal and individual risks they take. First-time researchers, in particular, should take care that there is no major risk involved, though all research involves some risks. Participants then must be informed throughout about the voluntary nature of participation in research and about the possibility of withdrawing at any stage. This should be shown in the written consent form required in most health research. Van den Hoonaard (2002), however, thinks that written consent is inappropriate in qualitative research, and Green and Thorogood (2004) even believe that the research relationship might be damaged through this. They argue that, although individuals are usually willing to participate, they often reconsider when asked to sign forms. However, these writers are sociologists and not health professionals, and the latter would have to ask for consent forms; otherwise they would not generally gain permission from ethics committees, however ethical their behaviour. Ethics committees generally request a consent form (see later in this chapter).

It is useful to anticipate potential problems in the course of the research and consider their solutions. The researcher must be aware that the research might threaten participants, superiors or institutions, even if it is intended to have a positive effect. Sim (1991) identifies a major dilemma of researchers: they experience conflict between the recognition of the rights of human beings and the wish to advance professional knowledge. Electronic mail and internet inquiry also pose particular problems as it is difficult to ascertain that the consent is truly given by the participants (Kralik *et al.*, 2005). Special measures need to be taken to safeguard people when the internet is used for research (see Further reading).

Anonymity and confidentiality

Qualitative healthcare research might be more intrusive than quantitative research; therefore, the researcher needs sensitivity and communication skills. Usually, anonymity is guaranteed, and a promise is given that identities will not be revealed. Qualitative researchers work with small samples and use thick description (see Glossary); it is not always easy to protect identities. Even a detailed job description or an unusual occupational title of an informant may destroy anonymity.

Researchers sometimes change minor details about the participants so that they cannot be identified. For instance, researchers may change the age of all participants by two or three years when age is not an important factor in the research (Archbold, 1986). This of course must be reported in the research account without giving exact particulars. Only the researcher should be able to match the real names and identities with the tapes, report or description; participants are given numbers or pseudonyms. Tapes, notes and transcriptions – important tools for the qualitative researcher – must be kept secure and names not located near the tapes. If other people, superiors, supervisors or typists have access to the information – however limited this might be – names should not be disclosed, participants' identities must be disguised and they should be asked for permission. It is also worth noting that, although undertakings of confidentiality are given, participants need to know that others might have access to the tapes for peer reviews for verification of the analysis.

Examples

1. Francesca, a registrar, wanted to show her supervisor some of her interview transcripts and the way she had analysed the data. The supervisor asked to listen to her tapes at the same time to hear the voice and intonation of the participants' narratives. The researcher had sought agreement from the participants when gaining permission for the research and assured them of the discretion of the supervisor and non-disclosure of their identities.
2. Jonathan, a nurse, wished to have his transcripts typed by a professional typist. He believed that he could use the time better by listening to the tapes. He realised that he had to gain the typist's written confirmation not to divulge the data or any detail that had been gleaned from transcribing them.
3. When Eva completed her data analysis, she decided to use 'peer debriefing' with some of her colleagues to find out whether her colleagues arrived at similar results of the analysis. She had taken this into account when writing the consent sheet by asking patients' permission to show the data to a small number of peers while keeping anonymity without identifying the participants.

The researcher's dilemma is to decide what information can be made public; if there is doubt or ambiguity, the decision depends upon the client's wishes.

Patton (2002) suggests that tapes should be erased a year after the research has been finished, but many ethics committees demand that they be kept for ten years; universities keep theirs often for five. At the participants' request, researchers sometimes erase the tapes after completion of the research, but this can only take place if approved by the REC. Visual data such as films, photos or videotapes are treated in the same way as other data. Covert image taking is not only unethical, it is also illegal (see Further reading).

Confidentiality is a separate issue from anonymity but also important. In research where words and ideas from participants are used, full confidentiality cannot be promised, especially as qualitative research contains quotes from the interview data. In these studies, confidentiality means researchers keep confidential that which the participant does not wish to disclose to others.

Patients, in particular, sometimes disclose intimate details of their lives which the researcher cannot divulge, although the information could be useful for the research.

The participant information sheet

The information for research participants needs to be clear, unambiguous and written in lay language. The researcher must confirm that the participation is voluntary. (More exact details can be found on the NRES website, Information Sheets and Consent Forms, pp. 14–47. Some of the elements in the information below are specific for qualitative research.)

The information sheet consists of a *short* summary:

- The title of the research
- Invitation to take part
- What is the purpose of the study (It is important to be as specific as possible)
- Why the participant has been asked to take part (How the participant was chosen, how many others in the research)
- Voluntary participation (Voluntary, right to withdraw at any time, no effect on standard of care)
- What happens if the participant takes part (How long is the research and the involvement of the participant, how often attendance is needed and how long, what will happen to the data, security and confidentiality of tape-recorded material)
- What are the disadvantages, benefits or risks
- What happens after the study (What happens to data such as tapes or fieldnotes)
- Issues of confidentiality, anonymity (Permission for use of quotes without identifying participant)
- Any involvement of others in the study (in qualitative research: the involvement of supervisors, peers for peer review, typists of interview scripts)
- What happens to the results (Will participants want to know about these, dissemination, publication)
- Who is funding and reviewing the study (self, funding body, university, etc)

The researcher also presents a consent form for signature when giving out the information sheet. This form is not the same for all participants but depends on the individual (adult, child, colleague, etc.) and the type of research. An example taking account of qualitative research is given below (p. 32 in Information Sheets and Consent Forms of NRES specifies more detail for research in general).

CONSENT FORM

Title of Research

Name and status of researcher (student, nurse, doctor, professional researcher)

Institutional affiliation

Contact address with telephone nr.

Date

Permission for research

I have read and understood the information sheet, and I am aware that I can ask questions about the research and receive satisfactory answers.

I know that the participation is voluntary and that I can withdraw at any time without giving a reason (and, for patients: without my care being affected).

I agree to take part in the interview (focus group, observation, etc) and give my permission for tape-recording this, and for the use of quotes, without my name being disclosed.

I understand that the data might be looked at by the researchers' supervisors or peers for reviewing without my identity being revealed.

I agree to take part in the research.

Name of participant

Name of researcher

(Information sheets for children, young people and guardians are given in section 3 of the NRES Information and Consent Sheet. The site is amended periodically.)

Researching one's peers

When carrying out research with one's peers, different problems arise. Although Platt (1981) suggests that in interview situations participants are often in a position of inequality, this is not so for colleagues, unless the researcher is in a position of authority as manager or senior colleague. When researchers interview and observe their peers, a more reciprocal relationship exists which makes it easier for participants to become equal partners in the research enterprise – the aim of most qualitative research relationships. Work colleagues and peers of the researcher can, however, become vulnerable. The relationship of trust that they have may be broken through unintended disclosures or subtle pressure 'for the sake of colleagueship'. Wiles *et al.* (2006: 294) put forward the idea that peers already know some of the 'tricks of the trade' when they take part in the research while patient participants do not have this knowledge or information. The peers' awareness of these issues might endanger honest disclosure. There may be common preconceptions which the researchers share with their peers; moreover, 'researching one's peers' may mean that researchers impose a framework which is based on their *assumption* of shared perceptions, and this does not allow participants to develop their own ideas. Coghlan and Brannick (2005) advise researchers not to become rigid in their views but be open to 'disconfirming' and challenging evidence.

The research relationship

Influence in research means a process of changing something whilst studying it. Researchers influence the research and its findings. Qualitative researchers acknowledge their subjectivity and make this explicit in their report. Thus, nurses and other health researchers must account for the influences of their own perspectives in the process and outcome of the research. They need to scrutinise their own actions throughout the research process and this includes the interpersonal and interactional aspects of the research (Guillemin and Gillam, 2004). This also suggests a quick response to 'ethical moments' which means managing critical issues when they arise.

The dual role

Health professionals have dual roles and responsibilities, that of professional and that of researcher, and they may experience problems of identity. On the one hand, they are committed to the research as they wish to advance health knowledge for the good of their clients and recognise that research is needed for the advancement of knowledge. On the other, as professionals they are dedicated to the care and welfare of clients. Nurses in particular who care so intimately for patients, and also other health professionals, cannot close their eyes to distress and pain because their professional training guides them towards caring and being advocates for their clients. If participants are threatened by the research or feel that they are, then the professional has to give up the researcher role.

In their professional role health researchers recognise the person as patient or client while in their researcher role they see the person as informant, as participant in the research. The different elements of the researcher identity – researcher/professional – cannot always be reconciled. West and Butler (2003) state that role conflict or confusion might prevent the researcher from performing either role well. Clients, too, do not always understand this duality and dichotomy in the health worker's role. They expect care and help from the person whom they perceive as a carer and who professes to be a researcher. Clients might recognise that professional intervention by the researcher is not always possible. Nevertheless, health professionals cannot completely detach themselves from their informants, particularly in the close relationship of the qualitative research process. They respond to distress and need, especially in emergency situations, or call on colleagues who perform appropriate roles in the setting. RECs will usually require a strategy for providing ongoing support, for example, carrying the names and addresses of self-help groups.

A research study requires both empathy and distancing. These traits appear contradictory. On the one hand, researchers are asked to be non-judgemental and must be aware of personal values that could influence the research. On the other, professionals often have empathy and feeling for their clients. The researcher, however, cannot allow preconceived attitudes or over-involvement to influence the data. This might be problematic because of the close relationship between researcher and participant.

Researchers must be able to put themselves into the informant's place; this helps to establish the rapport that is important in this type of approach but might also generate intense emotions in both. Qualitative research into sensitive topics generates these problems to a greater extent than any other type. The qualitative interview can in some cases resemble a counselling session in that the researcher is a non-judgemental listener. However, researchers who are also health professionals need to be careful to distinguish between research and therapeutic roles.

Research in the researcher's workplace

Writers on ethics always include a caution on carrying out research in one's own setting because it can be complex and difficult. As early as 1986, Archbold suggested that health professionals do not do research with people directly in their care, particularly because of the power relationship between the researcher and the researched. Nevertheless, many health researchers are interested in their own setting in particular and wish to understand the issues and solve the problems specific to their workplace. Qualitative researchers will experience some of the same dilemmas to those who carry out other types of inquiry, although some of the problems differ. Butler (2003) discusses some of these issues, such as recruitment, role conflict and issues of confidentiality.

The main problems are linked to the following:

Access and recruitment
The intimate nature of the relationship between participants and researcher
The dual role of the researcher

Gatekeepers such as managers or ethics committees sometimes deny access as they can foresee some of the problems. Even if gatekeepers understand the research and are sympathetic to it, dilemmas remain, as many are in a position of authority or care directly for the patient. Butler (2003) warns of the danger of implicit or subtle coercion and pressure; even if participants are assured that their participation is voluntary they might feel obliged to take part because they know the researcher as a professional on whom they are dependent to an extent. They might give different answers to a professional whom they know well, to avoid endangering their future care and relationship than to a researcher who is a stranger to them. The participants often disclose more about their lives than is necessary for the research. Not only might this special knowledge and information influence the researcher but it also adds to the danger of inadvertent disclosure in the research account. Researchers need special awareness and reflexivity (Coghlan and Brannick, 2005), always being conscious of and examining their own actions.

The role of research ethics committees

We have acknowledged the existence of ethics committees earlier in this chapter. Health Services (in most countries) and universities usually have their own ethics committees to scrutinise students' research to safeguard the participants, the researchers and the institution.

Guillemin and Gillam (2004) differentiate between 'procedural ethics' and 'ethics in practice'. Procedural ethics is linked to the process of gaining permission from ethics committees and review boards for the research. Ethics in practice is related to the considerations which arise in the process of carrying out the research such as day-to-day dilemmas that occur (see above). In this section we shall consider procedural ethics.

Procedural ethics includes completion of ethics forms which are requested by committees. Researchers try to convince these committees that they are competent and trustworthy. This means using language which is clear to readers (the committee includes lay members). Ethics Committees which, in the past were not always well informed about qualitative research, are now usually familiar with this type of inquiry.

West and Butler (2003) describe the review process of one such ethics research committee, and this might provide useful guidance for qualitative researchers. It focuses on general ethical issues and those specific to qualitative research which were discussed above, such as its emotional impact – on both researcher and participant – and the demands the researcher might make. The conflict or tension between the roles of researcher and health professionals should also be considered. Ethics committees are also concerned with the safety of the researcher. Many of these committees see interviews in people's homes as potentially problematic for the researcher and only permit them if safeguards are in place (such as mobile phones, information about timing of interviews and return to base, address left with colleague or supervisor). Indeed, committees advise researchers not to travel to dangerous locations.

> **Example**
>
> Carol, an experienced nurse researcher, wished to carry out a study in an area of the world that was seen as dangerous by the UK Foreign Office which cautioned against a visit to this country. The University Ethics Committee counselled against this research, even though Carol visited this part of the world every year for several months and argued that the research was important for the local population and health professionals alike.

An awareness of the emotional response helps researchers to deal with distress, stress or grief of the participants and indeed their own. Most ethics committees look for strategies that can potentially manage the emotional issues. Not all researchers are aware of the inconvenience or burden they place on participants, especially on those who are vulnerable. Qualitative interviews in particular can be very demanding in time and concentration. Ethics committees will mainly focus on the ethical elements of the research, but there are expectations for every application to be accompanied by a peer review (and the latter looks at the research in terms of 'good' science, that is, that the research design and procedures are appropriate and its aim worthwhile and credible). The *Research Governance Framework for Health and Social Care* (DH, 2005) demands quality standards in research; a bad research project could be considered unethical. (Different countries have different names for their ethics committees, for instance in the United States there are Institutional Review Boards (IRB), independent ethics committees which protect the rights and ensure the welfare of participants.)

Reviewing the research project

Walker *et al.* (2005) suggest some key ethical questions on which ethics committees will focus. Researchers themselves might reflect on these not only to get through the ethics committee review process but also to improve their own chances of acting within an ethical framework. Not all these questions have unambiguous answers but researchers reflect on them and are prepared to justify their actions. The following ethics checklist is given by Walker *et al.* (2005: 93–5):

Key ethical questions: Audiotaped interviews

Informed consent and the principle of respect for autonomy:

1. Is the recruitment strategy appropriate and acceptable?
2. Is the Participant Information Sheet (PIS) presented in a user-friendly way that reflects the person-centred nature of the interview process?

3. Does the PIS include information about the following?
   - The approximate length of the interview
   - Where and when the interview is arranged and how contact is to be made
   - What is expected of the participant
   - The possibility of eliciting distressing thoughts or memories and the availability of safeguards and follow-up supports in the event of this
   - Full details about confidentiality and possible limits to confidentiality
4. Does the application make it clear that consent is ongoing and will be reconfirmed at each stage of the research process?
   - Does the application include consent to use personal information once it has been collected/analysed?
   - Where focus groups are used, what action will be taken if one participant withdraws his or her consent following data collection (i.e. will all the data be discarded)?

Right to privacy/confidentiality:

1. Does the research location allow for privacy?
2. Does the applicant have appropriate strategies for dealing with the following potential problems or issues?
   - Legitimate complaints made during confidential disclosures
   - Concerns about the health, safety and/or well-being of the patient, based on confidential disclosures
   - Concerns about the safety or well-being of others, based on confidential disclosures
   - The protection of anonymity during writing-up/publication
3. Where the GP or other health professional is to be informed at any stage, will participants be asked for their consent?

Nonmaleficence/beneficence:

1. Is there any possibility that the interview might prompt distressing thoughts or memories?
   - If so, is this recognised and adequately addressed?
2. Do the interviews involve sensitive topics or potentially psychologically vulnerable groups?
   - If so, do the CVs of the research team indicate that the researcher is suitably qualified and adequately prepared to deal with the possible consequences?
   - Is the researcher adequately supported to deal with this?
3. How does the researcher intend to deal with participants' distress?
   - During interview
   - Following interview

- E.g. is there provision for professional support and/or follow-up services (including voluntary organisations), as appropriate?
4. Where a maximum time limit is imposed on the interview, has the researcher allowed sufficient time to deal with all possible eventualities, such as distress, questions etc., and achieve closure?

Fairness/Justice:

1. Does the information provided indicate that the power relationship between researcher and participant is suitably balanced to favour the needs of the participant?
2. Where applicable, is the involvement of the researcher as research tool adequately justified in terms of the potential for bias?
3. Is the exclusion of those from minority groups justified?
4. Is the sample adequately justified in terms of diversity according to such criteria as age, gender, disability and sexual orientation?

Safety of the researcher:

1. Are provisions in place to protect the safety of the researcher, particularly when interviewing in the home?
2. In the case of a sensitive topic, is support available to protect the emotional well-being of the researcher?

Data protection:

1. Are adequate steps identified to preserve confidentiality during transcribing and data storage?
   - Will transcribing be undertaken by someone outside the research team?
   - Does the storage of tapes/transcripts conform to local R&D policies and, where necessary, education institution requirements?

Key ethical questions: observation studies

Informed consent:

1. How will informed consent be obtained from all participants, particularly when observation is undertaken in a public setting?
   - Will information be provided individually or by public notice?
   - Is there a copy of the PIS and/or public information sheet, and is this suitable?
   - Is written or verbal consent to be obtained from each participant, or is consent presumed in the absence of dissent?
   - How will the researcher deal with those who fail to give, or subsequently withdraw, their consent?

- What special measures will be taken to gain consent from vulnerable groups and those with communication difficulties?
2. How will informed consent be obtained from consenting participants in closed (institutional) settings?
    - Will consent be ongoing?
    - Will participants have an opportunity to withdraw their consent to the use of the data after they have been collected?
    - What undertakings of confidentiality are given and are these realistic?
3. Are there any plans to use video extracts for demonstration or teaching purposes? [These data afford a powerful educational tool.]
    - If so, is this made explicit in the information sheet?

Rights to confidentiality:

1. What steps will be taken to preserve the confidentiality of the observation data, particularly *in vivo* data?
2. Does the applicant have an explicit strategy for dealing with observations that might require breach of confidentiality, such as malpractice, criminal behaviour, or concerns about the health, safety or well-being of participants?

Nonmaleficence:

1. Is there the potential to cause distress, embarrassment or other form of harm to an individual or organisation and how do the researchers intend to deal with this?
2. Are the research team members suitably qualified to undertake this type of work?
3. What mechanisms are there to deal with any observed malpractice or professional misconduct?

Fairness/Justice:

1. Is there any danger that participants might be under coercive influences to participate or maybe unaware that they are participating?
2. Is the study setting appropriate for the research question or aim?

Safety of the researcher:

1. Are provisions in place to protect the safety of the researcher if making observations in potentially insecure environments?

Data protection:

1. What measures are in place to store the data?
2. Does the storage of data conform to local R&D policies and, where necessary, education institution requirements?

Although consideration of these questions helps researchers to decide on the ethical content of their research, the answer does not automatically guarantee ethical behaviour throughout.

It can be seen that health researchers who attempt qualitative projects in clinical or social settings have to construct a complex ethical framework for the research which is all the more important when dealing with patients and clients. In all research situations the needs of the participants take precedence over those of the researcher.

Summary

- Researchers adhere to the principles and rules of the ethical framework.
- The 'dignity, rights, safety and well-being' of participants are paramount.
- Participation in research is voluntary.
- The researcher respects the rights to anonymity, confidentiality and privacy.
- In qualitative research the process of consent is ongoing.
- Vulnerable individuals and groups such as children, frail older or disabled individuals require particular ethical and legal considerations.
- The researcher should seek permission from the appropriate ethics committees.

References

Archbold, P. (1986) Ethical issues in qualitative research. In *From Practice to Grounded Theory* (eds W.C. Chenitz & J.M. Swanson), pp. 155–63. Menlo Park, Addison-Wesley.

Beauchamp, T.L. & Childress, J. (2008) *Principles of Biomedical Ethics*, 6th edn. New York, NY, Oxford University Press.

Butler, J. (2003) Research in the place where you work. *Bulletin of Medical Ethics*, **185**, 21–2.

Coghlan, D. & Brannick, T. (2005) *Doing Action Research in Your Own Organization*. London, Sage.

Cowles, K.V. (1988) Issues in qualitative research on sensitive topics. *Western Journal of Nursing Research*, **10** (2), 163–79.

Department of Health (2005) *Research Governance Framework for Health and Social Care*, 2nd edn. London, Department of Health.

Green, J. & Thorogood, N. (2004) *Qualitative Methods for Health Research*. London, Sage (next edition 2009).

Guillemin, M. & Gillam, L. (2004) Ethics, reflexivity and 'ethically important moments' in research. *Qualitative Inquiry*, **10** (2), 261–80.

Harris, R. & Dyson, E. (2001) Recruitment of frail older people to research: lessons learnt through experience. *Journal of Advanced Nursing*, **36** (5), 643–51.

Kralik, D., Warren, J., Koch, T. & Pignone, G. (2005) The ethics of research using electronic mail discussion groups. *Journal of Advanced Nursing*, **52** (5), 537–45.

Mander, R. (1988) Encouraging students to be research minded. *Nurse Education Today*, **8**, 30–5.

National Research Ethics Service website. http://www.nres.npsa.nhs.uk/

Nursing and Midwifery Council (2008) *The Code: Standards of Standards, Performance and Ethics for Nurses and Midwives*. London, NMC.

Patton, M.Q. (2002) *Qualitative Evaluation and Research Methods*, 3rd edn. London, Sage.

Platt, J. (1981) On interviewing one's peers. *British Journal of Sociology*, **32** (1), 75–91.

Rogers, K. (2008) Ethics and qualitative research: issues for midwifery researchers. *British Journal of Midwifery*, **16** (3), 179–282.

Royal College of Nursing (2005) *Informed Consent in Health and Social Care Research: RCN Guidelines for Nurses*. London, RCN.

Shaw, I. (2008) Ethics and the practice of qualitative research. *Qualitative Social Work*, **7** (4), 400–14.

Sim, J. (1991) Nursing research: is there an obligation on subjects to participate? *Journal of Advanced Nursing*, **16** (11), 1284–9.

Van den Hoonaard, W.C. (2002) Introduction: Ethical norming and qualitative research. In *Walking the Tightrope: Ethics for Qualitative Researchers* (ed W.C. Van den Hoonaard), pp. 1–16. Toronto, University of Toronto Press.

Van den Hoonaard, W.C. (2008) Re-imagining the "subject:" conceptual and ethical considerations on the participant in qualitative research. *Ciência Saúde Coletiva*, **13** (2), 371–9. Retrieved January 2009. http://www.scielosp.org/scielo.php?script= sci_arttext&pid=S1413-81232008000200012&lng=en&nrm=iso.

Walker, J., Holloway, I. & Wheeler, S. (2005) Guidelines for ethical review of qualitative research. *Research Ethics Review*, **1** (3), 90–6 (with permission from the editor).

West, E. & Butler, J. (2003) An applied and qualitative LREC reflects on its practice. *Bulletin of Medical Ethics*, **185**, 13–20.

Wiles, R., Charles, V., Crow, G. & Heath, S. (2006) Researching researchers: lessons for research ethics. *Qualitative Research*, **6** (3), 288–99.

World Medical Association Declaration of Helsinki (2008) *Ethical Principles for Medical Research Involving Human Subjects*. Seoul, WMA.

(**Further reading**)

Greig, A., Taylor, J. & McKay, T. (2007) *Doing Research with Children*, 2nd edn. London, Sage.

Hewitt, J. (2007) Ethical components of researcher–researched relationships in qualitative interviewing. *Qualitative Health Research*, **17** (8), 1149–59.

Li, J. (2008) Ethical challenges in participant observation: a reflection on ethnographic fieldwork. *The Qualitative Report*, **13** (1), 100–15. http://www.nova.edu/ssss/QR/ QR13-1/li.pdf.

Mishna, F., Antle, B.J. & Regehr, C. (2004) Tapping the perspectives of children: emerging ethical issues in qualitative research. *Qualitative Social Work*, 3 (4), 449–68.

Prior, L. (2008) Qualitative research design and ethical governance: some problems of fit. *J.NI Ethics Forum*, 4, 53–64.

Research Ethics Framework from the Economic and Social Research Council http://www. esrcsocietytoday.ac.uk/ESRCInfoCentre/Images/ESRC_Re_Ethics_Frame_tcm6–11291.pdf.

Wiles, R., Prosser, J., Agnoli, A. *et al.* (2008) *Visual Ethics: Ethical Issues in Visual Research*. ESRC National Centre for Research Methods Review Paper, Southampton ESRC National Centre for Research Ethics.

CHAPTER 5

The Issue of Supervision

(Although this book is an introductory text, some postgraduate students might like to be reminded of some of the supervision issues involved which are similar for all forms of inquiry.)

The supervisor is the most important support and critic during the research process. Supervisors oversee the dissertation or thesis and give advice on the research topic, methodology and other research issues as well as guiding and supporting students through the process and the rules of the university.

Although supervision may differ according to circumstances – that is the type of research, the topic as well as the level of study and experience of students – the principles remain similar for different students and types of research; the experience and expertise of the supervisors and their relationships with students will affect the success of the project. Delamont *et al.* (2004) stress the importance of the relationship between supervisor and researcher in the process; it can become close over the time of study but should stay within professional boundaries.

Supervisors have some responsibility for the quality and completion of the research project for ensuring that students define and achieve their aims, and an obligation to the student to support and advise as well as constructively criticise when necessary. On completion, it is important not to submit the work until the supervisors have given their approval for this. Although this is not mandatory, it is advisable, because an experienced supervisor would be able to judge whether the study is truly finished.

Students have and take responsibility for their research. While examining externally, the authors found that occasionally when students were questioned about an issue, they defended themselves by referring to the supervisor (I did this because my supervisor said...), but this is never a good idea, as students have to demonstrate that they can think for themselves and see the reasons for their arguments rather than following the supervisors' advice slavishly.

Sometimes students can choose their own supervisors from a given list of potential tutors after deciding on the research topic, but usually supervisors are allocated according to expertise in method and topic. There should be a match between student and supervisors, and they should feel comfortable with the topic and the relationship. Support and willingness to advise are the most useful criteria; postgraduate students in particular will become experts in their own research and their knowledge will often supersede the expertise of the supervisors, but undergraduates too will be able to speak authoritatively about the topic of their projects if they take time and effort to analyse the data carefully and link the relevant and appropriate literature to the findings.

The style of supervision will depend on student, supervisor and the research process. Some students, for example, like having a highly structured timetable and want to be strictly guided or organised by their supervisors, others are self-directed and see supervisors as an informal sounding board. The style of supervision has to be negotiated during the stages of the research. The stage of the research, whether at the start or towards completion, will make a difference as well as the level of research – both for undergraduates and postgraduates. This stage determines the amount of guidance and structure necessary. Undergraduates and novice researchers obviously need more guidance, while experienced researchers or doctorate students might need less, as one of the goals of the work is to demonstrate independence in thinking and managing the day-to-day process of the research. In qualitative inquiry, researchers need to be aware of the 'labour-intensive nature' of their studies which need careful time-management (Madill *et al.*, 2005).

The responsibilities of supervisor and student

Supervisors and students have a common aim: to achieve a study of high standard that will be completed on time. Both student and supervisor(s) should be committed to the contract of respectively carrying out and supporting the research. The supervisor generally guides and advises rather than directs, except in circumstances where the student acts contrary to ethical or research guidelines.

Supervisor and student will have to negotiate the relationship from the beginning of the study. The frequency of contact depends on the student's needs and the stage in the research process. This can be discussed at the beginning of the research and revised at intervals. Generally the student needs most help and support at the start and then again at the stage of writing up. Nevertheless, it is necessary for students to be in touch regularly rather than erratically. Some people need to see the supervisor often; others enjoy working on their own, though they too need feedback and constructive criticism. There should be a systematic and structured programme of work that forms the basis for the student–supervisor work relationship, but the instigation for this programme should come from students themselves unless it is their very first piece of research.

The responsibility for contacting supervisors rests largely with students; indeed Cryer (2006) suggests that legally the responsibility to inform the supervisor of problems and getting in touch with them is likely to be the student's. Telephone and e-mail contact can be useful, especially when a student experiences an academic or even a personal problem that affects the smooth process of the research.

Students should inform supervisors about problems that have occurred, preferably in advance of a meeting. This means that both student and supervisor are prepared for the meeting, saving precious time. Many students and supervisors keep written notes on the supervision meetings; this is useful as a basis for further appointments and makes meetings more systematic and methodical. The supervisor generally advises the student to come with questions and problems. Most supervisors become involved and interested in the students' research topics. Students have the right to expect this interest.

Often students are so enthusiastic about the research that they start data collection and analysis before becoming acquainted with the research methods. This can lead to inadequate interviewing and observation because methodological considerations have been neglected. Students must make sure that they are fully aware of the strategies, techniques and problems of their chosen research method, sometimes needing a break so they can reflect on methods and topic.

Students do not always want to start writing after the start of the data collection; they believe that much of the research is 'in their head'. In our experience this is a fallacy, and it is useful to start writing early. The supervisor sometimes asks for reflections or chapters on background, literature review and methodology, depending on the type of research. This ensures that students both understand the process and produce ideas that generate fresh motivation and interest, even though sections of the writing might have to be changed at a later stage. This way, students immerse themselves in the methodology, and some of the problems and pitfalls of the research become obvious and can be resolved at an early stage.

Writing and relationships

Students often find the writing up at the end an insurmountable task. The advice to start writing early will lessen this problem. The introduction, research strategies and writing up of ethical issues, might give direction to later chapters, and can be written quite early. If written work is sent to supervisors before a meeting, they are then able to give feedback and encouragement more easily. Students can expect that their supervisors have read the written work when they come for their prearranged supervision sessions, and that it will be criticised constructively. Sometimes supervisors email their comments to students before the meeting. Phillips and Pugh (2005) see the script as a basis for discussion. It is inadvisable to leave writing to the last stage of the research for two reasons: interesting and stimulating ideas will be forgotten and students might run out of time and hence panic. Seeing a chunk of the report in writing will motivate the student to proceed. All through the process, researchers make fieldnotes and memos as often as possible. The usefulness of carrying a small writing pad (as well as a field diary) to jot down ideas that arise cannot be underestimated.

Supervisors are not always gentle and diplomatic in their criticism; some students are hurt by this. The advice is best taken without seeing it as a personal attack but as an academic argument. In any case the relationship between supervisor and student develops over time as they learn about each other's weaknesses, strengths and idiosyncrasies, and both sides negotiate the process. The best supervisors are able to provide a supportive environment for students, draw out their ideas and are flexible and approachable (Phillips and Pugh, 2005), but direct and explicit in their critique of the research. Even if students lack this type of supervisor, they can still learn. As in everyday life sometimes it is necessary for students to work with individuals to whom they cannot relate on a personal level. This does not mean that the professional relationship need be problematic. Students do have some responsibility to try adapting to a style of tutoring with which they might not be familiar, just as supervisors need to do their best even for students with whom they have no particular friendly relationship.

Supervisors cannot always help their students because they do not have unlimited knowledge about all the facets of the research. Researchers often find other experts who can advise them, and on whose knowledge they can draw without offending the supervisor. Indeed, supervisors often know their own limitations and help students find other experts or advisors. It is useful, however, that students inform their supervisors when they seek advice from persons outside the supervisory relationship.

Students build up relationships with their supervisors on a one-to-one basis. Eventually the student becomes an independent researcher and expert in the field of study, and the supervisor acts as an adviser who takes a critical stance to the work.

Practical aspects of supervision

There are some other practical points that must be remembered. Students should make an appointment before coming to see their supervisors, if this is at all possible. Of course, open access to supervision is sometimes necessary and always valuable, but supervisors are busy with many other commitments, and an appointment system helps to save time for all parties. Students (and supervisors) should be available and punctual for a pre-arranged meeting, but if appointments have to be cancelled, the cancellation should be made as early as possible. If no other time for necessary supervision can be found, an occasional telephone session might do in an emergency. The main stress should be on regular and quality time of contact. For this, e-mail addresses and telephone numbers need to be exchanged. Sometimes supervisors are reluctant about revealing their home number, and the student should only use this in an emergency – and this is the same for the home telephone number of the student. University e-mails, however, can be very useful for academic exchanges between student and supervisor.

The following is a summary of the roles and tasks of supervisors and students (adapted from Holloway and Walker, 2000).

The responsibilities of supervisors:

- They support and advise students.
- They help to ensure that students adhere to ethical principles.
- They give feedback such as constructive criticism and motivating praise.
- They produce progress reports (if required).
- They introduce students to other experts or advisers (if needed).
- They make students aware of problems relating to progress and quality of the project.
- They encourage students throughout the research process.

The responsibilities of the students:

- They negotiate the process and style of supervision with the supervisor.
- They regularly submit written work to the supervisor (as negotiated), generally well before supervisory meetings.
- They give progress reports if required.
- They negotiate major changes and modifications in the research with the supervisor.
- They inform the supervisor of any problems which might interfere with the research project.
- They observe ethical principles (which include not plagiarising the work of others).

In addition to the above, postgraduates attend agreed research sessions or training programmes.

Single or joint supervision

Students have either one or two supervisors for their research studies. One supervisor could be an expert in research method, the other might have specialist knowledge in the field of study. Supervisors generally differ in their skills and knowledge but complement each other.

There are a number of arguments for joint supervision. For the student, continuity is ensured when one supervisor is absent or ill. The student's experience can be enhanced by the support of two supervisors. For the supervisors there is support from colleagues who can discuss the appropriateness of advice about which they are uncertain. New supervisors gain from the guidance of experienced colleagues.

Taught masters degrees in nursing and midwifery proliferate and recruit large numbers of students. Most part-time students work in the clinical setting and wish to carry out research in this environment in order to examine a problem or a major issue relevant to their work. Therefore the supervisor's experience and knowledge in the clinical setting can be useful.

Single supervision avoids the danger of the conflicting guidance from different people, however many universities see dual supervision in MPhil and PhD studies as important, though undergraduates and MSc/MA students often have a single supervisor.

When examining an educational problem, a student needs at least one supervisor with expertise in the educational field. Undergraduate students do not need several supervisors. As novices to the research process and relatively inexperienced in the clinical setting, they need guidance to the principles of research while the topic is of lesser importance, although it should reflect the student's interest and advance knowledge in a more limited subject area.

In PhD and MPhil research, students often have a supervisory team to assist continuity in supervision when one supervisor is absent for any reason. To avoid conflicting advice to students, it is, of course, important that joint supervisors have a common ideology about supervision, a similar view about the particular method and topic, and that they stay in contact with each other. Students must be aware of the pitfalls and problems in supervision, because ultimately the responsibility is theirs.

Students often propose ambitious projects in which they intend to use both qualitative and quantitative methods. For short student projects that take less than a year, mixed-methods study might be too time-consuming and the student is often advised to carry out single method studies (see Chapter 16).

Example

Maggie aimed to carry out a mixed-method study on students' experience of undergraduate project supervision. She managed good interviews and analysed these, but could not find the time or space to develop and handle a survey of a larger number of students in a short research project.

Supervisors have the task of asking questions about the particular circumstances, settings and people the students want to take into account when investigating the topic. Often they are able to advise students on relevant and useful method texts. Although students cannot be forced to listen to their supervisors, they will usually find it profitable to do so.

Trust and honesty are very important in establishing a supervisory relationship as supervisor and student are working collaboratively and in partnership (Rugg and Petre, 2004). In this process truth-telling is essential. There is an obvious duty for both to recognise the need to share all aspects of the study phases, be they positive or negative.

Supervisors are usually able to help because they have inside knowledge of the research and/or are experts in the chosen method. In general, supervisors have lengthy experience of a variety of student projects. This knowledge helps students to trust the advice given and be guided appropriately. Students have responsibility to the discipline and their profession to report the findings as truthfully and accurately as possible.

Problems with supervision

Students might have problems with their supervisors. Some are due to their own actions or inactions, others are the responsibility of the supervisor or the interaction between student and supervisor. Occasionally there may be a personality clash. The problems are more easily resolved at the beginning of the study, and it is important not to leave them for too long. Fortunately, there is rarely a major problem between researcher and supervisor. If it does occur, researchers, and particularly students who do research, can obtain advice from other members of the department or seek help from a senior staff member (such as the departmental research director, the departmental research degrees committee for research students, or the course tutor in the case of undergraduates) who will advise on an appropriate course of action. In most cases, negotiation with the supervisor(s) is not only possible but also desirable, and it resolves small problems.

Academic problems

The following problems may arise from time to time:

1. The supervisor is inaccessible or lacks time to see the student.
2. The supervisor gives too little guidance or is uncritical.
3. The supervisor is too directive or authoritarian.
4. The student cannot keep to the agreed timetable.
5. The supervisor leaves the university or is allocated a different role.

Students' most common complaints concern inaccessibility of supervisors. Supervisors are busy people who do not always see the student and supervision as their priority. Students can avoid this problem by making an appointment well before the supervisory session or by deciding on a future date at each meeting. It is important to inform the supervisor of cancellations. Students might supply supervisors with their home and (for part-time students) work telephone numbers so that they can cancel well before the meeting if they cannot attend.

When students have little guidance, feedback or criticism, they feel uninformed and unsure about their progress or the standard of their work. Students should not be afraid to ask for help. Most supervisors are willing to assist students in any way they can and have their interests at heart.

Students sometimes complain about too much guidance and over-direction. They may feel that the supervisor never allows them to make their own decisions and guides the work in a direction they do not wish to go. If the researcher is a novice, it is generally advisable to listen to the advice of the supervisor, particularly in the early stages. At a later stage, supervisors are generally open to academic argument and do not object to changes in direction as long as the student can justify these.

A problem sometimes occurs in joint supervision when supervisors have conflicting ideologies and different ideas about the research. Sometimes this is the outcome of misinterpretation. The situation can usually be negotiated. It is important for both researcher and supervisors to keep notes on meetings. It is also advisable for all parties to get together to discuss the research, but of course, this is not always possible.

One of the main problems is the timetable that has been negotiated with the supervisor and that the institution demands. Many students neglect this issue until it becomes urgent. It is most important to look at the date for completion at the very beginning and plan the research carefully so that the timetable can be kept. This means that students and supervisors have to be realistic (Delamont *et al.*, 2004). Qualitative research is particularly demanding during the analysis and writing stages, and takes more time than the student might have originally envisaged. Also, during this stage, students have to gain access to the literature connected with their themes or categories, and the articles often take much time to arrive at the library.

Occasionally supervisors change their roles or move on during the student's time at the university. They might be promoted and have little time for the student. They may have a sabbatical or a serious illness. In this case, joint supervision is valuable, and the department can add another supervisor if necessary. Also, telephone and e-mail tutorials are possible, and we have used these successfully. They cannot, however, replace face-to-face contact.

For postgraduates the guidelines for codes of practice of the National Postgraduate Committee (2001) might be useful. They can be found on the NPC website (http://www.npc.org.uk). The responsibilities of supervisors and postgraduate research students are made explicit on the guidelines.

Final notes

Throughout the study the student must keep in mind some major points linked to supervision.

1. *Consulting the supervisors:* Some students write many chapters of their study in well-motivated but misplaced haste before consulting their supervisors which means that occasionally they take an inappropriate path for the study.
2. *Consulting the regulations:* Each university or grant-giving body has its own regulations. Many students only consult these at the very end when most of the work has been completed. It is important to have an occasional read of the regulations from the very beginning of the study, so that they will be remembered throughout.
3. *Consulting the latest literature relevant to the study:* The student must be up-to-date with the latest research and important discussion on the research topic and also about the methodology.

The ultimate responsibility for the research lies with the students; they are in charge of their work.

Summary

The supervision process may be summarised as follows.

- Student and supervisor(s) have responsibility for and collaborate on the research project, but the main responsibility for the research lies with the student.
- Supervisors are chosen because of their knowledge in the area of methodology and topic.
- Negotiation between students and supervisors takes place early in the research when the ground rules are established.
- It is essential that close and regular contact is maintained between the student and the supervisor(s), and that they share ideas throughout the research.

References

Cryer, P. (2006) *The Research Student's Guide to Success*, 3rd edn. Maidenhead, Open University Press.

Delamont, S., Atkinson, P. & Parry, O. (2004) *Supervising the PhD: A Guide to Success*, 2nd edn. Maidenhead, Open University Press.

Holloway, I. & Walker, J. (2000) *Getting a PhD in Health and Social Care*. Oxford, Blackwell Science.

Madill, A., Gough, B., Lawton, R. & Stratton, P. (2005) How should we supervise qualitative projects. *The Psychologist*, **18** (10), 616–8.

National Postgraduate Committee (2001) *Guidelines for Codes of Practice for Postgraduate Research*. Updated 21 June (first written in 1992).

Phillips, E.M. & Pugh, D.S. (2005) *How to get a PhD*, 4th edn. Milton Keynes, Open University Press.

Rugg, G. & Petre, M. (2004) *Unwritten Rules of PhD Research*. Maidenhead, Open University Press.

Further reading

Biklen, S.K. & Casella, R. (2007) *Writing a Qualitative Dissertation*. New York, NY, Teachers' College Press (Selected chapters).

Gough, B., Madill, A. & Stratton, P. (2003) *Guidelines for the Supervision of Undergraduate Qualitative Research in Psychology. Higher Education Academy Network Support and Evaluation Series 3*. New York, NY, LTSN Psychology.

PART TWO

Data Collection

CHAPTER 6

Interviewing

Interviews as sources of data

In the last two decades, interviews have become the most common form of data collection in qualitative research. Novice health researchers often rely on interviews as their main form of data collection because they want to gain the inside view of a phenomenon or problem but also find observation difficult.

It is easily understandable why health professionals wish to interview clients and colleagues. In their professional lives, too, they have conversations with patients in order to obtain information. They counsel their clients and already possess many interviewing skills. Nursing or midwifery assessment, for instance, relies on skilful questions and includes interviewing to elicit information from patients or clients. It might therefore be assumed that research interviews are easy to carry out, but interviewing is a complex process and not as simple as it seems.

Beatrice and Sidney Webb who undertook social research around the turn of the last century used the term 'conversation with a purpose' when discussing interviews, and Rubin and Rubin (2005) too believe that researcher and informant become 'conversational partners', but the interview has only some of the characteristics of a conversation. Research interviews differ from ordinary conversations because the rules of the interview process are more clearly defined.

The one-to-one interview consisting of questions and answers is the most common form of research interview. Other types include focus group and narrative interviews (discussed more fully in Chapters 8 and 12).

Interview studies have contributed to the understanding of participants and of the wider culture. In health research, interviewing provides the basis both for exploring colleagues' perspectives and clients' interpretations. It is necessary, however, to warn researchers of 'anecdotalism' when they accept 'atrocity stories' from participants and do not always explore cases which contradict these (Silverman, 2006). If researchers apply high standards and rigour to the research, and search for contrary occurrences in the analysis of the interview data, their studies will represent – at least to some extent – the reality of most of the participants' perceptions and a description of the phenomenon under study.

The interview process

Unlike everyday conversations, research interviews are set up by the interviewer to elicit information from participants. The purpose of the interview is the discovery of informants' feelings, perceptions and thoughts. Marshall and Rossman (2006) maintain that interviews focus on the past, present and, in particular, the essential experience of participants. The interview can be formal or informal; often informal conversations or chats with participants also generate important ideas for the project. Depending on the response of participants, researchers formulate questions as the interview proceeds rather than asking pre-planned questions. This means that each interview differs from the next in sequence and wording, although distinct patterns common to all interviews in a specific study often emerge in the analysis. Indeed, for many research approaches it is necessary that researchers discover these patterns when analysing data.

One interview, however, does not always suffice. In qualitative inquiry it is possible to re-examine the issues in the light of emerging ideas and interview for a second or third time. Seidman (2006) sees three interviews as the optimum number, but these require much planning in the short time span available to undergraduates for their project, so this is only possible for postgraduates. Many novice researchers therefore use one-off interviews although postgraduates and other more experienced researchers sometimes carry out more than one with each participant.

Pilot studies are not always used in qualitative inquiry as the research is developmental, but novice researchers could try interviews with their friends and acquaintances to get used to this type of data collection. We found that we lacked confidence when we started, and a practice run proved very useful. In our experience students become more confident as interviews proceed.

Most qualitative research starts with relatively unstructured interviews in which researchers give minimal guidance to the participants. The outcome of initial interviews guides later stages of interviewing. As interviews proceed, they become more focused on the particular issues important to the participants and which emerge throughout the data collection. Most qualitative studies do not only explore commonalities and uncover patterns, but they also describe the unique experiences of individuals particularly in one-to-one interviews.

One-to-one interviews are the most common form of data collection although researchers also use group interviews (see Chapter 8).

Types of interview

Researchers have to decide on the structure in the interview. There is a range of interview types on a continuum, from the unstructured to the structured. Qualitative researchers generally employ the unstructured or semi-structured interview.

The unstructured, non-standardised interview

Unstructured interviews start with a general question in the broad area of study. Even unstructured interviews are usually accompanied by an *aide mémoire*, an agenda or a list of topics that will be covered. There are, however, no predetermined questions except at the very beginning of the interview.

Example

Tell me about your experience at the time you found out about your . . .

Aide mémoire
Feelings in the doctor's surgery
Interaction with different types of professionals
Coping with the condition and the associated pain
Being treated
Social support from other patients, relatives and friends
Practical support etc. (these are merely examples)

This type of unstructured interviewing allows flexibility and makes it possible for researchers to follow the interests and thoughts of the informants rather than follow their own assumptions. Interviewers freely ask questions from informants in any order or sequence depending on the responses to earlier questions. Warm-up and simple questions are generally asked first; however, if the interviewer leaves the essential questions till the end of the interview the participant may be tired and reluctant to discuss deeper issues.

Researchers also have their own agenda. To achieve the research aim, they keep in mind the particular issues which they wish to explore. However, direction and control of the interview by the researcher is minimal. Generally, the outcomes of these interviews differ for each informant, though usually certain patterns can be discerned. Informants are free to answer at length, and great depth and detail can be obtained. The unstructured interview generates the richest data, but it also has the highest 'dross rate' (the amount of material of no particular use for the researcher's study), particularly when the interviewer is inexperienced.

The semi-structured interview

Semi-structured or focused interviews are often used in qualitative research. The questions are contained in an interview guide (not interview schedule as in quantitative research) with a focus on the issues or topic areas to be covered and the lines of inquiry to be followed. The sequencing of questions is not the same for every participant as it depends on the process of the interview and the responses of each individual. The interview guide, however, ensures that the researcher collects similar types of data from all informants. In this way, the interviewer can save time, and the dross rate is lower than in unstructured interviews. Researchers can develop questions and decide for themselves what issues to pursue.

Example

Tell me about the time when your condition was first diagnosed. (Depending on the language use and understanding of the participant, this has to be phrased differently. For instance: What did you think when the doctor first told you about your illness?)

What did you feel at that stage?
Tell me about your treatment.
What did the doctor or nurses say?
What happened after that?
How did your husband (wife, children) react?
What happened at work?
and so on.

The interview guide can be quite long and detailed although it need not – should not – be followed strictly so that the participant has some control. It focuses on particular aspects of the subject area to be examined, but it can be revised after several interviews because of the ideas that arise. Although interviewers aim to gain the informants' perspectives, the former need to keep some control of the interview so that the purpose of the study can be achieved and the research topic explored. Ultimately, the researchers themselves must decide what interview techniques or types might be best for them and the interview participants. Our students and other researchers preferred good questions of medium length combined with the use of prompts and reported better results.

The structured or standardised interview

Qualitative researchers in general *do not use* standardised interviews as they are contradictory to the aims of qualitative research. In these, the interview schedule contains a number of pre-planned questions. Each informant in a research study is asked the same questions in the same order. This type of interview resembles a written survey questionnaire. Standardised interviews save time and limit the interviewer effect. The analysis of the data seems easier as answers can be found quickly. Generally, knowledge of statistics is important and useful for the analysis of this type of interview. However, this type of pre-planned interview directs the informants' responses and is therefore inappropriate in qualitative approaches. Structured interviews may contain open questions, but even then they cannot be called qualitative.

Qualitative researchers use structured questions only to elicit socio-demographic data, i.e. about age, duration of condition, duration of experience, type of occupation, qualifications, etc. Sometimes research or ethics committees ask for a predetermined interview schedule so that they can find out the exact path of the research. For the purpose of gaining permission, a semi-structured interview guide is occasionally advisable for health researchers.

Types of questions in qualitative interviews

When asking questions, interviewers use a variety of techniques. Patton (2002) lists particular types of questions, for example *experience*, *feeling* and *knowledge* questions.

Examples

Experience questions

Could you tell me about your experience of caring for patients with arthritis?
Tell me about your experience of epilepsy.

Feeling questions

How did you feel when the first patient in your care died?
What did you feel when the doctor told you that you suffer from...

Knowledge questions

What services are available for this group of patients?
How do you cope with this condition?

Spradley (1979) distinguishes between *grand-tour* and *mini-tour* questions. *Grand-tour* questions are broader, while *mini-tour* questions are more specific.

Examples

Grand-tour questions

Can you describe a typical day in the community? (To a community midwife)
Tell me about your condition. (To a patient)

Mini-tour questions

Can you describe what happens when a colleague questions your decision? (To a nurse)
What were your expectations of the pain clinic? (To a patient)

The sequencing of questions is also important.

Practical considerations

In qualitative studies questions are as non-directive as possible but still guide towards the topics of interest to the researcher. Researchers should phrase questions clearly and aim at the various participants' levels of understanding. Ambiguous questions lead to ambiguous answers. Double questions are best avoided; for instance it would be inappropriate to ask: How many colleagues do you have, and what are their ideas about this?

The researcher must be aware of practical difficulties in the data collection phase, particularly when interviewing in hospital. The routine of the hospital is disrupted by the presence of the nurse or midwife researcher whose activities might be viewed with suspicion by colleagues. A quiet place for interviews cannot always be found, and therefore the privacy of patients may be threatened. The ward might be full of noise and activity, and the researcher does not always find a convenient slot for interviewing without being interrupted by nursing activity, consultant round, cleaners, meals and so on. In the community, interviews are often interrupted by children or spouses and by the visits of friends or relatives.

Probing, prompting and summarising

During the interviews researchers can use prompts or probing questions. These help to reduce anxiety for researcher and research informant. The purpose of probes is a search for elaboration, meaning or reasons. Seidman (2006) suggests the term 'explore' and dislikes the word 'probe' as it sounds like an interrogation, and is the name for a surgical instrument used in medical or dental investigations and stresses the interviewer's position of power.

Exploratory questions might be, for instance: What was that experience like for you? How did you feel about that? Can you tell me more about that? That's interesting, why did you do that? Questions can follow up on certain points that participants make or words they use. The researcher could also summarise the last statements of the participant and encourage more talk through this technique.

> **Example**
> You told me earlier that you were very happy with the care you received in hospital. Could you tell me a bit more about that?

Participants often become fluent talkers when asked to tell a story, reconstructing their experiences, for instance a day, an incident, the feeling about an illness. Unfortunately the data from interviews are sometimes more fluent or extensive when the participants are articulate, and occasionally researchers may choose those who have language and interaction skills. This may create bias in the interviews however and is not a good strategy.

Example

A number of years ago one of our PhD candidates – an experienced midwife with good verbal and interactive skills – intended to interview clients about the nil-by-mouth policy of the maternity ward in which she wished to carry out research for her research diploma. She found that certain individuals only answered in very short sentences, could not be prompted and were generally in awe of the situation and the researcher. Also the policy was not an issue of interest to them – their concern focused only on the birth of their baby – but only for the midwives involved. The researcher had to abandon the topic area because she had not enough material for a long research study and also felt that there would be bias against less articulate and less confident clients.

The social and language skills of the researcher often make a difference to the outcome of the interview.

Non-verbal prompts are also useful. The stance of the researcher, eye contact or leaning forward encourages reflection. In fact, listening skills, which some nurses and midwives already possess from the counselling of patients, will elicit further ideas. Patients often give monosyllabic answers until they have become used to the interviewer, because they are reluctant to uncover their feelings or fear that judgements might be made about them. When participants do not understand the interview question, the researcher can rephrase them in the language they understand.

The social context of the interview

Interviews must be seen in the social context in which they occur; this affects the relationship between researcher and research as well as the data generated by it (Manderson *et al.*, 2006). The setting is of particular importance; if interviews take place in the home of the participants, they are more relaxed, the researcher might gain richer data and the participant is in some position of control. On the other hand, this setting can be a difficult choice for the researcher as there might be many distractions such as children or spouses who interrupt the proceedings. Sometimes a neutral place such as a corner in a café or park, or an academic environment can be appropriate.

The researcher has to reflect on time and location and the persons involved in the interaction. Experience, background and characteristics of the researcher, as well as the participants' group membership such as age, gender, class or ethnic group might also influence the interaction. Manderson *et al.* (2006) suggest that changes in any of these factors might generate different interview data as the social dynamics of the interview vary; indeed Roulston *et al.* (2003: 654) stress 'the socially constructed nature of interview talk'. When sensitive topics are discussed, researchers have to use their own judgement whether their gender or ethnic membership might interfere with the research relationship. In some situations it is more sensitive and even useful when researcher and participant are of similar background. This is by no means always so. One of our students, a very young woman, interviewed older people about their lives. This study elicited more data than would be usual. The participants provided very rich data and deep thoughts – perhaps because they did not feel threatened.

When patients are interviewed, they might ask the researcher about advice on their condition or treatment. It is best to separate the researcher and professional roles, although this cannot always be done. It is best to point out a professional source of information or put the participants in touch with an expert who can answer their questions. In the case of very vulnerable people and sensitive topics, the researcher might seek advisors or experts before the research starts and ask for permission to contact them if necessary. If an emergency occurs during the interview, the researcher has to adopt the best way to assist the patient.

Unexpected outcomes: qualitative interviewing and therapy

Certain commonalities exist between qualitative and therapeutic interviews. However, researchers and therapists have different aims; the researcher's aim is to gain knowledge while the therapist's aim is to assist in the healing process. Several studies have shown, however, that qualitative interviews might be beneficial for the participants, especially after they have gone through a traumatic experience (for instance, Colbourne and Sque, 2005 among others). Kvale (1996) argues that among other elements of interviews, interaction with others and remembering the past might be therapeutic.

Example

Colbourne and Sque (2005) report on research that included qualitative interviews with cancer patients. The outcome of these interviews showed them to have a beneficial effect on some of the participants. They suggest that nurse researchers as listeners could help participants gain more self-awareness and express repressed emotions among other factors. Just talking and interacting with others can be helpful. The research aim did not change through the process of the study, and the therapeutic impact was an unexpected – if welcome – outcome.

The researcher however, should not lose sight of the original purpose of the interview.

Length and timing of interviews

The length of time for an interview depends on the participants, the topic of the interview and the methodological approach. Of course, the researcher must suggest an approximate amount of time – perhaps an hour and a half – so that participants can plan their day, but many are willing or wish to go beyond this, some as much as three or four hours. Others, particularly elderly people or physically weak informants, may need to break off after a short while, say 20 or 30 minutes. Children cannot concentrate for long periods of time. Health researchers have to use their own judgement, follow the wishes of the informant and take the length of time required for the topic. One of our colleagues suggests that three hours should be the absolute maximum because concentration fails even experienced researchers or willing participants.

Phenomenological interviews focus on one phenomenon or a limited number of very specific phenomena. Because of the reflective character of the interviews, the participants may become tired as they uncover their feelings; hence the researcher may not be able to continue the research for long. Also, as the questions concentrate on the specific phenomenon, extraneous matters are not significant for the study, in contrast to ethnographic research for instance.

Stating an approximate time for the interview can ensure escape for the researcher who is pressed for time, although it is advisable to leave plenty of time for interviewing. For hard-pressed professionals this type of data collection is very time-consuming, however useful and therapeutic it may be for the informant. As stated before, researchers can, of course, re-interview one or more times.

Recording interview data

A number of techniques and practical points must be considered so that the data are recorded and stored appropriately.

Interview data are recorded in three ways

1. Tape-recording the interview
2. Note taking during the interview
3. Note taking after the interview

Tape-recording

Before analysing the data, researchers must preserve the participants' words as accurately as possible. The best form of recording interview data is tape-recording. Tapes contain the exact words of the interview, inclusive of questions, and researchers do not forget important answers and words, can have eye contact and pay attention to what participants say.

Researchers must ask for permission before taping. Some participants do not wish to be taped, and researchers have to respect this and either take notes or remember the gist of the interview and record it in their fieldnotes shortly after the interview. Occasionally informants change their minds about tape-recording, and their wishes should be paramount. The principle of respect for autonomy includes choice and free decision and must be considered first in terms of consent. This allows for the participants' right to refuse participation in research. This right can be exercised at any stage of the research process. Video-recording is more problematic, and many participants will refuse to be taped; this is their right. Some big programmes depend on video-recording (such as DIPEx[1]) but, again, the recording depends on the participants.

Initially the informants may be hesitant, but they will get used to the tape-recorder; a small recorder is easier to forget than a large one, but a larger recorder can be placed further away so it is not necessarily always visible or disturbing. By asking factual questions first, researchers allow the informants to relax and make them feel more secure. Some interviewees have soft and quiet voices, particularly if they feel vulnerable. Interviewers therefore place the tape-recorder near enough, but not so prominently that it intimidates the hesitant person. Lapel microphones allow a better quality of sound. A room away from noise and disturbances enhances not only the quality of the tape but also the interview itself; participants feel free to talk without interruption.

We have experienced some problems with tape-recorders. They sometimes break down, and it is advisable to try them out at the beginning of the interview and after it has been recorded. Researchers should remember to pack some extra batteries and tapes. A good recording device is available – a portable mini compact disc player made by Sony, but this is expensive. Each disc records 70 minutes and does not need to be turned over. Auto-reverse on tape-recorders is useful; standard cassettes need not be turned over (the quality of non-standard tape – for instance 120 minute tape – is not always very good). It is much better to use tape-recorders with conference facility, although we know that students often find them too expensive and have no access to them. The university often can supply tape-recorders to staff and students for the duration of the data collection.

The tape is dated and labelled. Only pseudonyms should appear on the tape or its transcription, and participants' names must be stored in a different place from the tapes. The transcription of data will be discussed in Chapter 17.

Note taking

Note taking is important but might disturb the participant during the interview. Contextual notes can be made before the interview; others immediately

---

[1] DIPEx is a website and data base of individual patients' experiences of health and illness website: formerly http://www.dipex.org; now www.healthtalkonline.org

afterwards when events and thoughts are still clearly in the mind of the researcher. Note taking is further discussed in Chapter 17.

The interviewer–participant relationship

The relationship between researcher and participant is based on mutual respect and a position of equality as human beings. The fallacy exists, however, that the interviewer and the person interviewed work together in a relationship of complete equality. Health researchers, by virtue of their professional expertise and skill in interviewing, are in a position of some power, however much they attempt to achieve a relationship of equality with the participant. Researchers can empower patients and colleagues by listening to their perspective and giving voice to their concerns. The interviewer also respects the way in which participants develop and phrase their answers (Marshall and Rossman, 2006); they are, after all, not passive respondents but active participants in an important social encounter. Trust is built up through involvement and interest in the perspectives of the patient. It must also be remembered, however, that the interviewer is not a blank screen (*tabula rasa*) but also an active participant in the interview and thus takes part in co-constructing meaning.

Indeed, Wengraf (2001) reminds researchers that intersubjectivity is an important issue in interviews: interviewer and participant inhabit a shared world and often a common culture. They have similar, though not the same, understandings of it and base interview questions and answers on shared meanings, but subjective ideas of both parties also must be taken into account. Interviews can be enjoyable for the participants: Lofland and Lofland (2004) suggest that there is often a *quid pro quo* in research. The researcher gains knowledge from informants who, in turn, find listeners for their feelings and reflections, and many indeed state that this is the first time for a disclosure of these thoughts.

Peer interviews

Many health professionals have an interest in the views and ideas of their colleagues. There are advantages and disadvantages in interviewing one's peers. Shared language and norms can be advantageous or problematic. A researcher who is involved in the culture of the participants more easily understands cultural concepts. Although there is less room for misinterpretation, misunderstandings can arise from the assumptions of common values and beliefs. Researchers do not always question ideas that are uncovered or constructs that arise from interviews with colleagues or they make unwarranted assumptions. This can be overcome by acting as 'cultural stranger', or 'naïve' interviewer, asking participants about their meaning and clarification of their ideas.

In many peer interviews, researcher and informant are in a position of equality (Platt, 1981), and the researcher is not distant or anonymous. The close relationship has the advantage that the participants will 'open up' and trust researchers, but there is the danger of over-involvement and identification with colleagues.

Coar and Sim (2006) reported on a study which included peer interviews and found that professionals often saw these as a test of their professional knowledge and felt vulnerable. The authors described the methodological issues involved in these peer interviews and showed that the interviews depended on the research relationship and the view of the professional identity of participants.

Students, however, sometimes interview friends and acquaintances for pragmatic and opportunistic reasons. Although this is useful to overcome the hurdles of getting to know informants and forming relationships, the selection from this group might create unease or embarrassment if the topic is a sensitive one. Informants and interviewers might hold assumptions about each other, which might prejudice the information. Therefore we suggest that students take great care in their choice of informants.

Problematic issues and challenges in interviewing

Interviews are often seen as easy by novice researchers. Roulston *et al.* (2003) give four specific challenges: unexpected participant behaviour, consequences of the researcher's own actions and subjectivities, phrasing and negotiating questions and dealing with sensitive issues. We shall give examples here: The people in the research are sometimes less articulate than the researcher assumes; they may be in an environment not conducive to interviewing, or they might not be able to concentrate. The researchers might not have explained their behaviour, and the participant is confused or worried; they might be too controlling in the interview and take over the talk or speak far too much. Sometimes this is linked to enthusiasm and interest, but nevertheless, too much talk from the interviewer is not appropriate. The questions might not be focused on the core of the study, or not open-ended enough. New researchers, in particular, often do not know how to phrase questions to put the participants at ease. People feel awkward to discuss sensitive issues, and particular skills are needed; whilst the participants might be willing to answer a nurse, they might feel uncomfortable being interviewed by a young student. Dealing with emotional situations is easier for some researchers, while it is more difficult for others.

Interviewing through electronic media

E-mail and other online research as well as telephone interviews have become more popular in all research in recent years. Computer-mediated research entails the direct use of computers in research. So far, not many health research studies exist which have used this form of inquiry but they are increasing, and telephone interviews are quite popular.

Online research and e-mail interviews

The use of computers for research is increasing. It is important to know about the possibilities of qualitative interviewing online and through e-mail correspondence where the researcher and the participant do not meet each other face to face. As in conventional one-to-one or focus group interviews, researchers seek special interest groups, or individuals with similar experiences or conditions, such as for instance a group of people in pain, supervisors of postgraduate students or patients with epilepsy, etc. Chat rooms and newsgroups can also be observed and their contents analysed. Denzin (1999), for instance, obtained access to a newsgroup of people recovering from alcoholism to examine the 'gendered narratives of self'.

There are two types of online one-to-one interviews: synchronous or asynchronous (Mann and Stewart, 2000). The synchronous interview takes place in real time and can be carried out with one participant or a group at the same time. This type of interview can proceed when researcher and participants read and write messages at the same time, using computers with software such as Internet Relay Chat (IRC). The researcher can ask questions and will receive an immediate response. The organisation of synchronous interviews is difficult because of differences in the time zones of various countries. It also limits the sample to those who own computers and use technology confidently, and without fear.

Morton Robinson (2001) suggests chat rooms as a source of data as dialogues and multiple conversations can take place; this type of interactive discussion might be seen as a focus group interview; it is shared by a number of participants. As more than one conversation often proceeds at the same time, chat rooms can be confusing. Bulletin boards are also useful as messages and replies are posted there, and they stay in place for a time.

Ethically, access to chat rooms and bulletin boards is problematic unless the messages are completely public. It is more ethical in every case that the researcher uncovers his or her research identity to those who write the messages. The researcher also has to be careful about the trustworthiness of the data, as they are often provided anonymously.

Often virtual focus groups are purposively established by a researcher. Kralik et al. (2006) discuss the use of computer mediated communication with groups of participants on e-mail which was the result of research with people who had chronic illnesses. The advantage of these types of conversations is 'regular, reflective contact' over a period of time (p. 214). This and other types of e-mail conversation afford the participants anonymity if they want it, and this is particularly important in research with vulnerable people.

Asynchronous or non-real time interviews are e-mail conversations. Data generation by e-mail correspondence entails asking a purposive sample of people with similar experiences to get in touch by e-mail and share these experiences with the researcher. These interviews enable correspondents to choose the best time for their writing. This technique is less intrusive than face-to-face interviews, but the researcher can still obtain the same rich data. Because correspondents never meet the researcher, they can be more open and honest about their condition or experiences. Status issues and hierarchical positions have less influence in this type of interview because the contact is not face to face. The procedure will only work fully, however, if the research is a process of ongoing dialogue over an extended period of time, sometimes as short as three months, sometimes as long as a year.

> **Examples**
> Orgad (2005) carried out e-mail as well as face-to-face interviews with individuals who had breast cancer. She also analysed breast cancer-linked websites. She wrote about this in a book which not only discusses the experiences of breast cancer and related matters but also internet communication.

The advantage for the researcher is the instant availability of typed text that can be accessed at any time after the interview. Researchers can respond to questions or seek more answers when they find time and have considered the correspondents' narratives. Participants are able to enter the correspondence from an environment of their choice, often their homes. Bodily presence is not essential for a 'good' interview. Mann and Stewart (2000) showed that it is useful for expressing emotions and being reflective about one's writing. Researcher and participant are able to get to know each other quite well over a period of time. These types of interview save travel, time and money. The e-mail interviewer can also avoid lengthy transcriptions as the message can be printed out immediately. In a geographical sense, the e-mail interview can widen the access to participants.

> **Example**
> In a global study Cheryl Tatano Beck conducted a piece of phenomenological research with 40 women in which she explored birth trauma. The data were generated through e-mail correspondence, and women sent their stories to the researcher over an 18-month period. In her article she discusses the benefits of this type of research (Beck, 2005).

Seymour (2001) lists several elements as important features of online research. She claims that 'the release of the interview from its imprisonment in time and space' makes it deeper, because the sites are open for longer periods of time and the response need not be immediate. Researchers can gain access to the participants in an ongoing process and clarify issues that are unclear, while participants too have the time to ask questions throughout the research process. The ongoing interaction, suggests Seymour, makes the position of the participants more egalitarian. There are also practical implications: The interviews need not be transcribed but are instantly available with little cost involved. Both researcher and participants have time to reflect on their answers. From a practical point of view, internet research is cheaper and more convenient in some ways, as it does not necessitate travelling costs or room booking and has fewer time constraints as the research is ongoing and fits into the time frame of both researcher and participant. Also there is a lack of assumptions that researchers have about the participants. As the latter are not visible and cannot be identified as members of particular groups with specific group membership, personality or outside appearance, they cannot be instantly labelled.

These interviews are not, of course, as spontaneous as face-to-face or even telephone interviews but they give the participants time to reflect on the questions. It must be remembered though, that researchers who use this form of inquiry automatically exclude those who have no access to computers, although they might be important groups. At the time of writing this text, e-mail interviews are possibly the most common form of research on the internet.

Telephone interviews

Telephone interviews are another effective way of interviewing. The telephone interview is immediate, and researchers and participants are able to respond spontaneously to each other.

Example

Breen et al. (2007) interviewed by telephone 21 general practitioners in the South of the UK to explore their attitudes to managing back pain as a biopsychosocial problem. From this they developed a series of vignettes to illustrate the study. They found feelings of frustration, mismatches in perceptions in the doctor–patient relationship and lack of resources among a variety of other important themes.

Telephone interviews are more convenient for health professionals or patients with little time for interviews but also save travel time for researchers who sometimes have to travel long distances and spend money on travel.

The advantages of telephone interviews are obvious. They include the immediacy of response, anonymity of participants and the effective use of time. Researchers need not travel to the participants' home or work location. The disadvantage is the lack of deeper interaction, as the interviewer does not get to know the participants. A telephone talk must be more structured, and this is in contrast to the tenets of qualitative research which is designed to elicit rich and deep data. It is, however, a useful way of obtaining data when other types of interview are not possible.

Ethical issues in interviewing

Ethical rules and principles that are considered in conventional forms of inquiry must also be considered in e-mail and other electronic research, for instance informed consent, confidentiality, the right not to be harmed or identified and the possibility of withdrawal at any time. Ethical issues are, however, particularly problematic in spite of the data protection law, as outsiders can gain access to the correspondence more easily than to tape-recorded interviews. It is therefore necessary that researchers inform the participants about the potential lack of security, and it is advisable to obtain written permission by post. Using e-mail, other online research and telephone interviewing means that the interviewer's words need to be more carefully considered and phrased, as they cannot be modified or accompanied by gestures and facial expressions like face-to-face conversations. Those obtaining access to a group site do not always ask for permission to 'listen in' or to use observations for research purposes, but we would suggest that health researchers inform the participants about the research and ask for this permission. In short, researchers must consider ethical issues most carefully and keep to ethical principles and procedures in electronic forms of inquiry.
(See also Chapter 4)

Strengths and weaknesses of interviewing

There is an ever-increasing use of interviewing as data collection. Atkinson and Silverman (1997) speak of 'the rhetoric of interviewing' where the assumption exists that researchers gain full access to inner feelings and thoughts, uncovering the private self. These writers question the overuse of the interview and claim that it is often seen naïvely or uncritically by researchers who take the words of the informants at face value and do not reflect or take an analytical stance; interviews do not have more privileged status than other forms of data.

There might also be inconsistency between words and actions – the old dilemma of 'what they say and what they do'. Therefore researchers need to observe situations and behaviour, so that they can collect data about social action and interaction. Observation is not only complementary to interviewing but is also a form of within-method triangulation. There are a number of critical comments about interviews listed by Kvale (1996: 292), which we will summarise. He suggests that much interview research

- centres on individuals and does not take social interactions into account;
- neglects the social and material context;
- does not take account of emotions;
- takes place in a vacuum and not in the real world;
- takes account of thoughts and experiences, not actions and focuses on verbal interaction;
- is atheoretical, trivial and ignores linguistic approaches to language.

These are not the only complex issues in interviewing. Researchers cannot know with certainty whether participants are telling the truth or if their memories are faulty. Generally however, they tell the 'truth' as seen from their perspective even if their memories are selective. The factual accuracy of the interview data are not as important as the motivations and thoughts of the participants (Holloway and Freshwater, 2007). Rarely the participant might tell lies but even these demonstrate their perspectives with roots in time and culture.

Researchers who interview will have to be aware of these issues to avoid the pitfalls in interviewing.

Advantages and limitations

One of the main features of qualitative interviewing is its flexibility. Researchers have the freedom to prompt for more information, and participants are able to explore their own thoughts as well as exert more control over the interview as their ideas have priority. This also includes opportunities for participants to react spontaneously and honestly to questions or to articulate their ideas slowly and reflect on them. Researchers can follow up and clarify the meanings of words and phrases immediately, but they can also take time so that trust can develop.

On the other hand, the collection and especially the analysis of interview data is time-consuming and labour intensive. Students who are very enthusiastic during the early data gathering process only realise when they are involved in transcribing and analysing how much time they need for the work.

The interviewer effect and reactivity

Participants sometimes react to the researcher and modify their answers to please or to appear in a positive light, consciously or unconsciously. For these reasons a monitoring process is necessary so that researchers recognise the interviewer effect and minimise it (Hammersley and Atkinson, 2007). This means spending time with the participant so that trust can develop. The interviewers too react to the words they hear. Within the framework of the research the researcher has different priorities from the participant. This has to be recognised so that both the insider's and the researcher's perspective can be made explicit in the research report. After all, health professionals are experts in care, informed about many health and illness issues and have their own perception of the phenomenon under study. Creswell (2007) warns against the possibility of misinterpreting the words of the participant. The interviewer effect is less noticeable in online interviews as interviewer and researcher do not see each other. Labelling or stereotyping is not likely, though it cannot be ruled out completely.

Summary

The in-depth interview is the most common form of data collection.

- Interviews can be face-to-face, online or by telephone.
- The qualitative research interview is relatively non-directive and depends largely on the participants whose ideas, thoughts and feelings researchers try to explore.
- The interviewer's agenda, the aim of the research and the research relationship influence the interview process.
- The advantage of the interview is obtaining the insiders' perspectives directly; its disadvantages are the problematic relationships between words and deeds and the change of participants' thinking over time.

References

Atkinson, P. & Silverman, D. (1997) Kundera's immortality: the interview society and the invention of the self. *Qualitative Inquiry*, **3** (3), 304–25.

Beck, C.T. (2005) Benefits of participating in internet interviews: Women helping women. *Qualitative Health Research*, **15** (3), 411–22.

Breen, A., Austin, H., Champion-Smith, C., Carr, E. & Mann, E. (2007) You feel so hopeless: a qualitative study of GP management of acute back pain. *European Journal of Pain*, **11** (1), 21–9.

Coar, L. & Sim, J. (2006) Interviewing one's peers: methodological issues in a study of health professionals. *Scandinavian Journal of Primary Care*, **24** (4), 251–6.

Colbourne, L. & Sque, M. (2005) The culture of cancer and the therapeutic impact of qualitative interviews. *Journal of Research in Nursing.*, **10** (5), 551–67.

Creswell, J.W. (2007) *Qualitative Inquiry and Research Design: Choosing Among Five Traditions*, 2nd edn. London, Sage.

Denzin, N.K. (1999) Cybertalk and the method of instances. In *Doing Internet Research* (ed. S. Jones). Thousand Oaks, CA, Sage.

Hammersley, M. & Atkinson, P.A. (2007) *Ethnography: Principles in Practice*, 3rd rev. edn. Abingdon, Routledge.

Holloway, I. & Freshwater, D. (2007) *Narrative Research in Nursing*. Oxford, Blackwell.

Kralik, D., Price, K., Warren, J. & Koch, T. (2006) Issues in data generation using email group conversations in nursing research. *Journal of Advanced Nursing*, 53 (2), 213–20.

Kvale, S. (1996) *InterViews: An Introduction to Qualitative Research*. Thousand Oaks, CA, Sage.

Lofland, J. & Lofland, L. (2004) *Analysing Social Settings*. 4th rev. edn. Belmont, CA, Wadsworth.

Manderson, L., Bennett, E. & Andajani-Sutjahjo, S. (2006) The social dynamics of the interview: age, class and gender. *Qualitative Health Research*, 16 (10), 1317–34.

Mann, C. & Stewart, F. (2000) *Internet Communication and Qualitative Research: A Handbook for Researching Online*. London, Sage.

Marshall, C. & Rossman, G.R. (2006) *Designing Qualitative Research*, 4th edn. Thousand Oaks, CA, Sage.

Morton Robinson, K. (2001) Unsolicited narratives from the internet: a rich source of data. *Qualitative Health Research*, 11 (5), 706–14.

Orgad, S. (2005) *Storytelling online: Talking Breast Cancer on the Internet*. New York, NY, Peter Lang.

Patton, M. (2002) *Qualitative Evaluation and Research Methods*, 3rd edn. Thousand Oaks, CA, Sage.

Platt, J. (1981) On interviewing one's peers. *British Journal of Sociology*, 32 (1), 75–91.

Roulston, K., deMarrais, K. & Lewis, J.B. (2003) Learning to interview in the social sciences. *Qualitative Inquiry*, 9 (4), 643–68.

Rubin, H.J. & Rubin, I.S. (2005) *Qualitative Interviewing: The Art of Hearing Data*, 2nd edn. Thousand Oaks, CA, Sage.

Seidman, I.E. (2006) *Interviewing as Qualitative Research*, 3rd edn. New York, NY, Teachers College Press.

Seymour, W.S., (2001) In the flesh or online. Exploring qualitative research methodologies. *Qualitative Research*, 1 (2), 146–8.

Silverman, D. (2006) *Interpreting Qualitative Data: Methods for Analysing Talk, Text and Interaction*, 3rd edn. London, Sage.

Spradley, J.P. (1979) *The Ethnographic Interview*. Fort Worth, TX, Harcourt Brace Johanovich College Publishers.

Wengraf, T. (2001) *Qualitative Research Interviewing: Biographic Narrative and Semi-Structured Methods*. London, Sage.

Further reading

Gubrium, J. & Holstein, J. (eds) (2001) *Handbook of Interview Research: Context and Method*. Thousand Oaks, CA, Sage.

Hamilton, R.J. & Bowers, B.J. (2006) Internet recruitment and e-mail interviews in qualitative studies. *Qualitative Health Research*, **16** (6), 821–35.

Kvale, S. & Brinkman, S. (2009) *InterViews: Learning the Craft of Qualitative Interviewing*. 2nd edn. Thousand Oaks, CA, Sage.

Markham, A. & Baym, M.K. (eds) (2008) *Qualitative Internet Inquiry: A Dialogue among Researchers*. Thousand Oaks, CA, Sage.

Sturges, J.E. & Hanrahan, K.J. (2004) Telephone and face-to-face qualitative interviewing. *Qualitative Research*, **41** (1), 101–7.

CHAPTER 7

Participant Observation and Documents as Sources of Data

Participant observation

Observation is a data source which researchers use to explore and understand the group or culture under study. In particular, it forms an essential element of ethnography and many other types of research, but not of approaches that are based on narratives or pure textual analysis, for instance, descriptive phenomenology or narrative analysis. Although interviewing is a more popular strategy for those undertaking qualitative inquiry, many qualitative researchers believe that it should complement interviews (Hammersley and Atkinson, 2007). Indeed, Strauss and Corbin (1998) see it as qualitative research *par excellence*. It provides access not only to the social context, but also to the ways in which people act and interact. In any case, for nurses and midwives it is important to observe patients, and this everyday practice in clinical settings might help them use participant observation in research. There are many opportunities to do so – perhaps on a ward, in a reception area, in the emergency department, a clinic or any other relevant location inside the hospital or the community.

Savage (2000) sees parallels between observation and clinical practice:

1. *Reliance on physical involvement:* The researcher is present in the setting. This means that health professionals need to be familiar with the location and learn about the behaviour and activities of the participants.
2. *Claims to experiential knowledge:* Whether they act as researchers or as professionals in clinical practice, health professionals experience the situation in similar ways although they interpret the situation differently when carrying out research or when performing their professional activities.
3. *Sharing of theoretical assumptions:* Similar underlying theoretical assumptions are shared both in research and clinical practice.
4. *Reciprocity of perspectives:* In both roles, health professionals attempt to empathise with patients and put themselves in their shoes. This is perhaps easier for the researcher than for the busy professional in clinical practice carrying out routine business. The relationship between observer and observed in a health setting is strong, and much meaning is shared.

When researchers decide to observe, they do not set up artificial situations but look at people in their natural settings. Qualitative researchers generally use the term 'participant observation', a phrase originally coined by Lindeman (1924) which he described as the exploration of a culture from the inside. As Jorgensen (1989: 15) states: 'Participant observation provides direct experiential and observational access to the insiders' world of meaning.' The social reality of the people observed is examined. The researchers will become an integral part of the setting they enter and, to some extent, a member of the group they observe.

There has been a debate about the nature of participant observation. Some see it as a research approach or methodology, others merely as a procedure or strategy for collecting qualitative data. The discussion here centres on observation as a data collection strategy within particular approaches to qualitative research such as ethnography, grounded theory, action research and others. Mulhall (2003) maintains that unstructured observation is an underused strategy in nursing research.

The origins of participant observation

Participant observation has its origins in anthropology and sociology. However, early travellers in ancient times wrote down their observation of cultures they visited, often as participants in those cultures, making it probably the earliest of all forms of data collection. From the early days of fieldwork, anthropologists and sociologists became part of the culture they studied, and examined the actions and interactions of people in their social context, 'in the field'. Studies in anthropology and sociology in particular used observation.

Immersion in culture and setting

Immersion in a setting can take a long time, often years of living in a culture. DeWalt and DeWalt (2002) stress that researchers need to be involved in the context for a prolonged period of time; they should learn the language used in the setting. For health professionals this is an easy task as they are already familiar with language, routines and people in the setting, although they must be aware that these vary for context and situation. However, extraordinary occurrences and critical events must also be observed as they are specific to the setting. DeWalt and DeWalt advise attention to detail which includes 'mapping the scene', observing patterns, arrangements and activities.

Participant observation sometimes proceeds over one or several years, although some observation does not take as long. Health professionals, of course, are already members of and familiar with the culture they examine. For these reasons they may not need a long introduction to the setting; they might, however, miss significant events or behaviours in the locale because of familiarity. This also means that they should suspend prior assumptions, so as not to miss important aspects or misinterpret the situation.

Prolonged observation generates more in-depth knowledge of a group or subculture, and researchers can avoid disturbances and potential biases caused by an occasional visit from an unknown stranger. Observation is less disruptive and more unobtrusive than interviewing. However, participant observation does not just involve observing the situation, but also listening to the people under study.

Example of immersion

Allan (2006) discusses a study in which she used participant observation and interviews in the conception and research clinics of a fertility unit of a teaching hospital. She collected the data over a period of two years visiting the clinics two or three hours each time. She immersed herself further in having informal conversations with staff and clients.

Focus and setting

The dimensions of social settings, according to Spradley (1980) focus on the features which catalogue some ideas about the foci of observation, although these depend on the particular research question.

Dimensions

Spradley classifies the dimensions of social situations as:

Space: the location in which the research takes place

Actor: the participants in the setting

Activity: what is being done

Objects: the material objects present in the setting

Act: single actions that persons in the setting carry out

Events: related activities and happenings

Time: sequencing and length

Goal: what people are aiming to do

Feeling: what people feel and how they express their emotions

(Adapted from Spradley 1980: 78 and 82.)

Nurse researchers and other health professionals centre particularly on the interaction of patients and professionals as well as the actions and activities of both groups. Not only are there descriptions of physical actions and interactions but also of the dialogue that goes on in the setting. The dimensions of the situation and context need detailed description and, eventually, interpretation by the researcher which often can only be developed through asking people about their behaviours and about the meanings of objects, routines and events. Hammersley and Atkinson (2007) argue that interviewing is part of participant observation.

Examples of observation

McGarry (2009) reported on her study with elderly persons in care provision to demonstrate the lack of power of this group. She used not only semi-structured interviews but also participant observation in the home setting to uncover the relationship and interaction between professionals and the elderly patients. The researcher became 'partial participant' in the settings by acting as shadower, observer and assistant. She observed during 47 working days including patient visits to health centres and general practitioners as well as management and team meetings also comprising various allied disciplines and administrators.

Randers and Mattiason (2004) carried out a study in a Norwegian hospital as a follow-up to the teaching of ethics to health professionals. They observed these professionals' behaviours and interactions with patients concerning autonomy and integrity. Observation periods were between four and five hours in duration at a time (both night and day).

Any appropriate setting can become the focus of the study. Participant observation varies on a continuum from open to closed settings. Open settings are public and highly visible such as street scenes, corridors and reception areas. In closed settings, access is more difficult and has to be carefully negotiated; personal offices or meetings in wards can be considered closed settings. It is useful to examine how people in the setting go about their routine and everyday business, how they act and interact with each other and how they relate to the space and the environment in which they are located. Rituals, routines and ways of communication can also be discovered. Gobo (2008) discusses two topics in observation: how to observe and what (whom) to observe. One of the answers to the first question is the matter of estrangement or alienation. Distancing from the setting (being a naïve observer) will generate surprise for the researchers and add a new lens through which settings and people can be observed. The question of what to observe can be answered more easily: Marginal groups are appropriate for observation; for instance, those who are ill are isolated from ordinary social interaction, and the researchers find it easier to suspend their assumptions. Some researchers study the adaptation of foreign nurses to a new culture, others observe learners on the hospital ward.

Researchers might observe critical incidents, dramatic events and examine language use, depending on location or topic, but they can also observe in detail exits and entrances of group members, body language, facial expressions and even choice of words (Abrams, 2000). In Gobo's (2008) words, 'social structure, talks and contexts' (p. 162) must be taken into account.

Observation provides a holistic perspective on the setting. Health researchers can observe as insiders and ask questions, which an outside spectator could not do. If they become deeply engaged and stay for a considerable time, participants will become used to them, and the observer effect will be minimal. The problems and unexpressed needs of the participants also can be observed. Although participants describe their experiences in interviews and reflect on events and actions, researchers will not have to rely only on participants' memories; they will be able to distinguish between 'words and deeds', 'what they say and what they do', which is not always the same. Observation, however useful and appropriate, is time-consuming; hence it is not generally used in undergraduate research, while postgraduates and health professionals in the clinical arena often include it.

Types of observation

Participant observers enter the setting without wishing to limit the observation to particular processes or people, and they adopt an unstructured approach. Occasionally certain foci crystallise early in the study, but usually observation progresses from the unstructured to the more focused until eventually specific actions and events become the main interest of the researcher.

Gold (1958) identified four types of (overlapping) observer involvement in the field which most qualitative researchers still describe:

1. The complete participant
2. The participant as observer
3. The observer as participant
4. The complete observer

The complete participant

The complete participant is part of the setting, a member of a group within it and takes an insider role that often involves covert observation.

Example of classic research with complete participant

Roth (1963), an American sociologist, was a patient in a tuberculosis hospital. While being part of the setting, he observed the interaction of patients with the health personnel, focusing on negotiation concerning time spent in and out of hospital. This is an early, classical observation study.

Pope and Mays (2006) argue that covert observation might be justified in research with patients to whom access is difficult, or when investigating sensitive topics. In spite of the value of some of these studies, complete participation generates a number of ethical problems. First of all, one would have to question seriously whether covert observation in care settings, without knowledge or permission of the people observed, is ethical. After all, this is not a public, open situation such as a street corner or rally, where individuals cannot be identified. In the public domain, observation is permissible and may produce valuable data. For health professionals who advocate caring and ethical behaviour, covert observation in closed settings would be inadvisable. We would not advocate this type of observation, and undergraduates or novice researchers should never attempt it (see also Chapter 4).

The participant as observer

Here, researchers have negotiated their way into the setting, and as participant observers they are part of the work group under study. This seems a good way of doing research, as they are already involved in the work situation. They might want to examine aspects of their own hospital or ward, for instance. The first stage is to ask permission from the relevant gatekeepers and participants and explain the observer role to them. The advantage of this type of observation is the ease with which researcher–participant relationships can be forged or extended. Researchers can move around in the location as they wish, and thus observe in more detail and depth. For new researchers, observation is more difficult than interviewing because of the ethical issues involved and the time needed for 'prolonged engagement'. For ethical reasons, the observers disclose their research role.

The observer as participant

An observer who participates only by being in the location rather than working there, is only marginally involved in the situation. In this case, researchers might observe a particular unit but not directly work as part of the work force; for instance, they might observe a location where they have not been previously. They must, however, announce their interest and their public role and go through the process of gaining entry and asking permission from patients, gatekeepers and colleagues. The advantages of this type of observation are the possibility of asking questions and being accepted as a colleague and researcher but not called upon as a member of the work force. On the other hand, observers are prevented from playing a 'real' role in the setting. Restraint from involvement is not easy, particularly in a busy situation where professionals must be protected from intrusion when working.

The complete observer

Complete observers do not take part in the setting and use a 'fly on the wall' approach. Being a complete observer when the observer is not a participant is only possible when the researchers have some distance from the setting and observe through a window, in a corner or through a two-way mirror where they are not noticed and have no impact on the situation or when they use static video cameras fixed on the ceiling.

There is no clear distinction however between some of these types of observation; they overlap.

Ethics issues in observation

Permission from participants should be requested in healthcare settings. Access and permission to observe is more difficult to achieve than in other forms of data collection. All within the setting are included for this permission and also those who have power to withhold and gain access, such as managers. When researchers have achieved the initial contact, it is important to establish rapport with the group or cultural members. Researchers must make it quite clear that they are not 'spies' for management in any of these situations.

Progression and process

Spradley (1980) claims that observers progress in three stages; they use *descriptive*, *focused* and finally *selective* observation. Descriptive observation proceeds on the basis of general questions that the observer has in mind. Everything that goes on in the setting provides data and is recorded, including colours, smells and appearances of people. Description involves all five senses. As time goes by, certain important areas or aspects of the setting become more obvious, and the researcher focuses on these because they contribute to the achievement of the research aim. Eventually observation becomes highly selective, centring on very specific issues only. Researchers adopt the strategy of progressive focusing.

LeCompte *et al.* (1997) give guidelines for observation, which we will summarise here.

The 'who' questions

Who and how many people are present in the setting or take part in the activities? What are their characteristics and roles?

Nurse and midwife researchers observe the situation and specifically focus on the many role performances and interactions.

The 'what' questions

What is happening in the setting, what are the actions and rules of behaviour? What are the variations in the behaviour observed?

Health professionals focus on the activities and behaviour of those involved.

The 'where' questions

Where do interactions take place? Where are people located in the physical space?

For health professionals this means looking at the ward, the clinic, the GP's surgery or meeting. Even discussions at the bedside or handovers are of importance.

The 'when' questions

When do conversations and interactions take place? What is the timing of activities?

Events, discussions and interactions take place at different times. Health professionals must ask whether there is any significance in the timing of these.

The 'why' questions

Why do people in the setting act the way they do? Why are there variations in behaviour?

The 'why' questions are self-explanatory. Researchers examine the reasons for the activities, behaviour or critical incidents. This does of course, often include interviewing participants.

Process

Mini-tour observation leads to detailed descriptions of smaller and more intimate units, while *grand-tour observations* are more appropriate for larger settings. After the initial stages, certain dimensions and features of observation become interesting to the researcher who then proceeds to observe these dimensions specifically. 'Progressive focusing', which was discussed earlier, is not just a feature of interviewing but also of observation.

The study becomes more focused as time progresses, because the observer notices important behaviours or interactions. Focused observations are the outcome of specific questions. From broader observations, researchers might proceed to observing a small unit. They could look for similarities and differences among groups and individuals. For this type of observation narrow focus and specificity are useful and necessary.

Marshall and Rossman (2006) argue that observation means systematic exploration of events and actions as well as noting the use and position of artefacts (objects) in the setting under study. Researchers observe social processes as they happen and develop. Participant observations can focus on events, processes and actions, but they cannot explore past events and thoughts of participants; this has to be done in interviews. Hammersley and Atkinson (2007) see interviewing as part of participant observation. The early classical work demonstrates this clearly, particularly the research by Becker *et al.* (1961). The participants, namely medical students, were observed in their interaction with patients, colleagues and teachers, and the researchers then asked questions about what they saw and heard. Hammersley and Atkinson (2007), in fact, propose that one might see all social research as participant observation to the extent that the researcher actively participates in the situation.

Researchers may be reluctant to carry out formal participant observation because of time and access problems; for instance, it is easier to interview colleagues or clients than to observe them. Observation might change the situation, as people act differently in the presence of observers, although they often forget being observed in long-term research. The latter, however, takes more time than is available in student projects and therefore it is more often used by postgraduates and experienced researchers who have a longer time span for their research.

When observations are successful, they can uncover interesting patterns and developments, which have their basis in the real world of the participants' daily lives, and the task of exploration and discovery is, after all, the aim of qualitative research.

As we have explained before, researchers sometimes triangulate within method. Triangulation enhances the trustworthiness and authenticity of the study (see Chapter 18).

Examples of within-method triangulation

Casey (2007) collected her data through observation and semi-structured interviewing. Her study explored the perceptions, understandings and experiences of nurses concerning health promotion. She observed nurses in practice and after this interviewed them on a one-to-one basis.

Gabbay and le May (2004) examined how general practitioners and practice nurses derived their healthcare decisions in two general practices. They used observation, semi-structured interviews and documents (practice guidelines and manuals among others) as sources of data.

The data gained from observation as those from interviews might be serendip-itous and generate unexpected findings.

Problematic issues

Observation, through familiarity with the culture under study, generates much information about settings and situations. However, there are also some prob-lems and disadvantages particularly for researchers who have time constraints; indeed interviewing is particularly popular in nursing and midwifery research because it is not quite as time consuming.

It is difficult to record the data during observation as scribbled notes take time and might cause reactivity from the people who are being observed. We would rarely advise video-recording as participants might become embarrassed or worried, and many professionals would not wish their actions to be on record on a tape. Often researchers have to base their recollections on memory rather than notes, and memories decrease over time. This means that notes which are not recorded in the location observed, need to be written immediately after the observation. As other types of data collection, observation relies on the researcher as the tool in the research whose assumptions can intrude. Indeed the researcher leaves assumptions and expectations behind when entering the setting. Ethical issues are paramount – as in all health research. The researcher must fade into the setting, show sensitivity and not be too obvious so that there is little observer effect. The presence and intentions of the researcher need to be disclosed to all participants.

Technical procedures and practical hints

A series of steps need to be taken, some of which are also described by Creswell (2007:134):

1. The setting for the observation is selected and permission for access obtained from gatekeepers.
2. The researcher obtains informed consent from participants.
3. Exact location, details and the most useful time and length of observation will be chosen and other decisions made about fieldwork and note taking.
4. Researchers decide on the roles in which they will adopt, from outsider to insider.
5. Physical settings, behaviours such as actions, interactions and reactions are observed and noted.
6. The researchers also note down their own feelings and reactions of the research by being reflexive.
7. The researcher disengages from the site and debriefs the participants while assuring anonymity.

Researchers might use cameras and video equipment to catch movements and expressions of participants more accurately, although video cameras could intimidate or disturb the participants and change their behaviour. If tape is used, it can be viewed over and over again so 'nothing is lost' (Abrams, 2000: 58). This also means, of course, that the tapes must be kept secure and confidential, and they cannot be shown to colleagues or friends, (for student projects, only to supervisors with permission of the participants).

Taking fieldnotes is an important task. Observations are translated into written records which researchers take while observing or immediately afterwards. These are detailed descriptions of the setting and the behaviour of participants. The researchers' own reflections on the situation and their feelings about it are also recorded in fieldnotes (see Chapter 10). Writing might be difficult at the time of observation, and participants might object. If not possible during observation, researchers need to write them soon afterwards. Mulhall (2003: 311) suggests that 'recording events as they happen' means that the memory of the researcher is fresh and details are not lost. In the first instance, of course, fieldnotes consist of jotting down quick notes which become expanded at a later stage.

Health researchers who are actively involved in patient care may not be able to observe as well as take notes at the same time. It is important to record impressions as soon as possible after the observation. Diagrams and charts also help in recording how people act and interact in the setting under observation.

Once researchers have collected the initial observational data, they start analysing them so that the collection and analysis of data interact and go in parallel. This way the observation can become progressively focused on emerging and interesting themes that are important to the research. Drawing maps of the location or indicating interaction through diagrams can be useful devices to help observation. (Some of the analysis of observation will be discussed in Chapter 17, but in general, it progresses in the same way as other types with the fieldnotes and memos as documents for analysis.) After creating ethnographic records, collecting interview answers, documents, images or other sources of data, Gobo (2008) suggests that the researcher goes through three main stages: those of deconstruction, construction and confirmation which are similar to the coding steps in grounded theory. When deconstructing, researchers break down the events that occur; in constructing they link the concepts found and generate stories about the phenomenon which is being studied; and confirmation follows particular core concepts in the data collection and confirms their presence in the observation, reports them and connects them to the theoretical ideas. This phase is more abstract and of higher 'generality' than earlier stages (see also Chapter 17).

Documentary sources of data

Documents which are written texts and records are also useful sources of data. Hammersley and Atkinson (2007) suggest that researchers use these because they give information for situations that cannot be investigated by direct observation or questioning. Also, documentary sources contain added knowledge about the group being studied. Typically they consist of autobiographies and biographies, official documents and reports, the latter ranging from informal documentary sources to formal and official reports such as newspapers or minutes of meetings. Timetables, case notes and reports can become the focus of nurses' investigation. The researcher treats them like transcriptions of interviews or detailed descriptions of observations; that is, they are coded and categorised. They act as sensitising devices and make researchers aware of important issues. Documents may be primary or secondary sources of data. Primary sources comprise documents which have been written by the people involved in the experience, action or event and can only be understood in the context of their time and locality.

Example of primary documents

Jones (2000) describes the case of an elderly man who had kept diaries for many years. She learnt that in these he had kept a record of symptoms and events while dealing with the health service and health professionals. Jones felt very fortunate to have this personal account of events that happened while the man had treatment for his condition. She saw the document as both authentic and meaningful.

Secondary documents have been written about these events at a later stage and might be comments on primary sources.

Example of secondary document analysis

In a case study, Green *et al.* (2006) explored the selection, implementation and outcomes of the approach to research capacity building in a department of nursing and midwifery at a university. As well as using interviews, they also carried out documentary analysis. The latter consisted of minutes of meetings and departmental documents and strategic plans.

Many of these texts exist before researchers start their work, others are initiated and organised by the researchers themselves. Historical documents, archives and products of the media exist independently from researchers while personal diaries might be written through their intervention or instigation; for instance Jacelon (2005) used participant diaries as a data source in her research with older people.

Scott (1990) differentiates between types of document by referring to them as *closed*, *restricted*, *open-archival* and *open-published*. Access to closed documents is limited to a few people, namely their authors and those who commissioned them. As far as restricted documents are concerned, researchers can only gain access with the permission of insiders under particular conditions.

> **Examples**
>
> Private documents might include patient complaints, their General Practitioner's or hospital notes for instance. Diaries and data belonging to specific people are closed documents. Historical documents are archival documents, and published documents could comprise published guidelines or White Papers.

Permission for access is asked from the living authors of diaries and keepers of other confidential documents. Open-archival documents are available to any person, subject to administrative conditions and opening hours of libraries. Published documents, of course, can be accessed by anybody at any time. There is no reactivity or observer effect in examining documentary data although researchers, of course, come to the reading with their own assumptions. They are useful and rich sources of information for researchers.

Qualitative researchers most often seek access to diaries – which are people's own accounts of their lives – and letters, but also to historical documents or the products of the media. Some researchers encourage participants to keep a diary for analysis. Jones (2000) lists two different forms of diary: *solicited* and *unsolicited*. The former are accounts of conditions or treatments kept by patients at the behest of researchers. Unsolicited diaries are the personal and informal records patients keep about their stay in hospital, about their condition, illness or care. A researcher cannot easily access these documents.

> **Example of diary research**
>
> Richardson *et al.* (2006) carried out research including eight participants who were experiencing chronic pain, and their families, whom they interviewed in depth based on a life grid. Some of these interviews were developed from seven participants' unstructured diaries. These diaries were kept over several weeks; participants recorded details of their pain and how it affected their daily lives.

Through documents, researchers in the health professions acquire a perspective on history which gives them insiders' views on past lives and attitudes; they can analyse contemporary documents – such as articles and comments in the press – and become aware of the significant features of issues or the dramatisation of particular events. Last, and most importantly, health professionals can trace the perspectives of diary or autobiography writers by collecting, reading and analysing these personal documents. Through this, researchers can gain knowledge of the experiences of others in a particular context and at a particular time.

Researchers must be concerned about four major criteria that determine the quality of the documents: *authenticity*, *credibility*, *representativeness* and *meaning* (Scott, 1990). To demonstrate authenticity for historical documents, questions about their history as well as their writers' intentions and biases must be asked. Credibility involves some of these questions too. Accuracy might be affected by the writer's proximity in time and place to the events described and also the conditions under which the information was acquired at the time. Representativeness of documents is difficult to prove because researchers often have no information of the numbers or variety of documents about a particular event.

Scott (1990) claims that the most significant aim of the document collection and analysis is their meaning and interpretation. It is far easier to analyse a personal document written in the recent past where the researcher is familiar with language and context than to assess the representativeness or authenticity of a historical document whose context can only be assumed. Therefore, the researcher can only try to interpret the meaning of the text in context, study the situation and conditions in which it is written and try to establish the writer's intentions.

As in other types of data, the meaning is tentative and provisional only and may change when new data present a challenge and demand reappraisal. Hammersley and Atkinson (2007) warn that documents may generate biases as they are often written by and for elites, or people in power. That in itself, however, might be useful because not many sources exist that give the ideas of these informants.

Images as sources of data

Images are increasingly becoming part of qualitative inquiry. Audiences sit in front of television or cinema screens or in the theatre. There is another reason for the low position of image-based research: researchers who work with visual data do not form a coherent group; they have not had a serious impact on qualitative research.

Loizos (2000) declares that images are important records of social reality. Visual information generates primary data or can be used to supplement other data collection methods, although care must be taken in its use. Videos in particular, can enhance and expand the data derived from initial observation (the ethical issues inherent in filming are problematic, however). Still photographs are not as useful – they freeze the situation in time and do not demonstrate its processual character.

Loizos gives some practical advice in his chapter on images, such as videos, photos or films. He also points to some essential reading for the use of images. He suggests, for instance, that researchers

1. log film rolls, cassettes, photos and other images immediately with written details of locations, people and dates;
2. get permission from informants to reproduce their images;
3. make sure to get good quality sound;

4. do not forget that the technology is just a means to an end;
5. only use films and other images when they really enhance the research as they may be expensive and disturb the participants in the situation.

(See also Performative Social Science in Chapter 15)

Summary

- Observation, documents and visual data are common sources of data and complement interviews.
- Observation, in particular participant observation is part of many qualitative approaches.
- There are different types of observation.
- Researchers need to record their observations and use 'thick description' for the writing up.
- Participant observation can pose ethical problems for the researcher.
- Documents such as diaries, historical writing or guidelines are popular sources of data.

References

Abrams, W.L. (2000) *The Observational Handbook: Understanding How Consumers Live with Your Product*. Chicago, IL, NTC Business Books.

Allan, H.T. (2006) Using participant observation to immerse oneself in the field: the role of emotions in nursing practice. *Journal of Research in Nursing*, **11** (5), 397–407.

Becker, H.S., Geer, B., Hughes, E. & Strauss, A.L. (1961) *Boys in White*. New Brunswick, NJ, University of Chicago Press.

Casey, D. (2007) Findings from non-participant observational data concerning health promoting nursing practice in the hospital setting focusing on generalist nurses. *Journal of Clinical Nursing*, **16** (3), 580–92.

Creswell, J.W. (2007) *Qualitative Inquiry and Research Design*, 2nd edn. Thousand Oaks, CA, Sage.

DeWalt, K.M. & DeWalt, B.R. (2002) *Participant Observation: A Guide for Field-workers*. Walnut Creek, CA, Altamira Press.

Gabbay, J. & le May, A. (2004) Evidence-based guidelines or collectively constructed 'mindlines': ethnographic study of knowledge management in primary care. *British Medical Journal*, **329** (7473), 1013–16.

Gobo, G. (2008) *Doing Ethnography*. Los Angeles, CA, Sage.

Gold, R. (1958) Roles in sociological field observation. *Social Forces*, **36** (3), 217–23.

Green, B., Segrott, J. & Hewitt, J. (2006) Developing nursing and midwifery research capacity in a university department: case study. *Journal of Advanced Nursing*, **56** (3), 302–13.

Hammersley, M. & Atkinson, P. (2007) *Ethnography: Principles in Practice*, 3rd revised edn. London, Routledge.

Jacelon, C. (2005) Participant diaries as a source of data in research with older adults. *Qualitative Health Research*, **15** (7), 991–7.

Jones, R.K. (2000) The unsolicited diary as a qualitative research tool for advanced capacity in the field of health and illness. *Qualitative Health Research*, **10** (4), 555–67.

Jorgensen, D.L. (1989) *Participant Observation*. Newbury Park, CA, Sage.

LeCompte, M.D. & Preissle, J., Tesch, R. (1997) *Ethnography and Qualitative Design in Educational Research*, 2nd edn. Chicago, IL, Academic Press.

Lindeman, E.C. (1924) *Social Discovery: An Introduction to the Study of Functional Groups*. New York, NY, Republic Publishing.

Loizos, P. (2000) Video, film and photographs as research documents. In *Qualitative Researching with Text, Image and Sound* (eds M. Bauer & G. Gaskell), pp. 93–107. London, Sage.

Marshall, C. & Rossman, G.R. (2006) *Designing Qualitative Research*, 4th edn. Thousand Oaks, CA, Sage.

McGarry, J. (2009) Defining roles, relationships, boundaries and participation between elderly people and nurses within the home: an ethnographic study. *Health and Social Care in the Community*, **17** (1), 83–91.

Mulhall, A. (2003) In the field: notes on observation in qualitative research. *Journal of Advanced Nursing*, **41** (3), 306–13.

Pope, C. & Mays, N. (2006) Observational methods, Chapter 6. In *Qualitative Research in Health Care* (eds C. Pope & N. Mays). Oxford, Blackwell.

Randers, I. & Mattiason, A. (2004) Autonomy and integrity: upholding older people's dignity. *Journal of Advanced Nursing*, **45** (1), 63–71.

Richardson, J.C., Ong, B.N. & Sim, J. (2006) Is chronic widespread pain biographically disruptive? *Social Science and Medicine*, **63** (6), 1573–85.

Roth, J.A. (1963) *Timetables*. Indianapolis, IN, Bobbs Merril.

Savage, J. (2000) Participant observation: standing in the shoes of others. *Qualitative Health Research*, **10** (3), 324–39.

Scott, J. (1990) *A Matter of Record: Documentary Sources in Social Research*. Cambridge, Polity Press.

Spradley, J.P. (1980) *Participant Observation*. Fort Worth, TX, Harcourt Brace Johanovich.

Strauss, A.L. & Corbin, J.M. (1998) *Basics of Qualitative Research: Techniques and Procedures of Developing Grounded Theory*, 2nd edn. Beverly Hills, CA, Sage.

Further reading

Angrosino, M. (2007) *Doing Ethnographic and Observational Research*. London, Sage.

Emerson, R.M., Fretz, R.I. & Shaw, L.L. (2007) Participant observation and fieldnotes. In *Handbook of Ethnography* (eds P. Atkinson, A. Coffey, S. Delamont *et al.*) pp. 352–68 London, Sage.

Sanger, J. (1996) *The Complete Observer? A Field Research Guide to Observation.* London, The Falmer Press.

Schensul, S.L., Schensul, J.J. & LeCompte, M.D. (1999) *Essential Ethnographic Methods: Observations, Interviews and Questionnaires.* Walnut Creek, CA, Altamira Press.

CHAPTER 8

Focus Groups as Qualitative Research

What is a focus group?

A focus group in nursing research involves a number of people – often with common experiences or characteristics – who are interviewed by a researcher (moderator, or facilitator) for the purpose of eliciting ideas, thoughts and perceptions about a specific topic or certain issues linked to an area of interest.

In the past, researchers have employed focus group techniques in the area of marketing and business research, but in the last decades they have become popular in social science and the caring professions. The ideas generated are normally analysed by qualitative methods, although focus groups can result in quantitative or multi-method research; for instance, they may generate findings to be used in the construction of a questionnaire, or employed as a way to obtain in-depth data at the end of a survey. The type of group and the number of interviews are determined by the research question. There is broad agreement between researchers in the definition of focus groups (see table by Freeman, 2006: 493). Researchers might use pre-existing groups whose members have the same experience – for instance a carer group of people with similar conditions or a support group – or they can establish their own group for which members are carefully and purposefully selected to achieve the functions of the particular type of research. Although focus group research can stand alone, focus group interviews are often just one source of data within a specific qualitative approach. Webb and Kevern (2001), however, discuss their incompatibility with phenomenology and grounded theory although they can be usefully employed in the latter if the character of grounded theory (GT) and the strategy of theoretical sampling are preserved.

The origin and purpose of focus groups

The first text on focus groups was written by Merton and Kendall (1946), as a result of these writers working with groups during and shortly after the Second

World War. In 1956 they expanded their knowledge into a book (Merton *et al.*, 1956). Business and market researchers had used this type of in-depth group interview since the 1920s. It became especially popular in market research in order to gather information about customers' thoughts and feelings about a product, though initially this type of research was not rooted in the qualitative tradition.

Today the focus group interview is used by a wide variety of researchers in the area of communications, policy, marketing and advertising. Focus groups in the social sciences and health professions have become fashionable since the growth of qualitative research methods in the 1980s. This approach does not rely merely on the ideas of the researcher and a single participant; instead, the members of the group generate new questions and answers through verbal interaction. Through these group interviews, researchers are able to discover the needs and feelings of their clients, the perceptions and attitudes of their colleagues, and they can examine the thoughts of decision makers. The cultural values and beliefs of people can also be explored this way.

Focus groups produce thoughts and opinions about a topic relevant to health care, treatment evaluation and illness experiences. Many examples are reported in nursing and social science journals.

Examples of focus groups

Research with two focus groups of nursing students was conducted in the UK by Pearcey and Elliot (2004) whose aim was the exploration of reasons for not wishing to enter a nursing career. The sample came from both second- and third-year students. Facilitator and researchers interviewed for 90 minutes taking into account each member's perceptions of the clinical experience.

In Australia five focus groups were interviewed over two hours by the same facilitator. The aim of the study was to investigate the view of nurses and doctors to incident reporting in order to improve the situation. One group each consisted of consultants, registrars, senior nurses, junior nurses and resident medical officers, a purposive sample from public hospitals. Both semi-structured and open-ended questions were used to stimulate talk between group members. The barriers to incident reporting were established.

(Kingston *et al.*, 2004)

Focus groups are characterised by interaction between the participants from which researchers discover how people think and feel about particular issues. It is not the intention to examine a wide variety of issues in one study; these groups are set up to explore a specific issue rather than general topics which are more often investigated in marketing or political focus groups.

> **Example**
>
> Norton (2008), a health education specialist, examined the sun-related behaviour of young adolescent women. She set up focus groups with students from a secondary school and a youth club, asking questions which were specifically related to behaviour in the sun.

Focus group members respond to the interviewer and to each other. The questions might start with eliciting knowledge about a specific condition, the use of a drug, a method of intervention, or by putting the members at ease but should soon go on to a discussion of feelings or thoughts. Different reactions stimulate debate about the topic because group members respond to each other. Discussions in groups might help not only in the development of ideas about problems and questions which researchers have not thought about before but also by finding answers to some of these questions and solutions to problems.

In nursing and other healthcare arenas, focus groups are used to

1. explore patients' experiences of their condition, treatment and interaction with health professionals;
2. evaluate programmes and treatment;
3. gaining understanding of health professionals' roles and identities;
4. examine the perception and efficacy of professional education;
5. obtain perspectives on public health issues.

These are just some of the functions of focus group interviewing. The ultimate goal for the researcher is to understand the reality of the participants, and not to make decisions about a specific issue or problem, although future actions may be based on the findings of the focus group interviews. Focus groups differ from individual interviews in that they depend on the stimulus that participants gain from each other, and that they discuss both unique and shared perceptions and experiences. Focus groups can be used as a single source of interview data or in conjunction with one-to-one interviews.

Sample size and composition

The sample is linked closely to the research topic. The people who are interviewed in a focus group usually have similar roles or experiences. They may be colleagues who share the same speciality, use the same technical equipment or nursing procedures or patients who suffer from the same condition. The purpose of the focus group generally determines its composition and size. Morgan (1998b) claims that a small group is better for controversial or complex topics, while larger groups tend to have lower levels of involvement with less highly intense topic areas. We have also found that in smaller groups individuals can be heard more clearly, though groups with larger numbers of participants might generate more ideas.

Morgan (1998a) suggests that well-defined criteria are needed for this selection. These might include demographic factors, gender, ethnic group membership and specific experiences or conditions. Participants in focus groups will have had common experiences, have the same condition or receive the same treatment. For instance, if a doctor wishes to interview a group of people with diabetes, she or he obviously involves individuals with this condition in the focus groups. A midwife might obtain the feelings and thoughts of pregnant women or new mothers by small focus groups. Colleagues who are interviewed generally share common interests, work in similar settings or perform similar tasks. If the interviewer wants the thoughts of colleagues from a psychiatric setting, for example, then the sample has to be composed of nurses with psychiatric experience. Students too can be interviewed in focus groups about perspectives on their education. Health promotion often is a topic for research.

The choice of the members of focus groups depends on a condition or experiences that potential participants have in common. Although group members share these, it does not mean that they all have the same views, or that they come from the same background or organisation. It might be useful to recruit members from naturally occurring groups such as antenatal classes, patient support groups or carers. While they have similar experiences, they are nevertheless heterogeneous in other ways, and so could illuminate the topic from all sides.

The number of focus groups depends on the needs of the researcher and the demands of the topic area. For one research project, the usual number is about three or four, but the actual number depends on the complexity of the research topic. If the sample of participants is heterogeneous, more groups are needed.

Examples

Pearcey and Elliott (2004) worked only two focus groups with nursing students, while Kingston et al. (2004) included five groups of doctors and nurses.

A study of the understanding of childhood asthma by mothers from three different ethnic groups had nine focus groups (Cane et al., 2001).

Studies with large focus groups and many informants are more difficult. Group sessions can last from one to three hours. We must stress, however, that three-hour interviews with patients would be far too long and demanding. In market research, participants are paid for their time and effort but not usually in healthcare research, because this would coerce the informants and squander resources. Much new information is gained in initial groups as the researcher can follow up the ideas obtained in subsequent interviews. As in other qualitative research, important themes emerge often at an early stage, although some serendipitous results might be found in a later phase.

Each group might contain between four and twelve people, but six is probably the optimum number as it is large enough to provide a variety of perspectives and small enough not to become disorderly or fragmented. Indeed, one of our colleagues found that in her experience, even a group of six was too large and that the optimum number of members in the group was three, but the number could of course vary depending on the topic or the background of group members. Greenbaum (1998), a market researcher, however, claims that group dynamics work better if the group is not too small. The larger the group, however, the more difficult the transcription becomes. When several people start talking together and the group is lively and noisy, it can be difficult to distinguish voices.

There may well be a difference between groups who come together for market research purposes and those who gather for health research. The former will feel much less vulnerable because the area of discussion is rarely threatening or sensitive. The nature of the topic area is of importance: focus groups in which sensitive topics are discussed are more difficult to facilitate.

Members of the group, although sharing common experiences, do not have to know each other. In a group of immediate colleagues or friends, private thoughts or ideas might not be revealed, although occasionally the opposite could be true. One individual is more likely to dominate others and the past history of the group may inhibit or lead individuals in a particular direction. In healthcare research, familiarity between participants, or participants and researchers could be useful because the 'warm-up' time – the time where informants get to know each other to facilitate interaction – is shorter, and the researcher can focus on the topic immediately. Stewart and Shamdasani (2007), for instance, believe that compatibility among group members is more productive than conflict or polarisation, although this too depends on the topic; sometimes conflict can generate new and different ideas.

Gender and age of the group members affect the quality and level of interaction and through this the data. For instance, evidence shows greater diversity of ideas in single sex groups than in those of mixed gender according to Stewart and Shamdasani. Mixed gender groups tend to be more conforming because of the social interaction between males and females; both groups sometimes tend to 'perform' for each other.

Conducting focus group interviews

Focus group interviews must be planned carefully. The informants are contacted well in advance of the interviews and reminded a few days before they start. As in other types of inquiry, ethical and access issues are considered. The environment for a focus group is important as the room must be big enough to contain the participants and the tape-recorder placed in an advantageous location, where they can all be heard and recorded. For focus group work, it is essential to have a top quality tape-recorder. Merton and King (1990) suggest a spatial arrangement of a circle or semi-circle, which seems the most successful seating arrangement.

The group interviews should have a clearly identified agenda otherwise they deteriorate into vague and chaotic discussions (Stewart and Shamdasani, 2007). Morgan (1997) believes in the importance of time management because both interviewer and informants have limited time. Time management is one of the tasks of the facilitator. Focus groups are more productive if the time for interchange is not too short. Usually focus group interviews last around $1^1/_2$ to 2 hours but this might depend on age, vulnerability or power of concentration of participants.

From the beginning the researcher establishes ground rules, so that all group members know how to proceed. Researchers plan the initial questions and prompts. When the interviews start, the interviewer puts the group at ease and introduces the topic to be debated. Strategies such as showing a film or telling a story related to the topic sometimes stimulate interaction. Kitzinger and Barbour (1999) also suggest such stimulus material as vignettes or photographs. Researchers often adopt the strategy of asking stimulus questions and generally proceed from the more general to the specific, just as in other qualitative interviews. Involving all the participants, rather than letting a few individuals dominate the situation demands diplomacy and would be easier with a smaller group. Extreme views in a group of people are balanced out by the reactions of the majority when debating questions. As suggested before, focus groups can be combined with individual interviews, observation or other methods of data collection but this is not essential.

In focus groups, as in all other research, ethical issues must be considered. Confidentiality, in particular, could be problematic in group interviews as members of the group might discuss the findings in other settings and situations. They should be reminded to keep the discussions confidential. Anonymity cannot be guaranteed, as members of the group might be able to identify other participants even when researchers only use first names. Participants may make remarks that are hurtful to others, or show prejudice, and the researcher has to find ways to deal with this.

The involvement of the interviewer

The interviewer becomes the facilitator or moderator in the group discussion although it could be useful to have another person who takes notes. In health research, the health professional is usually the interviewer (while in market research focus groups, professional moderators are employed). In a small project, a single interviewer usually facilitates the groups. The presence of a note-taker who can make fieldnotes, draw diagrams with the names of participants and generally help with practical matters, could be very useful. The researcher should have the particular qualities of the in-depth interviewer: flexibility, open-mindedness and skill in eliciting information. The creation of an open and non-threatening group climate is one of their initial important tasks.

Researchers must be able to stimulate discussion and have insight and interest in the ideas of the informants. The leadership role of the moderators demands abilities above that of the one-to-one interviewer. They must have the social and refereeing skills to guide the members towards effective interaction and sometimes be able to exert control over informants and topic without directing the debate or coercing the participants. If the group feels at ease with the interviewer, the interaction will be open and productive, and the participants will be comfortable about disclosing their perceptions and feelings. Researchers might experience difficulties with particular groups such as teenagers, while getting together groups of disabled people may present practical problems in the available space.

Morgan (1997) advises that the interviewers hold back on questioning if they want to examine the real feelings of participants; much of the discussion evolves from the dynamics of group interaction. Indeed Kitzinger (2005: 57) claims that 'a defining feature of focus group research is using the interaction between research participants to generate data and giving attention to that interaction as part of the analysis'. This non-directive approach has particular importance in exploratory research where perceptions are examined. High involvement of the interviewer leads more quickly to the core of the topic, but special facilitation skills are needed if the focus groups are going to be successful. The interviewers should not express their own biases or assumptions in the focus groups. A special relationship with a specific individual, an affirmative nod at something of which the interviewer approves, or a lack of encouragement for unexpected or unwelcome answers may bias the interviews too. Again, group behaviour is an important factor. Polarisation of views may generate a difficult group climate. Although conflicts of opinion can produce valuable data, the interviewer must defuse personal hostility between members, which demands good facilitating skills. Gestures and facial expressions have to be controlled to show members of the group that the interviewer is non-judgemental and values the views of all participants. Streubert Speziale and Rinaldi Carpenter (2007) argue that a good facilitator can help the group to avoid 'group think' and offence to some participants.

Analysing and reporting focus group data

The principles of qualitative data analysis are similar to those of other non-structured or semi-structured interviews. Most often the interviews are recorded, and initially the researcher listens several times to each tape before making transcripts. Although this method has been used in market research, it is difficult to identify individuals' voices on a tape. The problem of identification might be overcome with videotaping, but Sim (1998) suggests that this might inhibit participants, particularly when they discuss a sensitive issue.

All tapes, fieldnotes and memos are dated and labelled. A wide margin is left on the transcript for coding and categorising. The transcription should include laughter, notes about pauses and emphasis, and the researcher makes fieldnotes on anything unusual, interesting or contradictory and writes memos about theoretical ideas while listening, transcribing and reading. It is important to be clear about who says what, because this can identify those individuals who try to dominate the discussion. The interviewer could note this while listening to the tape. At the listening stage, major themes and patterns can already be found. It is important, however, that researchers focus on the context of group interaction not just on the comments of particular individuals but on all of them (Asbury, 1995). This interaction might stimulate thought in the participants but it could also intimidate some or encourage others.

Interviewers code paragraphs and sentences by extracting the essence of ideas within them and using labels which they put into the margin of the transcript. Through a reduction of these codes into larger categories, themes and ideas will be found. As in other types of qualitative research, the frequency of themes that are found is not as important as their significance; some obviously have priority over others for the specific study. The method of analysis in focus groups is similar to those of other approaches; in fact, focus groups can be analysed by thematic analysis (see Chapter 17) or another form of qualitative analysis.

The analyst repeats the process with each focus group interview and compares the transcripts. The major themes arising from individual interviews are then connected with each other; topics in one interview will overlap with those of other focus groups. Once these themes have been formulated, the patterns described and their meaning interpreted, the literature connected with these ideas is discussed. The appropriate literature becomes confirmation or challenge to the researcher's findings as in other qualitative research.

Researchers substantiate their work with relevant quotes from the participants, showing the data from which the patterns and constructs arise; excerpts from interactions are part of these quotes. Although patterns and consistencies are important for reporting, individual comments are also important as they might form an alternative response to the rest of the data. If there are many such deviant cases, it might be useful to add one-to-one interviews to explore these further.

To write up the study, the interviewers develop a storyline, that is, they must produce an account that is readable and clear. The main concerns of the participants have to emerge from the report as the most important parts of the story. The findings from the focus group interviews are often used as a basis for action.

Advantages and limitations of focus groups

In general the advantages and limitations in this approach are those of all qualitative interviews, but there are a number of strengths and weaknesses specific to focus groups (Stewart and Shamdasani, 2007). The main strength is the production of data through social interaction. The dynamic interaction stimulates the thoughts of participants and reminds them of their own feelings about the research topic. Informants build on the answers of others in the group. Second, on responding to each other's comments, informants might generate new and spontaneous ideas, which researchers had not thought of before or during the interview. Through interaction informants remember forgotten feelings and thoughts. Third, all the participants, including the interviewer, have the opportunity to ask questions, and these will produce more ideas than individual interviews. Kitzinger (2005) suggests that group interaction gives courage to the informants to mention even sensitive topics. The interview might empower participants because as group members they often feel more able to express their views.

The researcher has the opportunity for prompts and questions for clarification just like the other members of the group. These probes will produce more ideas than individual interviews, and the answers show the participants' feelings about a topic and the priorities in the situation under discussion. The researcher can clarify conflicts between participants and ask about the reasons for these differing views. Focus groups produce more data in the same space of time; this could make them cheaper and quicker than individual interviews. Some people dislike opening up their inner thoughts in public and may be reluctant to answer some questions – one of the reasons for careful selection of participants. Though the presence of others might inhibit disclosure, which is a disadvantage in these settings, it can also allow individuals to be quiet and obviate the need to respond if they do not wish to disclose something.

There are also some disadvantages. The researcher generally has more difficulty managing the debate and less control over the process than in one-to-one interviews. As group members interact throughout the interview, one or two individuals may dominate the discussion and influence the outcome or perhaps even introduce bias, as the other members may be merely compliant. The group effect may, as Carey and Smith (1994) suggest, lead to conformity or to convergent answers. They use the term 'censoring', by which they mean the critical stance of group members towards each other. The participants affect each other, while in individual interviews the 'real' feelings of the individual informant may be more readily revealed. A person who is unable to verbalise feelings and thoughts will not make a good informant in focus groups. Indeed, Merton and King (1990) stress the importance of educational homogeneity of the group. If group members have similar educational backgrounds, the chance for contribution from all members is greater. The status of a few well-educated individuals would inhibit the rest of the members in the group and might even silence them, and therefore similarity of social background is useful. The group members might know each other before the meeting, and it is important to take this into account. This means that sampling procedures which determine the composition of the group, are of paramount importance.

The group climate can inhibit or fail to stimulate an individual or it can, of course, be stimulating and lively and generate more data. Where a researcher feels certain that confrontation and conflict is likely to occur between potential group members, she or he has to be sensitive to group feelings and reconcile their ideas. Conflict can be destructive but can also generate rich data. In any conflict situation, ethical issues must be carefully considered. Sim (1998) identifies some problems with focus groups.

1. It cannot be assumed that there is conformity and consensus between the individual members of the group, although it may seem so.
2. Although some inferences may be drawn about the absence or presence of certain perspectives or feelings, the strength of the individual's emotions cannot be measured or assumed.
3. Focus group findings based on empirical data cannot be generalised, though theoretical generalisation is feasible as in other qualitative research.

In research with nurses and other health professionals, it is always difficult to establish focus groups because of the differences in time when they can be available or in the lack of a suitable location which has to be large enough to accommodate more than just two people. This is easier in the community than in hospitals.

Transcription can be much more difficult than in one-to-one interviews because peoples' voices vary, and the distance they sit from the microphone influences the clarity of individuals' contributions. As there are certain dangers of group effect and group member control, it is useful to analyse the interviews both at group level and at the level of the individual participants. The researcher must remember that the data must be seen within the context of the group setting (Carey and Smith, 1994). Fieldnotes should be made immediately after the session.

Critical comments on focus group interviews in healthcare

There is some criticism about the use of focus groups in nursing and healthcare. We would suggest that sometimes these interviews are used because researchers feel this is an easy and popular way of gaining access to a larger sample, and funding agencies seem to like it. The complexities of setting up and facilitating focus groups are often forgotten. In a search through the Cumulative Index of Nursing and Allied Health Literature (CINAHL), Webb and Kevern (2001) found rather unsophisticated and uncritical uses of focus group research in the years 1990–1999. Few articles contained empirical research, and furthermore, some of the discussions were superficial and non analytical. The writers suggest that researchers discuss the theoretical and methodological assumptions in their work and become more rigorous in their use of methodology. Webb and Kevern claim that the input from other disciplines, the social sciences in particular, would enhance and develop nursing knowledge.

Summary

- A focus group consists of a small number of people with common experiences or areas of interest.
- Several focus groups with a small number of individuals are involved in each study.
- Whilst the interviews are carefully planned, the interviewer must at the same time be flexible and non-judgemental.
- The dynamic of the group situation is intended to stimulate ideas and elicit feelings about the focus of the study.
- It is important that an open climate exists so that group members feel comfortable about sharing their thoughts and feelings.
- The data can be analysed by any qualitative analysis method as long as researchers have adhered to the principles of the particular approach.
- Not all qualitative approaches are compatible with focus group interviews.

References

Asbury, J. (1995) Overview of focus group research. *Qualitative Health Research*, 5 (4), 414–20.

Cane, R., Pao, C. & McKenzie, S. (2001) Understanding childhood asthma in focus groups: perspectives from mothers of different ethnic backgrounds. *BMC Family Practice*. http://www.biomedcentral.com/1471–2296/2/4

Carey, M.A. & Smith, M.W. (1994) Capturing the group effect in focus groups. *Qualitative Health Research*, 4 (1), 123–7.

Freeman, T. (2006) Best practice in focus group research: making sense of different views. *Journal of Advanced Nursing*, 56 (5), 491–7.

Greenbaum, T.L. (1998) *The Handbook for Focus Group Research*, 2nd edn. Lexington, MA, Lexington Books/DC Heath and Co.

Kingston, M.J., Evans, S.M., Smith, B.J. & Berry, J.G. (2004) Attitudes of doctors and nurses towards incident reporting: a qualitative analysis. *The Medical Journal of Australia*, 181 (1), 36–9.

Kitzinger, J. (2005) Focus group research: using group dynamics to explore perceptions, experiences and understandings. In *Qualitative Research in Health Care* (ed. I. Holloway), pp. 56–70. Maidenhead, Open University Press.

Kitzinger, J. & Barbour, R.S. (eds) (1999) Introduction: the challenge and promise of focus groups. *Developing Focus Groups Research: Politics, Theory and Practice*, pp. 1–20. London, Sage.

Merton, R.K. & Kendall, P.L. (1946) The focused interview. *American Journal of Sociology*, **51**, 541–57.

Merton, R.K. & King, R. (1990) *The Focused Interview: A Manual of Problems and Procedures*. New York, NY, Free Press.

Merton, R.K., Fiske, M. & Kendall, P.L. (1956) *The Focused Interview*. New York, NY, Columbia University Press.

Morgan, D.L. (1997) *Focus Groups as Qualitative Research*. Thousand Oaks, CA, Sage.

Morgan, D.L. (1998a) *The Focus Group Guidebook* (*The Focus Group Kit*), Vol. 1 (eds D.L. Morgan & R.A. Krueger). Thousand Oaks, CA, Sage.

Morgan, D.L. (1998b) *Planning Focus Groups* (*The Focus Group Kit*), Vol. 2 (eds D.L. Morgan & R.A. Krueger). Thousand Oaks, CA, Sage.

Norton, E. (2008) *An Exploration of Adolescent Sun–Related Behaviour: Comfort Matters*, Unpublished PhD thesis, Bournemouth University.

Pearcey, P.A. & Elliott, B.F. (2004) Student impressions of clinical nursing. *Nurse Education Today*, **24** (5), 382–7.

Sim, J. (1998) Collecting and analysing qualitative data: issues raised by focus groups. *Journal of Advanced Nursing*, **28** (2), 345–52.

Stewart, D.W. & Shamdasani, P.N. (2007) *Focus Groups: Theory and Practice*, 2nd edn. Thousand Oaks, CA, Sage.

Streubert Speziale, H.J. & Rinaldi Carpenter, D.R. (2007) *Qualitative Research in Nursing: Advancing the Humanistic Imperative*, 4th edn. Philadelphia, PA, Lippincott, Williams & Wilkins.

Webb, C. & Kevern, J. (2001) Focus groups as a research method: a critique of some aspects of their use in nursing research. *Journal of Advanced Nursing*, **33** (6), 798–805.

Further reading

Barbour, R. (2008) *Doing Focus Groups*. London, Sage.

Hennink, M.M. (2007) *International Focus Group Research: A Handbook for the Health and Social Sciences*. Cambridge, Cambridge University Press.

CHAPTER 9

Sampling and Site Selection

Sampling is the purposeful selection of an element of the whole population to gain knowledge and information. The question is: *whom* do the researchers choose and *how* do they choose (of course there is also other sampling such as time, location, etc. which is not discussed fully here). In qualitative inquiry it differs in several significant ways from the sampling strategies which quantitative researchers carry out; probability sampling, for instance, is inappropriate in qualitative research. Sampling is an important part of the research procedures and has to be suitable for the specific research topic and question. As in other forms of inquiry, researchers distinguish between the target population, the study population and the sampling frame (Procter and Allan, 2006). The accessible population that has the particular experience or knowledge of the phenomenon which the researcher is seeking to explore is the target population. The study population consists of the individuals to whom the researcher can gain access and who have the appropriate knowledge and experience, while the sampling frame is the population from which the sample is chosen. The terms mentioned above however are not often discussed in qualitative research though they hold for any type of research.

The researchers do not only describe the sampling strategies and justify the selection of the sample but also explain how they gained access to the participants in the research. Sampling is a complex process which is informed by the research question and theoretical considerations, and it is guided by the phenomenon of interest to the researcher.

Purposeful (or purposive) sampling

The sampling strategies of the qualitative researcher are guided by principles of ethics and the opportunity of gaining access to people whom they can observe and interview in-depth, and from whom they can obtain rich data. The selection of participants (settings, or units of time) is criterion-based, that is, certain criteria are applied, and the sample is chosen accordingly. Sampling units are selected for a specific purpose on which the researcher decides, therefore the term 'purposive' or 'purposeful' sampling is used. For instance, the researcher chooses a sample on the basis of group membership, on the basis of the experiences that participants have had or the type of treatment and care that they were given.

The group is specified in advance. Some researchers use the term 'criterion-based' sampling (Schensul *et al.*, 1999; Endacott and Botti, 2004), because most sampling strategies, even random or theoretical sampling, are highly purposive. However, *purposeful* or purposive is the term used by most qualitative researchers, and it is based on the judgement of the researcher. Purposeful sampling can also include the site or setting of the research.

At the start of the research, researchers must ask two questions: *what* to sample and *how* to sample. People generally form the main sampling units. The appropriate informant is chosen by the researcher or may be self-selected. Sometimes researchers can easily identify individuals or groups with special knowledge of a topic, occasionally they advertise or ask for informants who have insight into a particular situation or are experts in an area of knowledge. These voluntary participants selected for the research are often those that are most articulate because the researchers find it easier to communicate with them and elicit rich data, but this might lead to a neglect of certain individuals that are powerless or inarticulate and who should be included; indeed they might be very important as their voices are often marginalised.

Individuals are sampled for the information they can provide about a specific phenomenon, be it a condition, such as an illness, a treatment (for instance a particular medicine, manipulation, counselling), a type of care, professional decision-making, etc. They could be nurses who have cared for people under-going treatment, patients who have had day surgery or midwifery students who are interviewed about their clinical experience and so on. Identification of a particular population provides boundaries between those who are included in the study and those who stay outside it (inclusion and exclusion criteria). The members of the sample share certain characteristics. The sample is thus chosen on the basis of personal knowledge of the person selected about the phenomenon under study.

Useful informants would be people who have had experiences about which the researcher wants to gain information. For example, individuals who have diabetes might share experiences and the meanings that these have for them with the health researcher.

Informants with special knowledge or experience might consist of newcomers, people who are changing status, or those who have been in the setting for a long time. Individuals who are willing to talk about their experience and perceptions are often those persons who have a special approach to their work. Some have power or status; others are naïve, frustrated, hostile or attention seeking, although researchers must remember that the latter are not always the best informants because they may have a mainly negative perception of the organisation or institution under discussion – 'an axe to grind'. Ethically it is important that the persons in the sample are not jeopardised by 'confessing' to their practices (unless illegal) and uncovering their thoughts.

As in all research, the researcher needs to clarify the rationale for inclusion and exclusion of particular people or other sampling units.

Example of purposive sampling

Bisson *et al.* (2009) give an account of their qualitative research which aimed to gain the view of a variety of sufferers of Huntington's disease on decision-making on which they develop a care pathway for future decisions and powers of attorney. They used purposive sampling in order to gain a range of perspectives from various individuals such as sufferers, people with the gene, carers and clinicians in the field. They also included a lawyer, medical ethicists and advisors from the Huntington's Disease Association. This sample was chosen to gain a full range of perspectives from individuals. Theoretical sampling was also used to collect the views of both males and females, old and young participants.

Sampling types

There are various forms of sampling. We shall discuss only the most often used and important types. An overview of a whole range can be found in Patton (2002) and Kuzel (1999), although many sampling types overlap. The commonest methods are as follows:

- Homogeneous sampling
- Heterogeneous sampling
- Total population sampling
- Chain referral sampling (snowball sampling)
- Convenience or opportunistic sampling
- Maximum variation sampling
- Theoretical sampling

Homogeneous sampling

This involves individuals who belong to the same subculture or have similar characteristics. Nurses often use homogeneous sample units when they wish to observe or interview a particular group, for instance specialist nurses. Midwives may wish to examine the perspectives of community midwives on their role in the community. In these examples, a homogeneous group is being studied. The sample can be homogeneous with respect to a certain variable only – for instance, specific occupation, length of experience, type of experience, age or gender. The important variable would be established before the sampling starts.

Example of homogeneous sampling

Examples of homogeneous sampling would consist, for instance, of a group of adolescent schoolgirls between the ages of 13 and 15 who are being interviewed about a topic that is of importance to them, or a number of orthopaedic surgeons who have used a Taylor Spatial Frame. For the purpose of the specific studies, they would be homogeneous samples.

Heterogeneous sampling

A heterogeneous sample contains individuals or groups of individuals who differ from each other in a major aspect. For instance, nurses may wish to explore the perceptions of nurses, social workers and doctors who care for patients with HIV. The three groups form a heterogeneous sample. Heterogeneous sampling is also called maximum variation sampling (Patton, 2002) because it involves a search for individuals with widely differing experiences and for variations in settings.

Example for heterogeneous sampling

Researchers might wish to explore the perspective of people with a chronic illness and the ways they choose strategies for managing their condition. The heterogeneous sample might comprise males and females across a broad range of ages with different jobs and from a variety of different backgrounds. This sample would be chosen to maximise contrasts between the participants.

The sample might consist of people from a naturally occurring population – such as members of a local carers' group, a specific ward, a community of patients. Some sampling is based on early findings with a group and cannot be determined prior to the study. For instance, a midwife could sample women who have just given birth to their first child and find that it would be interesting to select older and younger primiparae because they might have different ideas about childbirth. Sometimes married couples are chosen as samples or people who live together. Occasionally the sample consists of focus groups, for instance self-help groups, or groups with similar conditions or experiences.

Total population sampling

A sample is called a total population sample when all participants selected come from a particular group; it is used infrequently in qualitative research. For instance, all the nurses with specific knowledge or a skill, such as those with training and experience in counselling, might be interviewed because the researcher focuses on this skill, and there might be few available with the particular expertise. There are some diseases where those who suffer from them are very small in number, and the researcher might interview all of these. All midwives in one midwifery unit might be observed, because the specific setting in which they work or the special techniques they adopt are seen as important. Not many qualitative studies carry out total population sampling.

Chain referral or snowball sampling

A variation of purposive sampling is chain referral or *snowball* sampling (the former is a term originally coined by Biernacki and Waldorf (1981)). A previously chosen informant is asked to identify other potential participants with knowledge of a particular area or topic, and these in turn nominate other individuals for the research. Researchers use snowball sampling in studies where they cannot identify useful informants, where informants are not easily accessible or where anonymity is desirable, for instance in studies about drug addiction or alcohol use. Penrod *et al.* (2003) suggest that chain referral sampling is useful in situations where people are vulnerable and when they are not easily accessible: this might include groups who are labelled negatively by society (for instance, those that suffer from sexually transmitted diseases), those with whom researchers discuss sensitive topics (such as sexual behaviour) or those individuals who fear being exposed or criminalised (i.e. substance users).

> ### Example of chain referral sampling
>
> A sample of Lesbian couples were interviewed by Spidsberg (2007) about maternity care. After initial recruitment through sending leaflets, snowballing took place through recruitment by women already interviewed through word of mouth information to friends who then volunteered to be interviewed

Convenience or opportunistic sampling

The terms *convenience* or *opportunistic* sampling are self-explanatory. The researcher uses opportunities to ask people who might be useful for the study and easy to access. To some extent, of course, most sampling is opportunistic and arranged for the convenience of the researcher. Researchers usually adopt this sampling strategy when recruiting people is difficult, though this is not the best way of sampling.

The researcher chooses individuals whose ideas or experiences will help achieve the aim of the research; occasionally variations in the sample have no specific influence on the phenomenon to be explored, and in this case a convenience sample can be selected.

> ## Example of convenience sampling
>
> Rodham *et al.* (2006) studied risk behaviours in adolescence. As a convenience sample for easy accessibility in their locality, they selected four schools from in the Bath area and asked for volunteers over 16 of the school population to participate in the study.
>
> Another convenience sample might consist of all midwives who work in a particular hospital because the researcher has easy access to them and they fit other criteria specified for the research.

Maximum variation sampling

Maximum variation sampling entails selecting a purposive sample of a wide variety of people and/or settings of interest to the researcher. It may include, for instance both genders, young and old, different nationalities, etc. The researcher intends to access a broad range of perspectives from many different people. This means that the sample will have to be relatively large. This type of sampling is not often used in qualitative research which is generally more specific.

Theoretical sampling

Glaser and Strauss (1967) advocate *theoretical sampling* in the process of collecting data. Theoretical sampling develops as the study proceeds, and it cannot be planned beforehand. Researchers select their sample on the basis of concepts and theoretical issues that arise during the research. The theoretical ideas control the collection of data; therefore researchers have to justify the inclusion of particular sampling units. At the point of data saturation, when no new ideas arise that are of value to the developing theory, sampling can stop. Coyne (1997) discusses qualitative sampling in depth and differentiates between purposive and theoretical sampling (Chapter 11), although she believes that theoretical sampling could be called 'analysis driven purposeful sampling'. Sandelowski (1995) also maintains that all sampling in qualitative research is purposeful; it is intended to achieve a specific aim. She claims that theoretical sampling is merely a variation of purposive sampling.

Other types of sample selection

Other methods of purposeful or criterion-based sampling sometimes overlap with those above and can be examples of purposive sampling (for a variety of these, see Schensul *et al.*, 1999: 236):

- Extreme case selection
- Typical case selection

- Unique case selection
- Deviant case selection

In *extreme case selection*, the researcher identifies certain characteristics for the setting or population. Extremes of these characteristics are sought and arranged on a continuum. The cases that belong at the two ends of this continuum become the extreme cases. For instance, nurses may study a very large or a very small ward. These can be compared with cases that are the norm for the hospital population.

In *typical case selection*, researchers create a profile of characteristics for an average case and find instances of this. They might exclude the very young or old, the almost healthy and the most vulnerable or any other participants at the end of a continuum. They would be those that are typical or normal for the investigation of a particular phenomenon.

When choosing *unique cases*, researchers study those that differ from others by a single characteristic or dimension such as people who share a particular condition but come from an unusual community, such as a sect or ethnic group. This type of sample consists of the uncommon and unique cases which are not normal or typical.

Deviant case selection is similar to the above and to extreme case selection. However, only those people are included who think in a very different way from other people whose ideas have been researched before, or those who have a different experience from others although they have had the same condition, treatment or care.

There are other terms for and types of sampling but the preceding are the most common. Kuzel (1999) lists five important elements of sampling which may occur in qualitative research:

1. Flexible sampling which develops during the study
2. Sequential selection of sampling units
3. Sampling guided by theoretical development which becomes progressively more focused
4. Continuing sampling until no new relevant data arise (sampling to saturation)
5. Searching for negative or deviant cases

Sampling decisions

Early in a research project, and depending on the research question and focus, researchers have to make their sampling decisions. Qualitative approaches demand different sampling techniques from the randomly selected and probabilistic sampling used by quantitative researchers. It is, however, just as important for qualitative researchers to make their sampling decisions on a systematic basis and on rational grounds. A sample in qualitative research consists of sampling units of people, time or setting. Nurse and midwife researchers have to select the individuals or group members (*whom* to sample), the time and context (*what* to sample) and the place (*where* to sample), because they cannot investigate everything. It must be remembered that the people and places must be available and accessible.

The sampling strategies adopted can make a difference to the whole study. The rules of qualitative sampling are less rigid than those of quantitative methods but the sampling needs to be criterion-based. Sampling need be both appropriate and adequate (Morse and Field, 1996). Appropriateness means that the method of sampling fits the aim of the study and helps the understanding of the research problem. A sampling strategy is adequate if it generates adequate and relevant information and sufficient quality data.

Sampling takes place after the research focus has been decided. Although qualitative researchers start selecting participants at this stage, they can continue the selection throughout the process if more are needed because of the changing focus or extension of ideas as the study progresses, especially in grounded theory and ethnography. In some cases it is not necessary to specify the overall sample and give an exact number of informants from the beginning of the study, although an initial sample should be stated. This sampling strategy differs from quantitative research where respondents are chosen before the project begins. A qualitative proposal could state, for instance, that the initial sample should consist of *x* (number of) informants. Grounded theory and ethnography favour this type of sampling while phenomenologists choose a sample without adding to it at a later stage. Ethics committees do not always accommodate the idea of theoretical sampling and wish to know the exact number and clear description of the sample.

Inclusion and exclusion criteria

When describing their sampling strategies, researchers describe inclusion and exclusion criteria. Inclusion criteria state what particular people are included in the research, while participants that are excluded – though meeting some of the inclusion criteria – might be too vulnerable to be interviewed or have certain traits that might make the research problematic. For instance, in Britain or the US, people who do not understand the English language might have to be excluded for practical or access reasons (although, of course, they might be the target population in other studies). Undergraduates are advised to exclude from their sample vulnerable people or those with mental health problems. In a study of the birth process, women with normal birth experience might be included while those with Caesareans or those with still-born babies might be excluded for ethical reasons. The exclusion and inclusion criteria depend, of course, on the aim of the particular study. One of the most important inclusion criteria is voluntary participation.

Sampling parameters

The investigators do not only decide on the participants in their study but also on the time and location of the research. The criteria for selecting must be clearly identified.

Woods (2006) suggests that sometimes 'naturalistic' sampling is appropriate, and the sample might consist of people, context and time. In an ethnographic study for instance, a particular subculture might be researched in different settings and situations. The people in the study are chosen for their experience and knowledge of the phenomenon under study. A particular phenomenon might be researched in a range of contexts in which it occurs. Different times of the day, year or stages in the process of care might also be a significant factor in the research.

The criteria for site selection, location and size also depend on the aim of the research. The setting can be small or large depending on the type of study; for instance it might be a ward, a general practice, the community or a hospital. For a multi-centre study it might be particular types of hospital or a number of clinics. The research might also take place during a particular important or critical time of the day.

> **Example 1:** *Setting and site*
> A nurse researcher has decided to examine the role of the critical care nurse. She chooses three different hospitals in the South of England as the setting for her study.

> **Example 2:** *Time*
> A district nurse might find that her patients are more anxious at particular times of the morning. She might then focus on a specific time in the afternoon to see whether patients behave in a similar way at that time.

Sample size

The sample may be small or large, depending on the type of research question, material and time resources as well as on the number of researchers. Generally qualitative sampling consists of small sampling units studied in depth. Sample size differs greatly in qualitative studies; a large sample is rarely necessary in qualitative research. However, researchers must be warned that some funding agencies and even some members of ethics committees do not have the appropriate knowledge of sampling and often reject the small sample that qualitative research entails.

Although there are no rigid rules; six to eight data units are seen as sufficient when the sample consists of a homogeneous group while between 14 and 20 might be needed for a heterogeneous sample. Most often, the sample consists of between 4 and 40 informants, though certain research projects contain as many as 200 participants and as few as 2. Qualitative studies that include a large sample do exist but are rare. Sample size, however, does not necessarily determine the importance of the study or the quality of the data.

Example of sampling size

Billhult *et al.* (2007) for instance, interviewed ten participants, while Kutash and Northrop (2007) only included six.

Aveyard and Woolliams (2006) describe their sample clearly: they had a larger sample of 30 registered nurses with at least one year experience from general medical wards in two teaching hospitals.

In an early qualitative study, Strong (1979) included as many as 1120 paediatric consultations, but the choice of a large sample is not only unusual, in many cases it might also be inappropriate. In this case however, it involved observations and the sample can be justified as it is based on observations in which immersion is necessary, rather than on interviews. Another large sample was selected by Benner (1984) in her study which included 109 participants.

A sample of just one participant was chosen by Todres *et al.* (2005). The research arose from a collaboration between a carer for a partner with Alzheimer's, and two researchers who wished to gain insight into the experience of caring.

There is rarely justification for a very large sample in qualitative research. Students or experienced researchers often choose these to appease funding bodies, which are used to large samples, or research committees which do not always know details of qualitative research. Often, qualitative researchers select larger samples because they are trained in quantitative research where generalisation is demanded, or because they are anxious that an external examiner might query the sample size. A large sample, however, is unnecessary and might result in less depth and richness as the researcher's intention is usually to research a specific setting and has a purposive sample. An overlarge sample might not capture the meanings participants ascribe to their experience, and it could result in the loss of the unique and specific. Even a sample of one can be meaningful (Todres *et al.*, 2005)

Saturation

Saturation indicates that everything of importance to the agenda of a research project will emerge in the data and concepts obtained; Lincoln and Guba (1985) call this 'informational redundancy'. *Data saturation* means sampling to redundancy. *Theoretical saturation* denotes that no new concepts or dimensions for categories can be identified which are important for the study. It does not mean that nothing new can be found at all. Indeed, Morse (1995) specifically states that frequency, quantity and repetition of ideas in the data do not signify saturation or data adequacy. Unfortunately, no specific rules or guidelines exist pertaining to saturation, so researchers have to decide for themselves when this has happened.

Many approaches aim for data or theoretical saturation but fail to achieve it. Bowen (2008) also deplores that researchers often state that saturation has been achieved but do not clarify what it means in the context of their own specific study. Often there are time constraints and other barriers to sample saturation; hence it is not always appropriate to confirm saturation.

Morse (1995) maintains that careful choice of sampling, and the cohesiveness of the sample can help in achieving saturation.

How shall we name them?

It is difficult for researchers to know what term to use for the people they interview and observe, especially as this name makes explicit the stance of the researchers and their relationship to those being studied. We favour the terms 'participant' or 'informant'. In surveys, both by structured interviews and written questionnaires, the most frequent term has been 'respondents', and indeed, many qualitative researchers and research texts still use it, but it seems less frequent now in qualitative research texts and reports.

Morse (1991) developed a debate about terms almost two decades ago, and her thoughts on sampling are still valid. She claims that 'respondent' implies a passive response to a stimulus – the researcher's question. It sounds mechanistic. Medical and business researchers still use this term often in qualitative research. Bio-medical researchers refer to 'subjects', again a word that expresses passivity of the people involved in a study. Interestingly it is used in legal documents and sometimes in ethical guidelines (see Chapter 4). West and Butler (2003) quote Margaret Mead who, decades ago, criticised the word 'subject' and maintains that research *with* informants would yield better data. In qualitative research it would be inappropriate. 'Interviewee' sounds clumsy and boring. The American Psychological Association now also uses the term 'participants' when discussing human beings involved in research (APA, 2003).

Anthropologists refer to 'informants', those members of a culture or group who voluntarily 'inform' the researcher about their world and play an active part in the research. Morse (1995) usually chooses this term, though she acknowledges the suggestion by some journal editors that it might be seen to have links to the word 'informant' as used by the police. Most ethnographers, however, still use the term and do not perceive it as negative. Generally, qualitative researchers prefer the term 'participant'; this expresses the collaboration between the researcher and the researched (DePoy and Gitlin, 2005) and the equality of their relationship, but the term could be misleading as the researcher, too, is a participant in the research. Van den Hoonaard (2008) debates the term 'human subject', its alternatives and ethical implications in his article; he too prefers the term 'participant' or 'informant' to the word 'subject' as it is more appropriate for social and interactive individuals although bio-medical researchers still talk of 'human subjects'.

In the end, however, the nurses or midwives must choose for themselves which term suits their research. In Morse's words: 'Subjects, respondents, informants, participants – choose your own term, but choose a term that fits' (1991: 406). We suggest that students use the terms 'participant' or informant in ethnographic studies, but never the word 'subject'.

Summary

The following are the important features of qualitative sampling:

- Sampling is usually purposeful and criterion-based, chosen specifically for the study.
- The sample of individuals in qualitative research is generally small.
- Sampling units can consist of people, time, setting, processes or concepts (the latter is called theoretical sampling).
- Sampling is not always wholly determined prior to the study but may proceed throughout (for instance in grounded theory).
- The individuals in the sample are usually called *participants* or *informants* (in qualitative research they should never be called subjects).

References

American Psychological Association (2003) *Code of Ethics 2002 (publ. 2003).* http://www.apa.org/ethics/homepage.html

Aveyard, H. & Woolliams, M. (2006) In their best interests? Nurses' experiences of the administration of sedation in general medical wards in England: an application of the critical incident technique. *International Journal of Nursing Studies*, **43** (8), 929–39.

Benner, P. (1984) *From Novice to Expert.* Menlo Park, CA, Addison-Wesley Publishing.

Biernacki, P. & Waldorf, D. (1981) Snowball sampling: problems and techniques of chain referral sampling. *Sociological Methods and Research*, **10** (2), 141–63.

Billhult, A., Stener-Victorin, E. & Bergbom, I. (2007) The experience of massage during chemotherapy treatment in breast cancer. *Clinical Nursing Research*, **16** (2), 85–99.

Bisson, J., Hampton, V., Rosser, A. & Holm, S. (2009) Developing a care pathway for advance decisions and powers of attorney: a qualitative study. *The British Journal of Psychiatry*, **194** (1), 55–62.

Bowen, G.A. (2008) Naturalistic inquiry and the saturation concept: a research note. *Qualitative Research*, **8** (1), 137–52.

Coyne, I.T. (1997) Sampling in qualitative research: purposeful and theoretical sampling: merging or clear boundaries? *Journal of Advanced Nursing*, **26**, 623–30.

DePoy, E. & Gitlin, L.N. (2005) *Introduction to Research: Multiple Strategies for Health and Human Services*. St. Louis, MO, CV Mosby.

Endacott, R. & Botti, M. (2004) Clinical research 3: sample selection. *Intensive and Critical Care Nursing*, **21** (1), 51–5.

Glaser, B. & Strauss, A. (1967) *The Discovery of Grounded Theory*. Chicago, IL, Aldine.

Kutash, M. & Northrop, L. (2007) Family members' experience of the intensive care waiting room. *Journal of Advanced Nursing*, **60** (4), 384–8.

Kuzel, A.J. (1999) Sampling in qualitative inquiry. In *Doing Qualitative Research* (eds B.F. Crabtree & W.L. Miller), 2nd edn, pp. 33–45. Thousand Oaks, CA, Sage.

Lincoln, Y.S. & Guba, E.G. (1985). *Naturalistic Inquiry*. Beverly Hills, CA, Sage.

Morse, J.M. (1991) Subjects, respondents, informants and participants [Editorial]. *Qualitative Health Research*, **1**, 403–6.

Morse, J.M. (1995) The significance of saturation [Editorial]. *Qualitative Health Research*, **5** (2), 147–9.

Morse, J.M. & Field, P.A. (1996) *Nursing Research: The Application of Qualitative Approaches*. Basingstoke, Macmillan.

Patton, M. (2002) *Qualitative Evaluation and Research Methods*, 3rd edn. Thousand Oaks, CA, Sage.

Penrod, J., Preston, D.B., Cain, R.E. & Starks, M.T. (2003) The discussion of chain referral as a method of sampling hard-to-reach populations. *Journal of Transcultural Nursing*, **14** (2), 100–7.

Procter, S. & Allan, T. (2006) Sampling. In *The Research Process in Nursing* (eds K. Gerrish & A. Lacey), 5th edn, pp. 173–88. Oxford, Blackwell.

Rodham, K., Brewer, H., Mistral, W. & Stallard, P. (2006) Adolescents' perceptions of risk and challenge. *Journal of Adolescence*, **29** (2), 261–72.

Sandelowski, M. (1995) Focus on qualitative methods: sample size in qualitative research. *Research in Nursing and Health*, **18**, 179–83.

Schensul, S.L., Schensul, J.J. & LeCompte, M.D. (1999) *Essential Ethnographic Methods 2: Observations, Interviews and Questionnaires*. Walnut Creek, CA, Altamira Press.

Spidsberg, D. (2007) Vulnerable and strong – lesbian women encountering maternity care. *Journal of Advanced Nursing*, **60** (5), 478–86.

Strong, P.M. (1979) *The Ceremonial Order: Parents, Doctors and Medical Bureaucracies*. London, Routledge & Kegan Paul.

Todres, L., Galvin, K. & Richardson, M. (2005) The intimate mediator: a carer's experience of Alzheimer's disease. *Journal of Clinical Nursing*, **12** (3), 422–30.

Van den Hoonaard, W.C. (2008) Re-imagining the subject: conceptual and ethical considerations on the participant in qualitative research. *Ciência and Saúde Coletiva*, **13**(2), 371–9. Retrieved January 2009, http://www.scielosp.org/scielo.php?script=sci_arttext&pid=S1413-81232008000200012

West, E. & Butler, J. (2003) An applied and qualitative LREC reflects on its practice. *Bulletin of Medical Ethics*, **185**, 13–20.

Woods, P. (2006) *Qualitative Research*. On website of University of Plymouth, http://www.edu.plymouth.ac.uk/resined/Qualitative%20methods%202/qualrshm.htm, accessed January 2008.

PART THREE

Approaches to Qualitative Research

CHAPTER 10

Ethnography

Ethnography is the direct description of a group, culture or community. Nevertheless, the meaning of the word ethnography can be ambiguous; it is an overall term for a number of approaches. Sometimes researchers use it as synonymous with qualitative research in general (for instance, Brewer, 2000), while at other times its meaning is more specific. In this chapter, we adopt the original meaning of the term, as a method within the social anthropological tradition. Ethnography can be qualitative and quantitative though ethnographers in the healthcare field adopt mostly qualitative procedures.

As the oldest of the qualitative methods, it has been used since ancient times; for instance, in the descriptions of Greeks and Romans who wrote about the cultures they encountered in their travels and wars. Deriving from the Greek, the term ethnography means a description of the people – 'writing of culture'. Ethnographers focus on cultural members, phenomena and problems in the context of culture and subcultures. Ethnographic data collection takes place mainly through observation, interviews and examination of documents (see Chapters 6 and 7).

Researchers stress the importance of studying human behaviour in the context of a culture in order to gain understanding of cultural rules, norms and routines. Ethnography does, however, refer both to a process – the methods and strategies of research – and to a product – the written story as the outcome of the research. People 'do' ethnography: they study a culture, observe its members' behaviours and listen to them. They also produce *an ethnography*, a written text (or, unusually, a performed piece of work) which is the ethnographic account; thus ethnography is both 'process' and 'product'.

The historical perspective

Modern ethnography has its roots in social anthropology and emerged in the 1920s and 1930s when famous anthropologists such as Malinowski (1922), Boas (1928) and Mead (1935), while searching for cultural patterns and rules, explored a variety of non-Western cultures and the life ways of the people within them. After the First and Second World Wars, when tribal groups in the traditional sense were disappearing, researchers wished to preserve aspects of vanishing cultures by living with them and writing about them.

In the beginning these anthropologists explored only 'primitive' cultures (a term that demonstrates the patronising stance of many early anthropologists). When cultures became more linked with each other and Western anthropologists could not find homogeneous isolated cultures abroad, they turned to research their own cultures, acting as 'cultural strangers', that is, trying to see them from outside; everything is looked at with the eyes of an outsider. Sociologists too, adopted ethnographic methods, immersing themselves in the culture or subculture in which they took an interest. Experienced ethnographers and sociologists, who research their own society, take a new perspective on that which is familiar. This approach to a culture known to them helps ethnographers not to take assumptions about their own society or cultural group for granted.

The Chicago School of Sociology, too, had an influence on later ethnographic methods because its members examined marginal cultural and 'socially strange' subcultures such as the slums, ghettos and gangs of the city. A good example is the study by Whyte (1943) who investigated the urban gang subculture in an American city. *Street Corner Society* became a classic, and other sociologists used this work as a model for their own writing. In some form, ethnography as a method is around a century old (Gobo, 2008) but its origins are much older.

A focus on culture

Anthropology is concerned with culture, and ethnography differs from other approaches by this emphasis. Culture can be defined as the way of life of a group – the learnt behaviour that is socially constructed and transmitted. The life experiences of members of a cultural group include a shared communication system. This consists of signs such as gestures, mime and language as well as cultural artefacts – all messages that the members of a culture recognise, and whose meaning they understand. Individuals in a culture or subculture hold values and ideas acquired through learning from other members of the group. The researchers' responsibility is to describe the patterns of beliefs and behaviour and the unique processes in the subculture or culture they study. It must be stressed, however, that the values and beliefs of cultural members depend on their location in the culture or subculture in which they live, on their gender, age or ethnic group. Indeed, sometimes conflicting value systems may exist.

Social anthropologists aim to observe and study the modes of life in a culture. This they do through the method of ethnography. They analyse, compare and examine groups and their rules of behaviour. The relationship of individuals to the group and to each other is also explored. The study of change, in particular, helps ethnographers understand cultures and subcultures. In areas where two cultures meet, they might focus on the conflict between groups if this is seen as important, for instance, in studies of interaction with doctors and other health professionals.

Applying ethnographic methods – especially observation – helps health professionals to contextualise the behaviour, beliefs and feelings of their clients or colleagues. Through ethnography, nurses and midwives become culturally sensitive and can identify the cultural influences on the individuals and groups they study. The goals of ethnographers in the health arena, however, differ from those of researchers in a subject discipline such as anthropology or sociology. Much ethnography in education, for instance, was intended to improve practice. Health professionals too, see the production of knowledge only as a first step; on the basis of this, they seek to improve their clinical practice.

Sometimes health researchers examine subcultures and situations with which they are familiar.

Examples

A nurse and a doctor in the accident and emergency department (A&E) might wish to study the culture of the A&E setting in the local hospital. They will closely observe the events, critical incidents and behaviour of patients and professionals in this setting in order to improve the system.

A midwife explores the work of the local midwifery unit. She observes the situation and asks her colleagues about the routine actions they perform. She also finds that some of the clients have problems with the way in which they are cared for and asks them about their feelings and perceptions.

Ethnographic methods

Researchers distinguish between several types of ethnography, some of which overlap. The main ways of using this approach is through the following:

- Descriptive or conventional ethnography
- Critical ethnography
- Autoethnography

Descriptive or conventional ethnography focuses on the description of cultures or groups and, through analysis, uncovers patterns, typologies and categories. This is used in most ethnographic studies.

Critical ethnography has its basis in critical theory and, as discussed by Thomas (1993), Carspecken (1996) and Madison (2005), it involves the study of macro-social factors such as power and examines common-sense assumptions and hidden agendas and is therefore more political. Thomas (p: 4) states the difference: 'Conventional ethnographers study culture for the purpose of describing it; critical ethnographers do so to change it'. Critical ethnography can be important for health researchers, particularly nurses, physiotherapists and midwives, because they are concerned with the empowerment of people. Indeed, Hardcastle *et al.* (2006) suggest that critical ethnography is used in healthcare research to address this issue of power in particular to emancipate the research participants. Using Carspecken's approach, the researchers studied renal nurses' decision-making and describe it.

Example of critical ethnography

The article by Blackstone (2009) explored the social construction of compassion by using critical ethnographic research in two areas, breast cancer and anti-rape movements. These studies focus on the participants' perceptions of 'doing good' and 'being good'. The researcher participated in and observed two sites in the Midwestern States of the United States, where she 'hung out' (her own words) for several years ('immersion in the setting'). She found that these two organisations had similarities. Fieldnotes provided a wealth of data. In this study, the findings were used to provide a framework for understanding in order to bring about change and empowering the women involved in these movements.

(For more detail see Blackstone (2009))

Autoethnography implies that researchers centre their studies on their own selves, their thoughts and feelings rather than focusing exclusively on others. Of course, any qualitative study is reflexive and takes into account the feelings and thoughts of the researcher, but in autoethnography they tell their own experiences rather than those of others. Anderson (2006) distinguishes between evocative and analytic autoethnography; the former focuses on the feelings and experiences of the researcher, the latter is more analytic than descriptive and designed to discuss social phenomena reaching beyond the researcher's own experience. The genre is often used in healthcare research (See discussion in Anderson (2006)).

Streubert Speziale and Rinaldi Carpenter (2007) cite many more specific types of ethnography, and they claim that there is no standard form. These approaches to ethnography might arise from different ideological or procedural bases, but they are similar in data collection and management.

Ethnography in healthcare

Ethnographic methods were first used in healthcare, specifically in nursing in the United States. One of the best known nursing ethnographers is Janice Morse who has written several well-known texts and is probably the best-known qualitative researcher in the nursing arena and has qualifications in anthropology. Leininger

(1985) uses the term 'ethnonursing' for the use of ethnography in nursing. She developed this as a modification and extension of ethnography. Ethnonursing deals with studies of a culture like other ethnographic methods, but it is also about nursing care and specifically generates nursing knowledge. Nurse ethnographers differ from other anthropologists in that they only live with informants in their working day and spend their private lives away from the location where the research takes place. Nurses, of course, are familiar with the language used in the setting, while early anthropologists rarely knew the language of the culture they examined from the beginning of the research, and even modern anthropologists are not always familiar with the setting, the terminology and the people they study.

Ethnography in the healthcare arena is applied research. Chambers (2000) uses this term in approaches that are linked to making decisions in the interest of clients and in the area of decision-making. In nursing and midwifery the method is used as a way of examining behaviours and perceptions in clinical settings, generally in order to improve care and clinical practice.

Example

Brown and McCormack (2006) carried out an ethnographic study to examine pain management processes for patients admitted to a colorectal unit of a hospital based on observation and pre- and post-operative interviews with patients and nurses. They found that pain management was not satisfactory in the acute surgical setting.

From their findings the researchers concluded that comprehensive pain assessment, appropriate documentation and effective communication were essential to improve pain management practice.

The ethnographic approach can also be a useful way of studying health promotion issues as it provides the social context and explores the social conditions in which participants live and by which they are influenced (Cook, 2005). In particular, critical ethnography offers an understanding of the differences and inequalities in the health of people.

Ethnographies in this field incorporate studies of healthcare processes, settings and systems. They are typified by observations of wards or investigations of patient perspectives or specific groups whose members have experienced a condition or illness. Socialisation studies are also important in the field of professional practice. They often examine the negotiation and interaction in the subculture of clinical practice or ward and classroom settings.

Schensul *et al.* (1999) give useful advice to ethnographers that might be adopted by nurse and midwife researchers too. They can take a number of steps:

- They describe a problem in the group under study.
- Through this, they understand the causes of the problem and may prevent it.

- They help the cultural members to identify and report their needs.
- They give information to affect change in clinical or professional practice.

Ethnographers do not always investigate their own cultural members. In modern Britain, health professionals care for patients from a variety of ethnic groups and need to be knowledgeable about their cultures. Culture becomes part of all aspects of healthcare because both professionals and clients are products of their group in a particular social context. Savage (2006) gives examples from the field of healthcare such as research carried out in hospice settings, studies on rules and rituals, pain and illness experience.

The main features of ethnography

The main features of ethnography are the following:

- Data collection through observation and interviews
- The use of 'thick' description
- Selection of key informants and settings
- The emic–etic dimension

Data collection through observation and interviews

Researchers collect data by standard methods, mainly through observation and interviewing, but they also rely on documents such as letters, diaries and taped oral histories of people in a particular group or connected with it.

As in other qualitative approaches, the researcher is the major research tool. Direct participant observation is the main way of collecting data from the culture under study, and observers try to become part of the culture, taking note of everything they see and hear as well as interviewing members of the culture to gain their interpretations. Huby *et al.* (2007) make the point that data can be collected both formally and informally, which is one of the advantages of being immersed in setting.

Health researchers commonly observe behaviour in clinical or educational settings. The decisions about inclusion and exclusion depend on the research topic, the emerging data and the experiences of the researchers. The participants and their actions are observed as well as the ways in which they interact with each other. Special events and crises, the site itself and the use of space and time can also be examined. Observers study the rules of a culture or subculture and the change that occurs over time in the setting. It does not suffice, however, to use the fieldnotes for description only and add a description of the interview data. The participants' accounts are transformed and translated by the researcher into more abstract and theoretical concepts as in most qualitative research reports.

Observations become starting points for in-depth interviews. The researchers may not understand what they see, and ask the members of the group or culture to explain it to them. Participants share their interpretations of events, rules and roles with the interviewer. Some of the interviews are formal and structured, but often researchers ask questions on the spur of the moment and have informal conversations with members. Often they uncover discrepancies between words and actions ('words and deeds') – what people do and what they say – a problem originally discussed by Deutscher (1970). On the other hand there may be congruence between the spoken work and behaviour. If any discrepancies exist, they must be explained and interpreted.

Ethnographers take part in the life of people; they listen to their informants' words and the interpretation of their actions. In essence, this involves a partnership between the investigator and the informants.

The use of 'thick description'

One of the major characteristics is *thick description*, a term used by the anthropologist Geertz (1973) who borrowed it from the philosopher Ryle. It is description that makes explicit the detailed patterns of cultural and social relationships and puts them in context. Ethnographic interpretation cannot be separated from time, place and events. It is based on the meaning that actions and events have for the members of a culture within the cultural context. Description and analysis have to be rooted in reality; researchers think and reflect about social events and conduct. Thick description must be theoretical and analytical in the sense that researchers concern themselves with the abstract and general patterns and traits of social life in a culture. Denzin (1989) claims that thick description aims to give readers a sense of the emotions, thoughts and perceptions that research participants experience. It deals with the meaning and interpretations of people in a culture.

Thick description can be contrasted with 'thin description', which is superficial and does not explore the underlying meanings of cultural members. Any study where thin description prevails is not a good ethnography.

Selection of key informants and settings

As in other types of qualitative research, ethnographers generally use purposive sampling that is purposive (criterion-based) and non-probabilistic. This means ethnographers adopt certain criteria to choose a specific group and setting to be studied, be it a ward, a group of specialists or patients with a specific condition. Some of researchers use samples from such subcultures as groups of recovering alcoholics and patients with myocardial infarction, or from professional education such as an investigation of mentoring. The criteria for sampling must be justified in the study and be explicit. Researchers should choose key informants carefully to make sure that they are suitable and representative of the group under study. Key actors often participate by informally talking about the cultural conduct or customs of the group. They become active collaborators in the research rather than passive respondents.

The sample is taken from a particular cultural or subcultural group. Ethnographers have to search for individuals within a culture who can give them specific detailed information about the culture. Key informants hold special and expert knowledge about the history and subculture of a group, about interaction processes in it and cultural rules, rituals and language. These key actors help the researcher to become accepted in the culture and subculture. Researchers can validate their own ideas or perceptions with those of key informants by going back to them at the end of the study and asking them to check the script and interpretation; this is called member check. (See also Chapter 18)

The bond between researcher and key informant strengthens when the two spend time with each other. Through informal conversations, researchers can learn about the customs and conduct of the group they study, because key informants have access to areas which researchers cannot reach in time and location. For instance, a midwife might wish to gain information about midwifery during the Second World War or a physiotherapist to discover the problems of working abroad, and have no access themselves to the past or the location. These researchers use informants who have this special knowledge, in these instances midwives who practised during the war or physiotherapists who have worked extensively abroad. Key informants may be other health professionals or patients. Patients are most often the cultural group being studied. They tell the nurses of their culture or subculture, and of the expectations and health beliefs that form part of it. Spradley (1979) advises ethnographers to elicit also the 'tacit' knowledge of cultural members – the concepts and assumptions that they have but of which they are unaware.

Fetterman (1998) warns against prior assumptions which key informants might have. If they are highly knowledgeable they might impose their own ideas on the study and the researcher; therefore the latter must try to compare these tales with the observed reality. There might be the additional danger that key actors might only tell what researchers wish to hear. This danger is particularly strong in the health system. Clients are aware of labelling processes and often want to please those who care for them or deal with them in a professional relationship. However, the lengthy contact of interviewer and informants and 'prolonged engagement' in the setting help to overcome this.

The emic–etic dimension

Ethnographers use the constructs of the informants and also apply their own scientific conceptual framework, the so-called *emic* and *etic* perspectives (Harris, 1976). First, the researcher needs an understanding of the emic perspective, the insider's or native's perceptions. Insiders' accounts of reality help to uncover knowledge of the reasons why people act as they do. A researcher who uses the emic perspective gives explanations of events from the cultural member's point of view. This perspective is essential in a study, particularly in the beginning, as it prevents the imposition of the values and beliefs of researchers from their own culture to that of another. The outsider's perspective, the etic view, has been prevalent for too long in health care and health research. Outsiders, such as health professionals or professional researchers, used to identify the problems of patients and described them rather than listening to the member's own ideas. Now, those who experience an illness are allowed to speak for themselves as they are 'experts' not only on their condition but also on their own feelings and perceptions; as Harris (1976: 36) states, 'The way to get inside of people's heads is to talk with them, to ask questions about what they think and feel'.

The emic perspective corresponds to the reality and definition of informants. The researchers who are examining a culture or subculture gain knowledge of the existing rules and patterns from its members; the emic perspective is thus culturally specific. For health researchers who explore their own culture and that of their patients, the 'native' view is not difficult to obtain because they are already closely involved in the culture. This prior involvement can be dangerous, because health professionals, by being part of the culture they examine, lose awareness of their role as researchers and sometimes rely on assumptions which do not necessarily have a basis in reality. Therefore reflection on prior assumptions is important.

Example

A ward sister carried out research on the emotional experience of people in hospital. She assumed that fear would be the most predominant aspect of the hospital experience. However, she found that embarrassment was a more strongly expressed emotion of many older people. This is a significant finding, because it confirms that embarrassment can disturb the stay of patients in hospital. Certain suggestions might be made to provide care that does not generate embarrassment.

Warren *et al.* (2000)

Of course, the etic view is important too. Etic meanings stress the ideas of ethnographers themselves, their abstract and theoretical view when they distance themselves from the cultural setting and try to make sense of it. Harris (1976) explains that etics are scientific accounts by the researcher, based on that which is directly observable. The researchers place individuals' ideas within a framework and interpret it by adopting a social science perspective on the setting. Emic and etic perspectives provide a partnership between researchers and participants. Not only do outsiders recognise patterns and ideas of which the people in the setting are not aware; they also translate the insights and words of the participants into the language of science.

The meaning of the participants differs from scientific interpretations. Researchers move back and forth, from the reality of informants to scientific interpretation, but they must find a balance between involvement in the culture they study and scientific reflections and ideas about the beliefs and practices within that culture. This can be described as 'iteration', where researchers revise ideas and build upon previous stages (Fetterman, 1998) (See also Chapter 1).

Fieldwork

The term fieldwork is used by ethnographers and other qualitative researchers to describe data collection outside laboratories. The major traits of ethnography have their basis in 'first-hand experience' of the group or community, and this usually, though not only, involves participant observation and interviewing (Atkinson *et al.*, 2007). Ethnographers gain most of their data through fieldwork. They become familiar with the community or group with whom they want to carry out research. Fieldwork in qualitative research means working in the natural setting of the informants, observing them and talking to them over prolonged periods of time. This is necessary so that informants get used to the researcher and behave naturally rather than putting on a performance. The observation of a variety of contexts is important. Spradley (1980: 78) provides a list in order to guide researchers when they observe a situation, although these guidelines cannot be seen as complete or all inclusive (see Chapter 7). The physical location of the researcher in the setting is necessary for observation in fieldwork.

The initial phase in the field consists of a time for exploration. Health researchers learn about an area of study and become familiar with it. This is not difficult, because they are already part of the community and well aware of patient and professional cultures. Acceptance need not be earned because health professionals have been part of these cultures, while anthropologists in foreign cultures must achieve entry through learning the ways of the group from the beginning. Fieldwork aims to uncover patterns and regularities in a culture which the people living in that community can recognise. There are several steps in fieldwork. In the first stage the researchers gain access to observe and study the culture in which they are interested and write notes on their observations. Secondly researchers start focusing on particular issues. They question the informants on the initial observations. In the third stage researchers realise that saturation has occurred, and they start the process of disengagement.

The best method of data collection in ethnographic research is participant observation, the most complete immersion in a culture. For instance, a nurse who intends to explore the work of a nursing development unit would either be a member of this unit or take part in it in order to observe the practices and reactions of the individuals within.

Micro- and macro-ethnographies

Micro-ethnographies focus on subcultures or settings such as a single ward or a group of specialist nurses. Fetterman (1998) claims that micro-studies consist of research in small units or focus on activities within small social settings. Ethnographers might select a setting such as a pain clinic, an operating theatre, a labour ward or a GP practice; two of our students, for instance, studied a mixed gender ward. Most students choose a micro-ethnographic study as it makes fewer demands on their time than macro-ethnography. It also seems more immediately relevant to the world of the health professional while policy makers would find macro-ethnography more useful.

There is a continuum between large- and small-scale studies, macro- and micro-ethnographies. A macro-ethnography examines a larger culture with its institutions, communities and value systems. This might be a hospital, or the nursing, midwifery or physiotherapy culture. A large-scale study means a long period of time in the setting and is often the work of several researchers. Both types of ethnography demand a detailed picture of the community under study as well as strategies for data collection and analysis. The type of project depends, of course, on the focus of the investigation and the researcher's own interests.

Ethnographic research can be very useful during changes in a culture. In a changing healthcare system, health professionals sometimes study developments not only in larger settings such as hospitals or communities but also in the smaller world of wards and theatres. Change – the transition from one stage or one ideology to another – can provide a useful focus for health or health policy research. Maternity wards, GP surgeries and other small units but also bigger sites and settings can be appropriate settings for ethnography.

Example of micro-ethnography

Cloherty *et al.* (2004) reported on ethnographic research in the postnatal ward of a maternity unit, involving observation and interviews with mothers and health professionals. The aim was to explore beliefs, expectations and experiences concerning supplementation of breastfeeding.

Example of macro-ethnography

The aim of a study by Fudge *et al.* (2008) was to explore the understanding of user involvement in health organisations and what influences them to put this involvement into practice. To achieve this aim, they used observation, interviews and documentary sources in a programme set up to improve stroke services in two London boroughs. Along with other findings, these researchers gained an understanding that the interpretation of the concept of user involvement is different in health professionals and service users. User involvement encompassed a large range of activities.

The ethnographic record: field and analytic notes

Researchers collect data by standard methods, mainly through observing and interviewing, but also rely on documents such as letters, diaries and the oral history of people in the culture they study. From the beginning of their research, ethnographers record what goes on 'in the field' – the setting and situation they are studying. This includes noting down fleeting impressions as well as accurate and detailed descriptions of events and behaviour in context. While writing notes and describing what occurs in the situation ethnographers become reflective and analytic.

Spradley (1979) lists four different types of fieldnotes in ethnography:

- The condensed account
- The expanded account
- The fieldwork journal
- Analysis and interpretation notes

Condensed accounts are short descriptions made in the field during data collection while expanded accounts extend the descriptions and fill in detail. Ethnographers extend the short account as soon as possible after observation or interview if they were unable to record during data collection. In the field, journal ethnographers note their own biases, reactions and problems during fieldwork. Researchers use additional ways to record events and behaviour such as tapes, films or photos, flowcharts and diagrams.

Fieldwork proceeds in progressive stages. Initially researchers gain the broad picture of the group and the setting. They observe behaviour and listen to the language that is used in the community they study. For nurses and midwives in a clinical setting this is not difficult because patients, colleagues and other health professionals trust them to record accurately and honestly. After initial observation, researchers focus on particular issues that seem important to them. Finally, writing becomes detailed analysis and interpretation of the culture under study.

Doing and writing ethnography

When writing up, researchers take all the stages of the process into account, and they form part of an ethnography. An ethnography is analytic as well as descriptive and interpretative. Ethnographers describe what they see and hear while studying a culture; they identify its main features and uncover relationships between them through analysis; they interpret the findings by asking for meaning and inferring it from the data. According to Stewart (1998) an ethnography is holistic in the sense that researchers create a portrait of the group under study. This also means that they take into account the social context in which the study takes place.

Description

As mentioned before, ethnography uses description. We must warn, however, that it is never as simple as it seems. Writers select specific situations for observation, disregard some events and interactions in favour of others and focus on particular issues that they perceive as relevant and significant. Not everything observed or heard is described but only that which is relevant for the study at hand. This involves analysis and interpretation.

Researchers describe by writing a story, which is a report of the actions, interactions and events within a cultural group. The reader should get a sense of the setting or a feel for it and understand what is going on there. The description is enhanced by the portrayal of critical events and ordinary life, as well as rituals and roles. Wolcott (1994) demands that during description the writer follow an analytical structure that gives a framework to the account.

Analysis

There are a number of ways in which qualitative ethnographic data can be analysed (see for instance: Gobo, 2008; LeCompte and Schensul, 1999; or the nursing text Roper and Shapira, 2000; Hammersley and Atkinson, 2007. There are also early foundational books such as Spradley (1979, 1980) and Agar (1980) which include analytic procedures). Analysis entails working with the data. To provide a simple overview: the researchers process the data by coding/labelling and transform the raw data through finding themes and by making linkages between ideas. This process will generate recognisable patterns. Analysis cannot proceed without interpretation but is more scientific and systematic; it brings order to disorderly data, and the researchers must show how they arrived at the structures and linkages. The informants' perspectives might be different, depending on their location in the hierarchy or their background and career, and this has to be taken into account and the question 'who says what?' is important. At the findings stage, other people's research connected with the emergent themes becomes part of the analytic process through comparison and integration in the study. It is important that the analysis accurately reflects the data. Whatever the analyst finds has to be related back to the data in order to see whether there is a fit between them and the analytic categories and themes.

Steps in the analysis

As in other qualitative research, data analysis takes place from the beginning of the observation and interviews. The focus becomes progressively clearer. In the data analysis the researcher revisits the aim and the initial research question. Analysis takes more time than data collection. In any type of ethnography mere description of behaviour and events is not enough as the aim of ethnography is analytic description of a culture or subculture. Ethnographers often start with domain analysis, that is, the area which they study and where they note specific events, incidents and activities.

The process of analysis involves several steps though ethnographers might explain this in different ways (see, for instance, the table in LeCompte and Schensul, 1999: 82–3):

1. Ordering and organising the collected material
2. Breaking the material into manageable – and meaningful – sections
3. Building, comparing and contrasting categories
4. Searching for relationships and grouping categories together
5. Recognising and describing patterns, themes and typologies
6. Interpreting and searching for meaning

These processes must not be seen necessarily as linear or sequential, and each step or stage can be revisited or repeated. There is also overlap between these activities. Spradley (1979: 92) claims that analysis involves the 'systematic examination of something to determine its parts, the relationship among parts, and their relationship to the whole'. Agar (1980) stresses the non-linear nature of the process: researchers collect data through which they learn about a culture, they try to make sense of what they saw and heard, and then they collect new data on the basis of their analysis and interpretation.

Researchers listen to their tapes, read the transcripts and fieldnotes from observation and note down significant elements. Of course they re-read and listen many times, and sometimes recognise differences between the first and the second reading and listening.

The data are scanned and organised from the very beginning of the study. If gaps and inadequacies occur, they can be filled by collecting more data or refocusing on the initial aims of the study. While this work goes on, researchers choose to focus on particular aspects which they examine more closely than others. While re-reading the data, thoughts and observations are being recorded, and a search for regularities can begin. The material is organised and broken down into manageable chunks. These pieces (of sentences, groups of words or paragraphs) are each given a meaningful label. This initial coding of data generates categories. The 'coding for descriptive labels' (Roper and Shapira, 2000) reduces or collapses the mass of data obtained.

For instance, the first interview – or the first detailed description of observation – is scanned and marked off into chunks, which are given labels. The second and third interview transcripts are then coded and compared with the first. Commonalities and similar codes are sorted and grouped together. This happens for each interview (or observation). Thematically, similar sets are placed together and grouped into categories. The researcher then tries to find the ideas that link the categories, and describes and summarises them. From this stage onwards diagrams are helpful because they present the links and patterns graphically.

The researcher compares the emerging categories and reduces them to (or collapses into) themes (major categories, constructs) and tries to find regularities. Broad patterns of thought and behaviour emerge. The patterns and regularities have their basis in the actual observations and interviews; they will be connected with the personal experiences of the researcher.

At that stage a dialogue starts with categories and themes drawn from the relevant and related literature. Ethnographic texts describe this 'taxonomic analysis' – analysis by classification or grouping of categories into an organised system which points to the relationship between these categories. They also might uncover a typology of participants: for instance, a midwife might recognise in the research on a maternity unit three 'types' of client, the 'dependent' the 'independent' and the 'controlling' client. A doctor might classify patients into passive and active individuals. These groupings generate a typology.

This does not present all the processes of ethnographic research. It also means searching for contrasts between categories, stating their dimensions and looking for conditions under which certain actions occur (see also Angrosino, 2007; Gobo, 2008).

Interpretation

Researchers take the last step, that of interpretation during and after the analysis, making inferences, providing meaning and giving explanations for the phenomena. While describing and analysing, they interpret the findings, that is, they gain insight and give meaning to them. Interpretation involves some speculation, theorising and explaining although it must be directly grounded in the data. It links the emerging ideas derived from the analysis to established theories through comparing and contrasting others' work with the researcher's own.

Eventually the story is put together from the descriptions, analyses and interpretations. LeCompte et al. (1997) compare this to assembling a jigsaw puzzle where a frame is quickly outlined and small puzzle pieces are collected together and placed in position within the frame. The difference is that one knows about the final picture of a jigsaw and has something to work towards, while in qualitative research one merely has an emerging picture where one can only imagine the outline which may change in the process of assembly.

Pitfalls and problems

There are a number of problems with ethnographic research in the health arena and elsewhere. First, it is difficult to examine one's own group and become a 'cultural stranger' questioning the assumptions of the familiar culture whose rules and norms have been internalised. Vigilance and advice from outsiders are very important. Second, because health professionals often have a background in the natural sciences and are taught to adopt a systematic approach to their clinical work, they sometimes may find it difficult to suffer ambiguity. It is better, however, to admit to uncertainty than to make unwarranted claims about the research. It resembles a diagnosis: signs and symptoms are examined for meaning but should never become once-and-for-all interpretation. Findings can be re-interpreted at a later stage in the light of reflection or new evidence.

Our students often write up their research, making statements that seem to be applicable to a whole range of similar situations. The findings from an ethnography cannot simply be generalised, however, and they are not automatically applicable to other settings though often theoretical ideas can be generalised. The researcher can compare with other specific situations similar to the case studied and can achieve typicality.

Novice researchers are often too descriptive and present raw data without analysis and interpretation. Even the quotes of the participants in the study are not raw data but purposefully selected by the researcher (see Chapter 17). Nevertheless, at the start of a research career, it is advisable to give more descriptive detail, clear analysis and to be careful with interpretation. With experience the balance might change. It is interesting that on revisiting the work at a later stage, many researchers start reinterpreting the data.

Summary

The main features of ethnography as a research method are as follows.

- Ethnographers immerse themselves in the culture or subculture they study and try to see the world from the cultural members' point of view.
- Data are collected during fieldwork through participant observation and interviews with key informants as well as through documents.
- Researchers observe the rules and rituals in the culture and try to understand the meaning and interpretation that informants give to them.
- They compare these with their own etic view and explore the differences between the two.
- Fieldnotes are written throughout the fieldwork about events and behaviour in the setting.
- Ethnographers describe, analyse and interpret the culture and the local, emic perspective of its members while making their own etic interpretations.
- The main evaluative criterion is the way in which the study presents the culture as experienced by its members.

Chapter 7 is particularly useful for ethnography.

References

Agar, M.H. (1980) *The Professional Stranger: Informal Introduction to Ethnography*. New York, NY, Academic Press.

Anderson, L. (2006) Analytic autoethnography. *Journal of Contemporary Ethnography*, **35** (4), 373–95.

Angrosino, M. (2007) *Doing Ethnographic and Observational Research*. London, Sage.

Atkinson, P., Coffey, A., Delamont, S., Lofland, J. & Lofland, L. (eds) (2007) Introduction to part one. In *Handbook of Ethnography*, pp. 9–10. London, Sage (paperback edn).

Blackstone, A. (2009) Doing good, being good and the social construction of compassion. *Journal of Contemporary Ethnography*, **38** (1), 85–116.

Boas, F. (1928) *Anthropology and Modern Life*. New York, NY, Norton.

Brewer, J.D. (2000) *Ethnography*. Buckingham, Open University Press.

Brown, D. & McCormack, B. (2006) Determining factors that have an impact upon effective pain management with older people, following colorectal surgery. *Journal of Clinical Nursing*, **15** (10), 1287–98.

Carspecken, P. (1996) *Critical Ethnography in Educational Research: A Theoretical and Practical Guide*. New York, NY, Routledge.

Chambers, E. (2000) Applied ethnography. In *Handbook of Qualitative Research* (eds N.K. Denzin & Y.S. Lincoln), 2nd edn, pp. 851–69. Thousand Oaks, CA, Sage.

Cloherty, M., Alexander, J. & Holloway, I. (2004) Supplementing breastfed babies in the UK to protect their mothers from tiredness and distress. *Midwifery*, **20** (2), 194–204.

Cook, K.E. (2005) Using critical ethnography to explore issues in health promotion. *Qualitative Health Research*, **15** (1), 129–38.

Denzin, N.K. (1989) *Interpretive Interactionism*. Newbury Park, CA, Sage.

Deutscher, I. (1970) Words and deeds: social science and social policy. In *Qualitative Methodology: Firsthand Involvement with the Social World* (ed. W.J. Filstead), pp. 27–51. Chicago, IL, Markham Publishing.

Fetterman, D.M. (1998) *Ethnography: Step by Step*, 2nd edn. Thousand Oaks, CA, Sage.

Fudge, N., Wolfe, C.D.A. & McKevitt, C. (2008) Assessing the promise of user involvement in health service development: ethnographic study. *British Medical Journal*, **306**, 313–17 Retrieved August 2008 from *BMJ*, doi:10.1136/bmj.39456.552257.BE (published 29 January 2008).

Geertz, C. (1973) *The Interpretation of Cultures*. New York, NY, Basic Books.

Gobo, G. (2008) *Doing Ethnography*. Los Angeles, CA, Sage.

Hammersley, M. & Atkinson, P. (2007) *Ethnography: Principles in Practice*. 3rd rev. edn. Andover, Routledge.

Hardcastle, M., Usher, K. & Holmes, C. (2006) Carspecken's five-stage critical qualitative method: an application to nursing research. *Qualitative Health Research*, **16** (1), 151–63.

Harris, M. (1976) History and significance of the emic/etic distinction. *Annual Review of Anthropology*, **5**, 329–50.

Huby, G., Hart, E., McKevitt, C. & Sobo, E. (2007) Editorial: addressing the complexity of health care: the practical potential of ethnography. *Journal of Health Services Research Policy*, **12** (4), 193–4.

LeCompte, M.D. & Preissle, J., Tesch, R. (1997) *Ethnography and Qualitative Design in Educational Research*, 2nd edn. Chicago, IL, Academic Press.

LeCompte, M.D. & Schensul, J.J. (1999) *Analyzing & Interpreting Ethnographic Data.* Walnut Creek, CA, Altamira Press.

Leininger M. (ed.) (1985) *Qualitative Research Methods in Nursing.* Philadelphia, PA, WB Saunders.

Madison, D.S. (2005) *Critical Ethnography: Method, Ethics and Performance.* Thousand Oaks, CA, Sage.

Malinowski, B. (1922) *Argonauts of the Western Pacific: An Account of Native Enterprise and Adventure in the Archipelagoes of Melanesian New Guinea.* New York, NY, Dutton.

Mead, M. (1935) *Sex and Temperament in Three Primitive Societies.* New York, NY, Morrow.

Roper, J.M. & Shapira, J. (2000) *Ethnography in Nursing Research.* Thousand Oaks, CA, Sage.

Savage, J. (2006) Ethnographic evidence: the value of applied ethnography in health care. *Journal of Research in Nursing*, **11** (5), 383–93.

Schensul, S.L., Schensul, J.J. & LeCompte, M.D. (1999) *Essential Ethnographic Methods: Observations, Interviews and Questionnaires.* Walnut Creek, CA, Altamira Press.

Spradley, J.P. (1979) *The Ethnographic Interview.* Fort Worth, TX, Harcourt Brace Johanovich College Publishers.

Spradley, J.P. (1980) *Participant Observation.* Fort Worth, TX, Harcourt Brace Johanovich College Publishers.

Stewart, A. (1998) *The Ethnographer's Method.* Thousand Oaks, CA, Sage.

Streubert Speziale, H.J. & Rinaldi Carpenter, D. (eds) (2007) Ethnography as method. In *Qualitative Research in Nursing: Advancing the Humanistic Imperative*, 4th edn. Philadelphia, PA, Lippincott Williams & Wilkins.

Thomas, J. (1993) *Doing Critical Ethnography.* Newbury Park, CA, Sage.

Warren, J., Holloway, I. & Smith, P. (2000) Fitting in: maintaining a sense of self during hospitalisation. *International Journal of Nursing Studies*, **37**, 229–35.

Whyte, W.F. (1943) *Street Corner Society: The Social Structure of an Italian Slum.* Chicago, IL, University of Chicago Press.

Wolcott, H.F. (1994) *Transforming Qualitative Data: Description, Analysis, and Interpretation.* Thousand Oaks, CA, Sage.

Further reading

Hodgson, I. (2000) Ethnography and health care: focus on nursing. *Forum: Qualitative Research*, **1** (1). Online journal (in English and German) at: http://qualitative-research.net/fqs/fqs-eng.htm, accessed February 2008.

LeCompte, M.D. & Schensul, J.J. (1999) *Designing and Conducting Ethnographic Research*. Walnut Creek, CA, Altamira Press.

Pope, C. (2005) Conducting ethnography in medical settings. *Medical Education*, **39** (12), 1180–7.

Year 2006, Vol. 35 (4) of the *Journal of Contemporary Ethnography* deals exclusively with auto-ethnography and there is a debate between those who adhere to evocative and the defenders of analytic autoethnography.

CHAPTER 11

Grounded Theory

Grounded theory (GT) has been used in healthcare research and particularly in nursing for decades and is still popular; indeed Cutcliffe (2005: 421) states that it has become 'a global phenomenon'. It is an approach to collecting and analysing data. The finished product is also called a GT – it is a development of theory directly based and grounded in the data collected by the researcher. From its very start, this approach has been modified, not only by the main protagonists themselves but also by researchers who adopted and adapted it during its application to their own inquiry. In this chapter, we will describe the main features of GT and trace development and changes over time.

This approach has its origin in sociology, particularly symbolic interactionism (SI), and was initially developed in the collaboration of the sociologists Barney Glaser and Anselm Strauss who were trained respectively in quantitative and qualitative methods. Indeed, GT can comprise both qualitative and quantitative procedures but is most often allied to qualitative research. GT is not tied, however, to a specific discipline or even to a particular form of data collection – there are studies in psychology, healthcare, business management and other fields. GT, like other qualitative approaches, is often adopted by researchers where not much knowledge exists about the phenomenon under study.

Data sources can be varied, such as interviews, observations or documents, and visual and oral presentations or events. Health researchers particularly appreciate the systematic and organised way of the GT process. Caring is an interactive process, hence the focus in GT on interaction, communication and active engagement in social situations, suits most health professionals.

History and origin

GT originated in the 1960s by Barney Glaser and Anselm Strauss, who worked together on research about health professionals' interaction with dying patients in 1965. From research, writing and teaching, the classic text *The Discovery of Grounded Theory* (Glaser and Strauss, 1967) emerged. Four other books on GT followed – *Field Research: Strategies for a Natural Sociology* (Schatzman and Strauss, 1973), *Theoretical Sensitivity* (Glaser, 1978), *Qualitative Analysis for Social Scientists* (Strauss, 1987); *Basics of Qualitative Research* (Strauss and Corbin, 1990, 1998) was an attempt by Strauss and Corbin (Corbin is a researcher with a nursing background) to modify earlier ideas on GT. The last book on which Strauss (who died in 1996) worked, is a clear and practically useful book on GT; it describes an approach which has been tried and developed. In 2008 Corbin followed this up with a later book. Although at times called formulaic and prescriptive, the 1990 and 1998 editions have helped many nurse researchers as handbooks to find certain elements on GT such as theoretical sampling and saturation (this will be explained later). The book edited by Chenitz and Swanson (1986) discussed GT in relation to nursing research. Strauss and Corbin (1997) edited a book in which they show how researchers have applied GT in practice. In the early nineties Glaser (1992) criticised the approach taken by Strauss and Corbin and asserted that what they described was not true GT but 'conceptual description'. Since then, Glaser has written prolifically – including various Readers on GT – and developed his own perspective in books and website. He founded his press (Sociology Press, Mill Valley, CA), established a 'Grounded Theory Institute' and now publishes the international journal *The Grounded Theory Review*. The ideas of Glaser and Strauss diverged in later years. Recently Kathy Charmaz (2006) developed a constructivist GT from earlier work which led to an edited handbook (Bryant and Charmaz, 2007).

In nursing and healthcare the GT approach has been popular from its inception; Benoliel, (1996: 419–21) lists the GT research studies that have been carried out in nursing between 1980 and 1994 and gives a good overview of the history of GT. There are chapters in Munhall's (2006) edited book and in particular Morse's publications in the United States. Melia in the eighties and nineties and recently Cutcliffe (2000, 2005) in Britain are some of the better known nurse researchers who have used and/or discussed GT approaches. Schreiber and Stern (2001) edited a GT text specifically for nurses.

Symbolic interactionism

The theoretical framework for GT has its roots in SI, focusing on the processes of interaction between people exploring human behaviour and social roles (although it must be said that Glaser has now a somewhat different perspective and sees SI as just one of the contributions). SI explains how individuals attempt to fit their lines of action to those of others (Blumer, 1971), take account of each others' acts, interpret them and reorganise their own behaviour. Mead (1934) established the philosophical framework, and Blumer contributed to GT the idea that human beings are active participants in their situation rather than passive respondents. Jeon (2004) shows the debt GT owes to SI; the notion of self as ever changing and adapting is central to this.

Mead, the main proponent of SI, sees the self as a social rather than a psychological phenomenon. Members of society affect the development of a person's social self by their expectations and relationships. Initially, individuals model their roles on the important people in their lives, 'significant others'; they learn to act according to others' expectations, thereby shaping their own behaviour. The observation of these interacting roles is a source of data in GT, and individual actions can only be understood in context.

SI focuses on actions and perceptions of individuals and their ideas and intentions. The Thomas theorem states: 'If men [sic] define situations as real, they are real in their consequences' (Thomas, 1928: 584), thereby claiming that individual definitions of reality shape perceptions and actions. Participant observation and interviewing trace this process of the 'definition of the situation'. Researchers should see the situation from the perspective of the participants rather than their own. Qualitative methods suit the theoretical assumptions of SI. Researchers use GT to investigate the interactions, behaviours and experiences as well as individuals' perceptions and thoughts about them. The intention of the research is 'the idiographic study of particular cases rather than the nomothetic study of mass data' (Alvesson and Sköldberg, 2000: 13).

The main features of grounded theory

The main aim of GT is the *systematic* generation of theory from the data collected by researchers. Existing theories can be modified or extended through GT. Researchers start with an area of interest, collect and analyse the data and allow relevant ideas to develop, without preconceived theories to be tested for confirmation. Glaser and Strauss (1967) advised that rigid preconceived assumptions prevent development of the research; imposing a framework might block the awareness of major concepts emerging from the data. The approach seeks explanation rather than being descriptive.

The theory generated through the research must be applicable to a variety of similar settings and contexts. GT researchers are able to adopt alternative perspectives rather than follow previously developed ideas. For this, they need flexibility and open minds, qualities related to the processes involved in nursing. The following gives an example of the use of GT and the need for flexibility by researchers.

Example 1

MacIntosh (2003), a nurse educator, examined the socialisation of nurses in a nursing education programme through open-ended interviewing of experienced nurses and gaining their perceptions of the process of becoming professional and the problems inherent in this process. She justified her use of GT in this study by pointing to the lack of previous research about the influences of socialisation and perceptions of professional development. The researcher followed the tenets of GT by revising and reworking ideas when new data emerged from the interviews. The development of the study was not linear but flexible and changed direction when the need arose.

This research demonstrates that GT research is not a simple and orderly process, though it is systematic.

The GT style of research uses constant comparison. The researcher compares each section of the data with every other throughout the study for similarities, differences and connections. Included in this process are the themes and categories identified in the literature. All the data are coded and categorised, and from this process, major concepts and constructs are formed. The researcher takes up a search for major themes that link ideas to find a core category for the study.

Strauss (1987) sees the processes of induction, deduction and verification as essential in GT, and he believes that the approach should be both inductive and deductive. GT does not start with a hypothesis though researchers might have 'hunches'. After collecting the initial data, however, relationships are established and provisional hypotheses conceived. These are verified by checking them out against further data. Glaser (1992) however, questions the process of verification as discussed later in this chapter and stresses the inductive element and the 'emergence' of theory. Theoretical sampling, one of the main features of GT, is discussed below.

Grounded theorists accept their role as interpreters of the data and do not stop at merely reporting them or describing the experiences of participants. Researchers search for relationships between concepts, while other forms of qualitative research often generate major themes but, generally, do not develop theories.

Data collection, theoretical sampling and analysis

Data collection

Data are collected through observations in the field, interviews of participants, diaries and other documents such as letters or even newspapers. Researchers use interviews and observations more often than other data sources, and they supplement these through literature searches. Indeed, the literature becomes part of the data that are analysed. Everything, even researchers' experience, can become sources of data; Glaser (1978) believes that 'everything is data'. The work is based on prior interest and problems that researchers have experienced and reflected on, even when there is no hypothesis. Data collection and analysis are linked from the beginning of the research, proceed in parallel and interact continuously. The analysis starts after the first few steps in the data collection have been taken; the emerging ideas guide the collection of data and analysis. This process does not finish until the end of the research because ideas, concepts and new questions continually arise which guide the researcher to new data sources and concepts. Researchers collect data from initial interviews, observations or documents and take their cues from the first emerging ideas to develop further interviews and observations. This means that the collection of data becomes more focused and specific as the process develops (progressive focusing).

The researcher writes fieldnotes from the beginning of the data collection throughout the project. Certain occurrences in the setting, or ideas from the participants that seem of vital interest, are recorded either during or immediately after data collection. They remind the researcher of the events, actions and interactions and trigger thinking processes.

According to Glaser (1978) the following are necessary for GT:

- Theoretical sensitivity
- Theoretical sampling
- Data analysis: coding and categorising
- Constant comparison
- Literature as a source of secondary data
- Integration of theory
- Theoretical memos and fieldnotes
- The core category

Theoretical sensitivity

Researchers must be theoretically sensitive (Glaser, 1978). Theoretical sensitivity means that researchers can differentiate between significant and less important data and have insight into their meanings. There are a variety of sources for theoretical sensitivity. It is built up over time, from reading and experience which guides the researcher to examine the data from all sides rather than stay fixed on the obvious.

Professional experience can be one source of awareness, and personal experiences, too, can help make the researcher sensitive.

Example 1: Professional experience

A specialist nurse, an expert on anorexia nervosa, explores this condition from the perspectives of those who suffer from it. He has expert knowledge in the field gained in his long professional career. His professional experience makes him sensitive to patients' feelings and perceptions (Newell, 2008).

> **Example 2:** Personal experience
> A general practitioner has had diabetes from an early age. When she observes or interviews patients about their condition, she might include questions on the feelings patients had on the diagnosis of diabetes or their thoughts about living with this condition.

The literature sensitises, in the sense that documents, research studies or autobiographies create awareness in the researcher of relevant and significant elements in the data. Strauss and Corbin (1998) believe that theoretical sensitivity increases when researchers interact with the data because they think about emerging ideas, ask further questions and see these ideas as provisional until they have been examined over time and are finally confirmed by the data.

Theoretical sampling

Sampling guided by ideas with significance for the emerging theory is called *theoretical sampling*. In theoretical sampling 'the emerging theory controls the research process throughout' (Alvesson and Sköldberg, 2000: 11). One of the main differences between this and other types of sampling is *time* and *continuance*. Unlike other sampling, which is planned beforehand, theoretical sampling in GT continues throughout the study and is not planned before the study starts. Cutcliffe (2000) shows that the initial data collection and analysis guides the direction of further sampling.

At the start of the project researchers make initial sampling decisions. They decide on a setting and on particular individuals or groups of people able to give information on the topic under study. Once the research has started and initial data have been analysed and examined (one must remember that data collection and analysis interact) new concepts arise, and events and people are chosen who can further illuminate the problem. Researchers then set out to sample different situations, individuals or a variety of settings, and focus on new ideas to extend the emerging theories. The selection of participants, settings, events or documents is a function of developing theories.

Theoretical sampling continues until the point of data and theoretical saturation. Students do not always understand the meaning of the concept 'saturation', and believe it to be a stage when no new information or concepts are obtained through data collection and analysis. For Glaser and Strauss (1967) 'theoretical saturation' has occurred when no more data emerge that can be used to find dimensions and develop properties of the categories the researcher has established and not when a concept is mentioned frequently and is described in similar ways by a number of people, or when the same ideas arise over and over again. Instead, it only occurs when no new data of importance for the developing theory and for the achievement of the aim of the research emerge.

It is very difficult to reach saturation; indeed, one might ask if it can ever truly be established, but the attempt at saturation is necessary. Saturation occurs at a different stage in each research project and is difficult to recognise. Draucker *et al.* (2007) present a sampling guide to assist in both systematic decisionmaking and category development.

Theoretical sampling, though originating in GT, is occasionally used in other types of qualitative analysis.

Data analysis: coding and categorising

Coding and categorising goes on throughout the research. From the start of the study, analysts *code* the data. Coding in GT is the process by which concepts or themes are identified and named during the analysis. Data are transformed and reduced to build *categories* which are named and given a label. Through the emergence of these categories theory can be evolved and integrated. Researchers form clusters of interrelating concepts, not merely descriptions of themes. Sometimes these codes consist of words and phrases used by the participants themselves to describe a phenomenon. They are called *in vivo* codes (Strauss, 1987). A new recruit to the profession might declare in an interview: 'I was thrown in at the deep end', for instance. The code might be 'thrown in at the deep end'. *In vivo* codes can give life and interest to the study and can be immediately recognised as reflecting the reality of the participants. In this process of analysis, the first step is concerned with open coding which starts as soon as the researcher receives the data. Open coding is the process of breaking down and conceptualising the data.

In GT, all the data are coded. Initial codes tend to be provisional and are modified or transformed over the period of analysis. At the beginning of a project or a study, line-by-line analysis is important, although it may be a long drawn-out process for analysts. Codes are based directly on the data, and therefore the researcher avoids preconceived ideas. An example of an interview with a nurse tutor gives some idea of level 1 coding.

Example

Well I suppose most people get fed up with doing the same things year in, year out.	Getting bored
I really felt like a change.	Desire for change
Regular hours are important to me.	Wish for regularity
I hadn't been promoted to the level to which I could function.	Lack of promotion

---

The analyst groups concepts together and develops categories. At the start a great number of labels are used, and after initial coding, analysts attempt to condense (or collapse) codes into groups of concepts with similar traits which are categories. Hutchinson (1993) called these level 2 codes. These categories tend to be more abstract than initial codes and are generally formulated by the investigator. These are examples of level 2 codes.

Example

I had this fear that I was not going to survive.	Fear of dying
Nobody, but nobody was there to help me and I felt that I was completely alone.	Lack of support Feeling isolated
We all need somebody close to be with us when we're ill.	Need for significant other

---

The broken down data must be linked together again in a new form. The main features (properties) and dimensions of these categories are identified.

Level 3 constructs are major categories which, although generated from the data and based in them, are formulated by the researchers and rooted in their professional and academic knowledge. These constructs contain developing theoretical ideas and themes and through building these constructs, analysts reassemble the data. Categories are linked to subcategories. This process of reassembling the data is called *axial coding* by Strauss and Corbin. There is no reason, however, why researchers cannot use the categories that others have discovered. For instance, Melia (1987) borrows the term 'awareness context' from Glaser and Strauss, but usually health researchers develop their own useful categories. In developing the relationship between categories, researchers have to take the six c's into account (Glaser developed these and other theoretical coding families in 1978): causes, context, contingencies, covariances, consequences and conditions for each category.

1. **Causes** are reasons for or explanations for the occurrence of a category.
2. **Context** is the setting and factors surrounding the phenomenon.
3. **Covariance** occurs between the given category and others (i.e. a category changes with change in another).
4. The development of a category is affected by certain **conditions**.
5. **Contingency** means that the given category has an impact on another category.
6. **Consequences** are the outcomes or functions of a given category.

Glaser advises that most GT research fit into a causal model, a consequence model or a condition model. Even if the GT method is modified by researchers, it is useful to keep this in mind.

Although there is no initial hypothesis in GT, Strauss and Corbin (1998) (though not Glaser) suggest that during the course of the research, working propositions or hypotheses are generated. These must be based in and indicated by the data. The process of testing and verification for the hypotheses which link the categories goes on throughout the research in the Straussian version of GT. Researchers also seek deviant or negative cases which do not support a particular working proposition. When these are found, the researcher must modify the proposition or find reasons why it is not applicable in this particular instance.

The process of coding and categorising only stops when:

- no new information on a category can be found in spite of the attempt to collect more data from a variety of sources;
- the category has been described with all its properties, variations and processes;
- links between categories are firmly established (Strauss and Corbin, 1998)

The core category

The researcher must discover the *core category*. In GT, the major category which links all others is called the core category or core variable. Like a thread the category should be woven into the whole of the study; it is part of the overall pattern. The linking of all categories around a core is called selective coding. This means that the researcher uncovers the essence of the study and integrates all the elements of the emergent theory.

> **Example:** *Core category*
> Fenwick *et al.* (2008), (with Fenwick as the researcher), wrote an article on how women achieve normality after having had a baby by Caesarean section. They claim that 'achieving normality' is an important factor in the status passage to motherhood after a Caesarean section and hence became the core category.

The core category is the basic social–psychological process (BSP) involved in the research. The BSP is a process that occurs over time and explains changes in behaviour. It represents the ideas that are most significant to the participants.

> **Example of basic social–psychological process**
> A project about the perceptions of young people with epilepsy shows in essence that they want to be seen as normal by their peers. Thus, 'being normal' may be a core category. On the other hand, the study might show that these young people, after discovering that they have epilepsy, want to be seen as they were before the diagnosis and try to achieve this by a variety of means. 'Reclaiming a normal self' could be identified as a BSP.

Strauss (1987) claims some major characteristics for the core category:

1. It must be the central element of the research related to other categories and explain variations.
2. It must recur often in the data and be part of a pattern.
3. It connects with other categories without a major effort by the researcher.
4. The core category develops in the process of identifying, describing and conceptualising.
5. The core category is usually fully developed only towards the end of the research.

Constant comparison

Coding and categorising involves constant comparison. Initial interviews are analysed and codes and concepts developed. By comparing concepts and sub-categories, researchers are able to group them into major categories and label them. When they code and categorise incoming data, they compare new categories with those that have already been established. Thus, incoming data are checked for their 'fit' with existing categories. Each incident of a category is compared with every other incident for similarities and differences. The comparison involves the literature. Constant comparison is useful for finding the properties and dimensions of categories. It helps in looking at concepts critically as each concept is illuminated by the new, incoming data. Strauss and Corbin (1998: 4) stress that they do not offer prescriptions but 'essentially guidelines for suggested techniques'. However, it is useful if researchers are completely familiar with the main features of the GT approach.

Using the literature

The place of the literature in a GT study is problematic; experts have different perspectives on this. Some purists believe that there should not be an initial literature review of the specific topic to be researched but an overview of the more general area. The reason for this is that researchers would not be directed to particular issues in their field, but that their own data retained priority in the study. Others feel that an initial review sensitises the researcher to issues related to the topic and stimulates questions to be asked. One can give arguments for and against a long literature review before collection and analysis of data begins. Researchers must be able to justify their study, and therefore they need to find out the type and extent of knowledge that already exists in the field. They should not, however, generate a focus from other people's studies but rather from their own data which have priority.

Strauss and Corbin (1998) list a number of points about the use of the literature.

1. Concepts from the literature can be compared with those deriving from the study.
2. The literature can stimulate theoretical sensitivity. It can make researchers aware of existing ideas.
3. The literature can generate questions and problems.
4. Knowledge of existing theories can be useful in influencing the stance of the researcher.
5. The literature can be used as an added source of data although these do not have priority over the researchers' own data.
6. Researchers have to consider why the literature confirms or refutes their own ideas or data.
7. Even before the study starts, initial questions can help develop conceptual areas.
8. During the analysis process more questions can be generated, especially when the researchers' data and the findings of the literature show a discrepancy.
9. The literature can guide theoretical sampling. It can help decide where to go next. Ideas might arise which increase the chance of developing further the emerging theory.
10. The literature can be used to validate the researcher's categories. Concepts in the literature may confirm or refute the findings of the researcher.

The dialogue with the literature is critical in the process of theory development. Glaser speaks of several levels of literature and suggests that researchers initially read in the general area, while not studying the specifics related to their own research. The latter should not be carried out until fieldwork, coding and categorising is well under way, otherwise researchers might rely on ideas by others rather than develop their own. We suggest that the grounded theorists trawl the literature initially to find the gap in knowledge where they can contribute to the field, without studying it in detail or being directed to specific ideas, otherwise they might lose the primacy of their own data and be constrained by others' writing.

Most grounded theorists believe that the literature becomes a source for comparison. When categories have been found, researchers trawl the literature for confirmation or refutation of these categories. They try to discover what other researchers have found, and whether there are any links to existing theories. Researchers can also use the literature to compare their own theories with those previously developed.

Integration of theory

To be credible the theory must have 'explanatory power', that is, establish a causal relationship. This is different from descriptive qualitative research. In a good project, categories are connected with each other and tightly linked to the data. Researchers do not describe static situations but take into account and develop processes.

Glaser and Strauss (1967) state that two types of theory are produced: substantive and formal. Substantive theory emerges from the study of a particular context or setting – such as a ward, or patients with myocardial infarction, or professional education – hence this type of theory is very useful for health researchers. It has specificity and applies to the setting and situation studied; this means that it is limited. Formal theory, however, is generated from many different situations and settings, and it is conceptual. It might be a theory about vocational education, general experiences of suffering or being a mother, for instance. The 'career' of the dying patients in hospital, the stages through which patients proceed, which Glaser and Strauss investigated is substantive theory. When this is linked to the concept of 'status passage' which can be applied to many different situations, it becomes formal theory. This type of theory has general applicability, that is, it holds true not just for the setting of the specific study but also for other settings and situations, and it is not speculative but based in the data.

In a small student project, it would be difficult to produce a formal theory with wide applications, but substantive theories can still be important and have general implications for the work of the nurse. Another example can be given from nursing:

Example: *A substantive grounded theory*

Sandgren *et al.* (2006) carried out research in the field of palliative cancer nursing through interviews and participant observation. The findings of their research showed that there was emotional overload through their work which they sought to reduce. Nurses adopted a variety of strategies to survive the emotional stress of the setting. Emotional shielding, emotional processing and emotional postponing were the strategies that they adopted to achieve emotional survival. Striving for emotional survival through adopting a number of strategies such as emotional shielding, processing and postponing, etc. became the substantive theory.

The theory developed is generalisable in the sense that it can be applied to other, similar situations. Other events and situations can be understood through the knowledge acquired in building the theory.

Theoretical memos and fieldnotes

While going through the process of research, the researcher writes fieldnotes and memos. When observing and interviewing, the investigator writes fieldnotes from the beginning of the data collection. Certain occurrences or sentences seem of vital interest and they are recorded either during or immediately after data collection. They remind the researcher of events, actions and interactions and trigger thinking processes. There can be descriptions of the setting too to act as triggers for remembering.

Strauss and Corbin (1998: 110) define memos as 'records of analysis, thoughts, interpretations, questions and directions for further data collection', and they should be dated and detailed. Every GT researcher should write memos. They are meant to help in the development and formulation of theory. In theoretical memos, the researcher discusses tentative ideas and provisional categories, compares findings, and jots down thoughts on the research. Initially, memos might contain notes to remind the researcher 'don't forget...' or 'I intend to...'. Later they encompass micro-codes, and later still, major emergent categories, hunches, implications and concepts from the literature; memos become more varied and theoretical. Ideas for follow-up, related issues and thoughts about deviant cases become part of these memos.

Strauss (1987) suggests that memos are the written version of an internal dialogue that goes on during the research. Diagrams in the memos can help to remind the researcher and structure the study. Memo writing continues throughout the whole of the research, it goes through stages and becomes more complex in the process. Memos and diagrams provide 'density' for the research and guide the researcher to base abstract ideas in the reality of the data. Eventually, memos become integrated in the writing.

Pitfalls and problems

Wilson and Hutchinson (1996) discuss some of the common mistakes made in GT. They list six of these:

1. Muddling method (or method slurring)
2. Generational erosion
3. Premature closure
4. Overly generic analysis
5. The importing of concepts
6. Methodological transgression

Some of these are discussed further in other chapters, as they are common to several approaches. There are also problems with building a GT. Many researchers, particularly students in dissertations, projects and even theses, give good conceptual descriptions but do not develop a theory or even theoretical ideas. The difference between conceptualisation and description is significant. It is not enough to describe the perspectives of the participants or discuss 'themes' to develop a truly 'grounded' theory.

The term 'emerging categories' (or 'emerging theory') is problematic as they can only be achieved by hard work. This problem is linked to theoretical sampling. Often researchers use selective (or purposive) sampling procedures. Coyne (1997) differentiates clearly between purposeful and theoretical sampling. While the researcher decides on purposeful sampling beforehand according to certain criteria, dimensions and settings, for GT research this type of sampling is necessary but does not suffice. The decisions about theoretical sampling are not made on the basis of initial criteria but throughout on the basis of emerging concepts, because of the inductive nature of the research.

A number of computer programmes for qualitative research do exist (see Chapter 17). Becker feels that computers might prevent sensitivity to the data and the discovery of meanings. Computers distance researchers from the data. Although this need not be so, we realise that in health research, where emotional engagement and sensitivity is necessary, the use of computers could be problematic. Charmaz (2000) also maintains that in a study in which the researcher is deeply involved with the participants, computer analysis has an undesirable distancing effect.

Generalisability and replicability of GT research are often discussed. Of course, it is difficult to match the original situation and context. Each researcher has a personal approach and a relationship with the participants which cannot be exactly reproduced. However, if nurses and midwives make procedures explicit and clearly describe the original conditions and setting, others can follow the same rules and procedures and discover the same general scheme. Strauss and Corbin (1998) maintain that the findings of a GT study become more generalisable if the study is systematic, relies on theoretical sampling and examination of special conditions and discrepancies. A range of similar theoretical concepts from a variety of sources can become cumulative.

Glaser's critique and further development

Several versions of GT can be distinguished. The ideas of Strauss and Glaser, for instance, have diverged in the last decade. Glaser (1992) wrote a book in response to the book by Strauss and Corbin (1990), criticising the authors for distorting the procedures and meaning of GT. Glaser claims that their book does not truly describe GT. He accuses the authors of 'forced conceptual description' (p. 5). He exhorts researchers not to impose their research problem but start with an interest and a questioning mind so that they see their informants' perspectives with no preconceptions. Thus, the researcher does not start with a research question but with a research interest. Although agreeing that Strauss and Corbin have described a research method, Glaser denies that its roots have much in common with the original 1967 volume. The new method, he claims, results in conceptual descriptions rather than in the emergence of concepts and formation of the links between them that explain variations in behaviour.

The difference between the ideas in Strauss and Corbin's text and the original development lies in the way in which concepts are generated and relationships explained. Glaser states that GT should not be verificational but inductive, it does not move between inductive and deductive thinking (although the 1967 book does mention verification). Deduction is rarely used except for reasons of conceptual guidance; this differs from the ideas of Strauss and Corbin who include the element of verification by suggesting that researchers test working propositions or 'provisional hypotheses' during their research.

Glaser also argues that participant observation does not suffice for a truly GT; interviews which explain the meanings of the participants are always necessary (many researchers see interviews as an integral part of participant observation in any case). Other differences exist between the two camps: Annells (1997) claims that Strauss and Corbin see theory as a construct 'cocreated' by the researcher and participants, while Glaser believes that theory is 'emerging' from the actual data. It is interesting that Glaser, who started out as a survey researcher, seems to have become more flexible and less structured over time, while Strauss develops a more prescriptive way of researching.

Glaser (1992) believes that any initial literature review on the specific topic would contaminate the data and denies the need for it because it might direct researchers to irrelevant ideas. This he had also stated in his earlier book (Glaser, 1978). However, he too suggests that the literature can be integrated in the developing concepts. Discrepancies between concepts developed from the researchers' original data and the data from the literature may be discovered and the reasons for them investigated. Theoretical sensitivity helps to generate ideas and relate them to theory.

Glaser also advises against taping and transcribing interviews as he believes it a waste of time. We believe, however, that taping interviews might help those who are forgetful or those who have difficulty writing fieldnotes while interviewing. Of course, listening to interviews after taping is of great importance. We would argue that the memory of researchers might not be accurate and lead to misinterpretation. Mills *et al.* (2006) suggest naming the branches of GT 'traditional' (Glaser, who himself calls it 'classic'), 'evolved' (Strauss and Corbin) and 'constructivist' (Charmaz uses this term).

Constructivist grounded theory

Charmaz (2006) criticises some of the early ideas in the GT approach and argues that it has developed from a more prescriptive and positivist style of research to a flexible way of thinking. She claims that the methods have developed in a number of different ways depending on researchers' perspectives. She sees this as developmental and she welcomes the move towards a more constructivist GT. As Charmaz suggests (p. 187) that the 'interpretation of the studied phenomenon is in itself a construction.' and that 'people . . . construct the realities in which they participate'. This means that researcher, participants and readers co-construct the research. Reality emerges or is discovered in the context of interaction. Indeed constructivists sometimes suggest that 'truth', and reality, are socially constructed (many researchers would acknowledge the influence of context on research). Constructivist GT is hence more relativist and subjective.

An informative list of the differences between the approach of Strauss and Corbin and that of Glaser can be found in MacDonald (2001).

Which approach for the health researcher?

The varied approaches within GT seem to be based on different epistemological and methodological perspectives, though we would claim strong similarity between them. The development of GT itself has illuminated its elements and aspects in different ways.

Researchers can make up their own minds on which approach to follow when doing GT as long as they are knowledgeable about it and can explain why they have adopted a particular stance or followed specific processes. In any case, many researchers adapt methods during the process of research or use elements which they find useful. For a study to be called a 'Grounded Theory' the major features of GT should be included; most importantly the researcher must develop a theory, grounded in the data and with 'explanatory power'.

Summary

- The aim of the GT approach is the generation or modification of theory.
- Data usually are collected through non-standardised interviews and participant observation but also by access to other data sources.
- Data collection and analysis interact.

- Researchers code and categorise transcripts from interviews or fieldnotes.
- The researcher has a dialogue with the literature when discussing categories.
- Throughout the analytic process, constant comparison and theoretical sampling takes place.
- Memos – theoretical notes – provide the researcher with developing theoretical ideas.
- The theory that is generated has 'explanatory power' and is grounded in the data.

References

Alvesson, M. & Sköldberg, K. (2000) *Reflexive Methodology: New Vistas for Qualitative Research*. London, Sage.

Annells, M. (1997) Grounded theory method, part 1: within the five moments of qualitative research. *Nursing Inquiry*, **4** (2), 120–9.

Benoliel, J.Q. (1996) Grounded theory and nursing knowledge. *Qualitative Health Research*, **6** (3), 406–28.

Blumer, H. (1971) Sociological implications of the thoughts of G.H. Mead. In *School and Society* (eds B.R. Cosin *et al.*), pp. 11–17. Milton Keynes, Open University Press.

Bryant, A. & Charmaz, K. (eds). (2007) *The Sage Handbook of Grounded Theory*. London, Sage.

Charmaz, K. (2000) Grounded theory: objectivist and constructivist methods. In *Handbook of Qualitative Research* (eds N.K. Denzin & Y.S. Lincoln), 2nd edn, pp. 509–35. Thousand Oaks, CA, Sage.

Charmaz, K. (2006) *Constructing Grounded Theory: A Practical Guide through Qualitative Analysis*. London, Sage.

Chenitz, W.C. & Swanson, J.M. (eds). (1986) *From Practice to Grounded Theory: Qualitative Research in Nursing*. Menlo Park, CA, Addison-Wesley.

Coyne, I.T. (1997) Sampling in qualitative research: purposeful and theoretical sampling: merging or clear boundaries? *Journal of Advanced Nursing*, **26**, 623–30.

Cutcliffe, J.R. (2000) Methodological issues in grounded theory. *Journal of Advanced Nursing*, **31**, 1476–84.

Cutcliffe, J.R (2005) Adapt or adopt: developing and transgressing the methodological boundaries of grounded theory. *Journal of Advanced Nursing*, **51** (4), 421–8.

Draucker, C.B., Martsolf, D.S., Ross, R. & Rusk, T.B. (2007) Theoretical sampling and category development in grounded theory. *Qualitative Health Research*, **17** (8), 1137–8.

Fenwick, S., Holloway, I. & Alexander, J. (2008) Achieving normality: a key to the status passage to motherhood after a caesarean section. *Midwifery*, **25** (4), e5.

Glaser, B.G. (1978) *Theoretical Sensitivity*. Mill Valley, CA, Sociology Press.

Glaser, B.G. (1992) *Basics of Grounded Theory Analysis*. Mill Valley, CA, Sociology Press.

Glaser, B.G. & Strauss, A.L. (1967) *The Discovery of Grounded Theory*. Chicago, IL, Aldine.

Hutchinson, S.A. (1993) Grounded theory: the method. In *Nursing Research: A Qualitative Perspective* (eds P.L. Munhall & C. Oiler Boyd), pp. 180–212. New York, NY, National League for Nursing Press.

Jeon, Y.H. (2004) The application of grounded theory and symbolic interactionism. *Scandinavian Journal of Caring Sciences*, **18** (3), 249–56.

MacDonald, M. (2001) Finding a critical perspective in grounded theory. In *Using Grounded Theory in Nursing* (eds R.S. Schreiber & Stern, P.N.), pp. 113–57. New York, NY, Springer.

MacIntosh, J. (2003) Reworking professional nursing. *Western Journal of Nursing Research*, **25** (6), 725–41.

Mead, M. (1934) *Mind, Self and Society*. Chicago, IL, University of Chicago Press.

Melia, K. (1987) *Learning and Working: The Occupational Socialisation of Nurses*. London, Routledge.

Mills, J., Bonner, A. & Francis, K. (2006) The development of constructivist grounded theory. *International Journal of Qualitative Methods*, **5** (1), Article 3. Retrieved January 2008 from http://www.ualberta.ca/~iiqm/backissues/5_1/pdf/mills.pdf

Munhall, P.I. (ed.) (2006) *Nursing Research: A Qualitative Perspective*, 4th edn. Sudbury, MA, Jones and Bartlett.

Newell, C. (2008) *Recovery in Anorexia Nervosa: The struggle to develop a new identity*. Unpublished PhD, Bournemouth University.

Sandgren, A., Thulesius, H., Fridlund, B. & Peterson, K. (2006) Striving for emotional survival in palliative cancer nursing. *Qualitative Health Research*, **14** (1), 79–96.

Schatzman, L. & Strauss, A.L. (1973) *Field Research: Strategies for a Natural Sociology*. Englewood Cliffs, NJ, Prentice Hall.

Schreiber, R.S. & Stern, P.N. (eds). (2001) *Using Grounded Theory in Nursing*. New York, NY, Springer.

Strauss, A.L. (1987) *Qualitative Analysis for Social Scientists*. New York, NY, Cambridge University Press.

Strauss, A.L. & Corbin, J. (1990) *Basics of Qualitative Research: Grounded Theory Procedures and Techniques*. Newbury Park, CA, Sage.

Strauss, A.L. & Corbin, J. (eds). (1997) *Grounded Theory in Practice*. Thousand Oaks, CA, Sage.

Strauss, A.L. & Corbin, J. (1998) *Basics of Qualitative Research: Techniques and Procedures for Developing Grounded Theory*, 2nd edn. Thousand Oaks, CA, Sage.

Thomas, W.I. (1928) *The Child in America*. New York, NY, Alfred Knopf.

Wilson, H.S. & Hutchinson, S.A. (1996) Methodologic mistakes in grounded theory. *Nursing Research*, **45** (2), 122–24.

Website of Glaser's Grounded Theory Institute www.groundedtheory.com

Further reading

Annells, M. (1997) Grounded theory method, part 2: options for users of the method. *Nursing Inquiry*, **4** (3), 176–80.

Corbin, J. & Strauss, A.L. (2008) *Basics of Qualitative Research: Techniques and Procedures for Developing Grounded Theory*, 3rd edn. Los Angeles, CA, Sage.

McCann, T. & Clark, E. (2003a) Grounded theory in nursing research: part 1 methodology, *Nurse Researcher* **11** (2), 7–18.

McCann, T. & Clark, E. (2003b) Grounded theory in nursing research: part 2 – critique, *Nurse Researcher* **11** (2), 19–28.

McCann, T. & Clark, E. (2003c) Grounded theory in nursing research: part 3 – application, *Nurse Researcher* **11** (2), 29–39.

Morse, J.M., Stern, P.N., Corbin, J., Charmaz, K., Bowers, B. & Clarke, A.E. (2008) *Grounded Theory: The Second Generation*. Walnut Creek, CA, Left Coast Press.

CHAPTER 12

Narrative Inquiry

The nature of narrative and story

Stories are reflections on people's experience and the meaning that this experience has for them. Narrative research is a useful way of gaining access to feelings, thoughts and experience in order to analyse them. For many decades, health research had focused on the decisionmaking and thoughts of professionals and their measurement of the treatment outcomes, while the feelings and ideas of the patient, the 'insider', tended to be neglected. This changed with the advent of qualitative health research. The perspectives of patients are uncovered through their stories.

Many researchers apply the terms 'narrative' and 'story-telling' interchangeably, although others make a distinction. Frank (1995) uses the concepts of story and narrative differently: He cites the term 'story' when discussing the tales people tell, and narrative when referring to 'general structures' that encompass a number of particular stories. Paley and Eva (2005) claim that story integrates plot and character – both need to be present – while narrative comprises both sequence of events and causal links between them. However, the line between story and narrative is blurred, and we shall occasionally use these terms interchangeably. Even Frank admits that a distinction between the two is difficult, and Riessman (2008) too sees these terms as ambiguous.

Researchers refer to life stories, biographies or narratives; Labov (1972), one of the first sociologists to carry out research through narratives, sees the term narrative as more specific – as events in the past that are being retold. First person narratives provide much material for research. It must be remembered, however, that their content emerges from memory, and that people's memories are selective (Skultans, 1998). Nevertheless, the remembered events, as well as the experiences people choose from their vast store of memory, focus on the significant aspects of their social reality.

Narrating helps people to make sense of their experience. It unveils the intentions and motives of human beings to the researcher. Individuals remember an experience, tell the story sequentially as they perceived it happening and seek explanations for events and actions while interpreting and reflecting on them. However, narrators prioritise; some events and experiences carry more importance than others; according to the specific social context or the people to whom they speak, they emphasise different aspects of the story. They might neglect or fail to mention some issues or events, or they might exaggerate others, depending on their perspective or the audience to whom they speak.

> ## Examples of narratives and narrative analysis
>
> Carter (2004) illustrates the value of children's narratives of pain and how they can influence clinical practice by allowing professionals to hear children's voices and have empathy for them.
>
> An Australian study of the mental health of men in rural areas used narrative inquiry (Gorman *et al.*, 2007). These men's stories of resilience and survival showed how they coped with problems.
>
> McIlfrick *et al.* (2007) used narrative analysis to explore patients' experiences of chemotherapy in a day hospital. These patients viewed their experiences as both negative and positive, the former relating to the dehumanising aspects of treatment and the latter to social relationships with other patients and the maintenance of a sense of normality. The researchers used an in-depth analysis of patients' narratives.

Narratives are not only used in research but also in psychotherapy and in clinical and developmental psychology, mostly in the form of life stories. In sociology and anthropology too, narrative is seen as useful for examining culture, society or social and cultural groups. They are popular in medicine or nursing to gain the patient perspective. Charon (2006), a doctor, discusses the 'practice of narrative medicine' to which we can add 'the practice of narrative nursing', meaning that health professionals witness the lived experiences of illness, and they become more aware of the suffering and pain of their clients.

Lieblich *et al.* (1998) maintain that it is natural for people to tell stories. Researchers can use this talent to elicit stories from their participants. Participants affirm their identities through narratives. Ricoeur (1984, 1991) also affirms the ability of human beings to integrate actions and thoughts into a coherent narrative and create a link between past, present and future. Narrators create and affirm their identities through telling their tale. While sociologists such as Arthur Frank, Julius Roth and others have written portrayals of their illness and told their own story, lay people tell of the process and progress of their condition. Riley and Hawe (2005) stress the processual, dynamic and culture-bound nature of narratives; thus time and context are essential elements which researchers need to take into account.

Narrative research

Narrative research is a broad term and can incorporate other approaches – a narrative study may be an ethnography, take a phenomenological approach or use discourse analysis, but it can also stand as an approach on its own. It refers to 'any study that uses or analyses narrative material' (Lieblich *et al.*, 1998: 2). In this chapter it is used as an approach which is separate from other qualitative forms of inquiry.

A few narrative researchers believe, as Elliott (2005) does, that narrative inquiry can be quantitative as well as qualitative; however, to have lengthy stories from participants needs a more flexible approach and open questions and for these quantitative methods are inappropriate.

Narratives in health research

Although the use of narratives for research and other purposes has gone on in an informal way for a while, it is relatively recent in health research (Frid *et al.*, 2000). Narratives develop and increase professional knowledge, and through the acquisition of this knowledge they can improve care. Stories enable professionals to understand their clients and gain access to their experience and the meaning they give to this experience. For clinical and professional practice it means 'the focus of narrative will enable nursing [and other health professions] knowledge to be grounded in concrete situations' (Frid *et al.*, 2000: 3). It is not easy for health researchers to abandon their own assumptions and focus on the stories of ill people. Frank (2000) gives examples of this. He also refers to the difficulty professionals have to listen to the voice of patients, to hear what is relevant to those who suffer, because professionals have more skills to respond to patients as 'medical *subjects*' rather than 'ill *persons*' (our italics).

Narrative accounts in healthcare can be obtained from a number of different groups:

- Patients or clients
- Caregivers and relatives
- Colleagues and other professionals

Narratives from the point of view of the patient can be seen in several ways.

Patients, for instance, might tell their experience of an illness or a chronic medical condition or of care and treatment by professionals. Ill people tell stories to show what it means to be sick. New mothers tell stories about the meaning of childbirth. Old people tell stories about the meaning of old age in the context of this society. Narratives can also be a reaction to care and medical treatment, or as a counterperspective to that of health professionals. Through narratives and narrative interpretations, patients and clients may also attempt to justify their own actions and behaviour. As long as patients tell their stories, they might feel that they have some control. In addition, they use these narratives to achieve an attempt at normality: they compare their ill selves to their normal social, physical and psychological condition. Holloway and Freshwater (2007) summarise some of the reasons for storytelling which many authors have discussed, for instance Kellas and Manusov (2003), Riessman (2008) and others.

Through storytelling people have the possibility to

- give meaning to experiences, in particular suffering;
- interpret and verbalise important events and share them with others;
- present a holistic view of experience and perspective;
- try to find adjustment when conditions are unalterable;
- confirm group membership in a shared culture;
- attribute blame or responsibility to themselves or others;
- take control over their own lives.

Many authors have shown that telling stories also has healing functions (for instance Pennebaker, 2000 or Brody, 2003), though narrative inquiry has a different purpose, and healing or alleviating suffering and pain are unintended consequences – though of course welcome.

McCance *et al.* (2001) use narrative methodology to explore caring in nursing practice. They use it as a means to 'tap into the patient experience'. It is not easy to gain access to people's feelings and thoughts but eliciting a narrative may help in this process. Telling stories about specific experiences rather than giving general accounts or thinking in general terms is 'real' for patients; they often tell the story sequentially along temporal dimensions. Greenhalgh and Hurwitz (1998: 45) claim that narratives used in healthcare research can

- set a patient-centred agenda;
- challenge received wisdom;
- generate new hypotheses.

Through their stories, patients help health professionals to focus on their perceptions and experiences rather than applying a professional framework immediately. If professionals truly listen to patients, they might also hear the unexpected and will be able to change their own assumptions if necessary.

Relatives are narrators of their care-giving experience as it happened and seek explanations for their own behaviour, for the patients' reactions and for professional care and treatment. Through this, they are able to justify their own thoughts and actions to professionals and researchers. Caregivers of patients with Alzheimer's disease, for instance, tell the sequence of events and discuss the behaviour of their relatives and their own reaction towards them. Essentially, caregivers attempt to share what caring means to them.

Researchers and health professionals use patient narrative to locate the sufferer at the centre of his or her illness. They see the narrative as a useful path to the understanding of sick people and the illness experience, as interpreted by patients in a specific cultural framework. Professionals – be they individual professionals in interaction with particular patients or professional groups who define specific conditions or illnesses within a biomedical framework – give different versions from patients. Both versions are valid and together might give the full picture. Sakalys (2000), in particular, addresses the question of culture in a discussion of narratives and claims that the social and cultural interpretation defines the illness experience and the sick role for the individual. Narratives also demonstrate the conflicts and dilemmas between individual meanings and healthcare ideologies.

In professional education and practice, narrators might tell the story of interaction in specific situations and of learning or teaching experiences. The researcher's aim is the understanding of the essence of that experience in the context of the participants' lives. Josselson (1995) claims that empathy and narrative show the way to people's reality; understanding of this can be achieved through qualitative research. Kleinman (1988) also urges 'empathic listening'. Health professionals need both empathy for and stories from their clients. Nurse and midwife teachers, in particular, often use narratives to teach students reflection and clinical decisionmaking as well as empathy.

Example

The following research shows the value of narratives. An exploration of how people with motor neurone disease talk about living and coping with their condition demonstrates how survival is the essential element in the findings. Brown and Addington-Hall (2008) carried out longitudinal narrative interviews over 18 months with 13 individuals. Although the participants' narratives were unique, they also contained common elements. Brown and Addington-Hall point out that storylines are 'organising threads' that help professionals to understand and help these individuals and their families.

Types of narrative

Jovchelovitch and Bauer (2000) list the two dimensions of narrative and story-telling: the chronological dimension where narratives are told in sequential form with a beginning, a middle and an end, and the non-chronological, which is a plot constructed as a coherent whole from a number of events – small tales which combine into a big story. According to Paley and Eva (2005), certain conditions need to be fulfilled in the configuration of a plot:

1. The plot contains a central character.
2. This character encounters a problem.
3. A link exists between character and explanation.
4. The plot and its configuration elicits an emotional response in the listener.

It depends on the storyteller what he or she wishes to communicate to others or what to leave out of the story. People organise their experience through narratives and make sense of them, not least by relating them to time. Indeed, Bruner (2004: 692) states that the only way to account for 'lived time' is in the form of narrative. Narratives allow access to a person's perceived reality in many different ways. Richardson (1990) describes many of these types of stories:

1. Everyday stories
2. Autobiographical stories
3. Biographical stories
4. Cultural stories
5. Collective stories

Often, narratives contain a number of overlapping stories. We shall illustrate these by examples (real, but not necessarily literal, comments):

The everyday story

In the everyday story, people tell how they did everyday things and carry out their normal tasks: '... And then I went out into the garden and did some work, and then I came inside and sat down.' Most patients import these everyday stories into the history of their condition, care and treatment.

> **Example**
> When researching people's experience in hospital, one of our students found that their narratives always tended to start at a time before they arrived. 'We were watching television, I had just made a cup of tea when it happened... and then my wife called the ambulance, I could hardly walk, and then they went through the night with all lights blazing and a lot of noise.'

Autobiographical stories

In an autobiographical story people link the past to the present and future: 'I used to go dancing, but now I can't dance any more, I shall probably never dance again because of my pain.' Through autobiographical stories people also justify and explain their actions: 'Because I had such an awful pain in my back I could not have regular work.' In autobiographies in which individuals tell their illness history, they demonstrate that they see their own stories as unique and quite separate from those of others. The storyteller can link together various disparate events through narrative (Polkinghorne, 1995): '... And then I went

into the garden, and I did some work, and then my back went...and that's why
I am unemployed now.'

Example of autobiographical tale

Sparkes (1996) draws on his own experiences to illustrate the power of narrative.
He connects his own story of 'the fragile body-self' with the experiences of others
and their 'biographical disruptions'. Speaking of 'identity loss', chronic illness
and feelings about masculinity, he links his discussion to the cultural and social
context.

Biographical stories

Biographical stories, however, link individuals with each other. Reading and
listening to biographical stories enables them to share and compare their experiences. The stories guide beyond the subjective to intersubjective understanding
and empathy by living in a shared world. By writing accounts of others' stories,
researchers help readers understand the feelings and vulnerability of others.
An element of the autobiographical or biographical tale is the victory story in
which individuals demonstrate how they overcame adversity by describing their
feelings and actions (Sandelowski, 1996).

Cultural stories

Through the cultural story participants tell, they make visible and demonstrate
meanings in a particular cultural context, for instance the meaning of death
or the understanding of disease: 'I had epilepsy. In our society people don't
understand that, and I was labelled as not quite normal.' Or 'My back pain
is invisible, nobody believes that it exists, if I had a broken leg I would not
be labelled lazy or work shy.' Or 'Everybody wants you to have the baby
in hospital, in an earlier time, you could have it at home. Luckily times are
changing again.'

Collective stories

In research the collective story is significant. By retelling a number of stories, for
instance of patients, professionals or students, researchers reflect the thoughts
and paths of a group or collective of people with similar experiences and give
a portrayal of a condition or patterns of experience. For instance, a person
suffering from pain might mention that others are much worse off, or that new
mothers tell stories that are embedded in the culture of motherhood. Collectivity

creates a *Gestalt* or whole picture of the condition or experience. For nurses and midwives this means that they might recognise the needs of the group members and improve their care.

Illness narratives

Kleinman's (1988) *The Illness Narratives* is probably the best known example of narrative in the health and illness arena though not in research.

Patients use narratives to seek meaning and make sense of their suffering, and they want to share this with 'significant' others. The researcher on the other hand, re-tells stories in order to give voice about participants' feelings and thoughts. It is questionable, however, that the account is always the authentic voice of the participants because researchers translate and interpret the narrators' tales. Paley and Eva (2005) query the concept of truth as it is sometimes applied to narrative. They believe that 'truth' in the factual sense is irrelevant and that meaning and interpretation are important, not whether the story is factually 'real'. Sandelowski (1996: 122) also criticises the naïve notions of stories as either true or false. Nevertheless, researchers make an attempt to represent the ideas of the participants. Although the narration may be true in its meaning, it is not always based on fact or objective reality but is a social construction and perception of what has happened to the narrator. At a time when people have little power to act – for instance when they have experienced an illness, breaking up of a relationship or another trauma in their lives – they attempt to explain this in a different language from that of those in power. To paraphrase Bruner (1991: 11): the patient tells the tale in 'life talk' (that is, in ordinary language) while the professional listens to it and translates it into professional language.

People often tell stories about their illness, particularly when the condition threatens their lives such as in an acute illness or when it restricts their daily activities and intrudes on normal life. Through illness and suffering, individuals often have an impaired sense of self, and on this they reflect. As it is of such importance to them, they attempt to tell their story to their significant others such as family and friends, employers and work colleagues. They tell it also to the health professionals, doctors and nurses. For each of these groups, ill people adopt different ways of telling.

Illness narratives differ from other stories in that they have an altered temporality while in ordinary tales the present connects effortlessly to the past and future. The future of those telling about their illness is sometimes uncertain and occasionally non-existent.

Frank (1995) proposes three different forms that narratives can take:

1. The *restitution* narrative
2. The *chaos* narrative
3. The *quest* narrative

> **Example**
>
> Whitehead (2006) demonstrates how people who live with myalgic encephalo-myelitis (ME) interpret their lives and conditions. Their stories about living with this condition reflect the restitution, chaos and quest narratives that were discussed by Frank. Their restitution narrative indicated the orientation of patients towards better health in the future; the chaos narrative focused on lack of control over their own fate; the quest narrative showed challenge, movement towards change and adaptation to the condition.

The different types of the narrative are not always distinct. Frank's justification for differentiating between narratives is to create 'listening devices' – the wish to sort out narrative threads in order to help listeners attend these stories, not to question the uniqueness of an individual's tale nor to give a unifying view of experience. In any case, most stories combine elements of all three forms of narrative. Each of these forms is a reflection of both the culture and the person of the storyteller.

The restitution narrative

The restitution narrative permeates the tale of those who have been ill. This includes the wish to get well soon. It can be connected with the concept of Parsons' (1951) sick role. Individuals are sick – they receive treatment and care – it is seen as their duty to get better – they will be better in the future. People emphasise not only their desire to get better, but they often claim that they are well and have achieved the state of normality: 'I am OK now'. Most restitution tales reflect Parsons' ideas about the sick role: the person inhabiting the role is not at fault; the patient is exempt from normal role responsibilities; he or she is expected to ask for expert help, comply with the advice and make every attempt to get better.

The restitution narrative reflects the predominant Western culture. Indeed, Frank claims that 'it is the culturally preferred narrative'. It takes the machine as a model: the machine breaks down, one takes it to a repair shop, and it is repaired. It is reconstructed, almost 'as good as new'. It also implies that people have control over their bodies and minds, and that the future is, to some extent, predictable.

> **Excerpt from restitution tale**
>
> My husband did all the housework
> Because I couldn't
> I had to leave my paid employment
> I was in such pain

> But I went to the doctor's
> He told me not to stay in bed all the time
> He prescribed some painkillers
> And then it got better
> Very slowly
> (paraphrased and condensed from an interview)

The chaos narrative

The chaos narrative suggests that the person will not ever get well again and encompasses his or her suffering in words and silences. This tale is not always tolerated in the predominant culture that focuses on cure (the 'machine' can be fixed or repaired). Perhaps a chaos narrative is easier to listen to for nurses because they focus on care. This narrative has no order and little structure, and it is told by people who have a serious chronic condition, or a life-threatening or terminal illness. This tale is more difficult to understand because it is never linear; it does not have a proper beginning, middle and end nor does it follow the same direction.

For the story to be effective, the storyteller must have some distance from it as the person in the middle of an experience finds it difficult to talk about it. There is iteration with narrators going backwards and forwards much of the time. The chaos narrative implies the narrators' lack of control over their lives. The illness generates complete 'biographical disruption'. Frank claims that health professionals should not hurry patients on when they are telling the tale as this denies the patients the right to their experience. He advises professionals to have tolerance for chaos within a story.

Excerpt from a chaos story

They don't know what it's like to be trapped in your own home for weeks on end and not be able to go anywhere. I only half accept it. My mind is telling me 'you should be doing this and that', but my body is telling me the exact opposite. I almost think it makes you become two people. (Holloway *et al.*, 2007)

The quest narrative

The quest narrative is told by people who are on a mission, who accept the challenge to learn something from their experience and feel that they are on a journey during which they change their identity. People think they must transmit to others what they have learned. They tell the story chronologically. Disability stories often contain the element of challenge and mission. We have all read of people with a serious illness who tell their story to the newspapers or on television 'to help others'. They often maintain that the illness has transformed them; the narrative has a moral dimension. Even though the condition may not improve, the ill person has control over his or her life.

Example of quest narrative

Thomas-MacLean (2004) demonstrates all three types of narratives and claims that in her research, the quest narrative is rare. She gives examples of the determination to experience life as much as possible by people who realise they have cancer, the different priorities they now have, and how they attempt to assist others in the same position.

Narrative interviewing

To obtain a narrative from participants, researchers use narrative interviews in which individuals can tell of their experience. The tale is not the experience itself but a representation of the experience as it is stored in the memory of the individual. Ochs and Capps (2002: 127) suggest 'remembering is a subjective event'; but participants see it as true, although it cannot necessarily be corroborated or verified. Nevertheless, the perception of the 'truth' of the event, treatment or care determines, or at least influences, both perception and action.

Narrative interviewing does not break a story into pieces and take it out of context, which other types of interview sometimes do; the latter 'often fracture the text' (Riessman, 1993: 3). Narrative interviewing has a main area of deep interest to participant and researcher. A stimulus or reminder provides the trigger for the story. Riessman does stress that narratives differ distinctly from other types of discourse such as question and answer interviews.

Jovchelovitch and Bauer (2000) state that the topic area must be both familiar and also experiential to the participant. The initial question must be broad enough to trigger a long story. For instance, 'Tell us about your time in hospital' might encourage patients into narrating a lengthy tale about what happened to them in the hospital setting. If the interviewer interrupts this story continually, it cannot flow. When the narrative is completed, however, the interviewer might ask some questions to develop the story by including the words of the participant. For instance: 'You said to me that time hung heavily while you were in hospital, can you tell me more about that?' Narrative interviews, like all other forms of interview, are affected by the relationship between the researcher and the participant, perhaps even more so as the researcher does not just ask questions to receive some answers but gives the participants control of the interview and as much time as they need to tell their story. Narrative interviews sometimes contain elements of question and answer exchange but mostly sections of narrative. It is not always possible to draw boundaries and discover where the narrative starts and finishes. There is a worrying tendency to carry out semi-structured interviews and call these narrative interviews, but in true narrative interviews, there is little interruption by the researcher.

Narrative interviews often focus on life histories or life stories as they show development of experience and perspective over time. One colleague for instance explored the experiences of international students who were studying for a master's degree at a university in Britain, to show whether there had been cultural adaptation and change for these students (Brown, 2008).

Narrative analysis

This whole chapter is about narrative analysis and what it implies. Riessman (2008) does not acknowledge a specific standard set of procedures for analysing the data but offers a choice to researchers. The actual data analysis of narratives is similar to that in other types of qualitative research and depends on the methodological framework. Polkinghorne (1995: 15) defines narrative analysis as 'the procedure through which the researcher organizes the data elements as into a coherent and developmental account'. The main steps include data transcription and reduction. The first step is the verbatim transcription of the narrative data (see the section on transcribing and sorting, in Chapter 17).

There are different approaches to analysing narrative data such as, for instance, thematic, structural and dialogic/performance analysis according to Riessman (2008) but other ways of analysing narratives are also legitimate.

Thematic or holistic analysis

The researcher analyses a narrative as a whole. In this type of analysis it is important to identify the main statements – the core of the experience that reflects and truly represents the narrators' accounts, even though they might not have given the story in a sequential and ordered way. It centres on the contents of the participants' story and the meanings inherent in it. The units of text in the transcription are reduced to a series of core sentences or ideas. The core statements of the experience integrate its various elements. This essence of experience is highly auditable in the examples below.

Example
Your life is pain
It stops you doing . . .
Going out

> Just trying to be a normal person
> I don't feel like doing anything
> All you want to do is to dwell on your own suffering
> Pain becomes an obstacle
> To any type of performance
> (excerpt from participants' tales in a pain experience study)

The essence of these statements and the core of the experience is that 'the pain takes over'. Other themes can be linked to this statement. Both Riessman and Elliott advocate this type of analysis in applied research, particularly for novice researchers; Riessman calls it thematic analysis and claims that it is the most straightforward. In this, researchers interpret and theorise from the whole story and its meaning, rather than breaking it into categories. The attention focuses on the contents, on 'what' is in the story, rather than 'how' it is told. Unlike analysis in grounded theory, the story is not taken apart but kept together for interpretation. (For further advice see Riessman 2008: 53–76.)

The term thematic analysis is not unambiguous in qualitative inquiry; here it is described the way Riessman uses it in her book.

Structural analysis

This type of analysis has its origin in the work of Labov and Waletzky (1967). It does not focus on contents but on form, 'how' the story is told, and it is tied to the text of the story. These sociologists developed a structural model of narrative in which they broke down the story and analysed its elements. These six elements are the following (adapted from Riessman 2008: 84; Elliott, 2005: 42. They describe the Labov/Waletzky model):

1. *Abstract:* The summary of the story matter
2. *Orientation:* The time, place, situation and participants
3. *The complicating action:* The sequence of events, i.e. the plot with its inherent crisis
4. *Evaluation:* The appraisal of the story and its meaning for the storyteller
5. *Resolution:* The outcome of the plot
6. *Coda:* The return to the present time

(For a detailed discussion see Riessman 2008: 77–103.)

Dialogic/performance analysis

The last of Riessman's approaches to analysis of data is that which she calls dialogic/performance analysis which is a 'broad and varied interpretive approach'

(Riessman, 2008: 105) to narrative. It investigates the emergence of interactive talk. This seems to be similar to conversation or discourse analysis where the focus is not only on the content and form but also on the people involved and to whom they orient their talk. She calls this a 'hybrid' form of analysis which takes components from other approaches. We would not recommend this type of analysis to novice researchers.

Visual analysis

The last type of Riessman's narrative analysis focuses on visual images. This is becoming popular and useful in illness narratives, in particular photographs, but sometimes also other images such as painted work, film or theatre (see also Chapter 15). The images can be specifically generated for a topic area or researchers might use existing images from the past or the present (photographs of medical conditions; films of interaction between health professionals and clients; paintings of disfigured people). Lorenz (2007) presented a paper of her work with a survivor of traumatic brain injury. In this she explored the story of a woman who took photographs of living with her injury over a period of five years. The woman showed her pictures to Lorenz and told her what they meant to her. A participant's story can, of course, be told with images, thus having a great visual impact, but the researcher's scholarly work needs analysis and interpretation, and this generally does involve some writing.

Problematic issues

One of the issues in narrative research is that of 'truth'. For the researcher it is difficult to decide on the veracity or falsehood of stories as they are retrospective and also rely on memory. Is the truth being told, or 'the truth as the participants see it'? Hidden motives might underlie the way the narrator tells the story. There are inconsistencies and tensions that lie within it. These problems need reflection and discussion. If the stories fit into the social context and framework, they become more credible, but of course the researcher may never know whether the story was accurate. These issues and the debates about it can become a topic of exploration. People select from their memory banks what they wish to remember, or they might forget what 'really' happened. However, the way the story is told, what is withheld or included, what is dramatised or forgotten, is important for the data analysis. Even ostensible 'untruths' might become significant.

The narratives of people and the storytelling by the researcher can be problematic in other ways. On the one hand, Lieblich et al. (1998) state that narratives are often seen more as art than as science because they are rooted in intuition and experience. On the other, they argue for a structured and coherent approach to storytelling.

Atkinson (1997) highlights three major issues:

1. Narratives of health and illness play an important part in medical sociology and anthropology (and we would add in nursing and healthcare).
2. Sometimes these narratives are based on inappropriate assumptions and on mistaken methodological and theoretical claims.
3. Narrative analyses must be systematic and should not be seen as single solutions to problems.

Atkinson criticises the unexamined assumptions that underlie these narratives in which researchers take a simplistic view of this form of research; the link between narratives and experiences is complex and they should not be seen as individualistic and romantic constructions of self but located within the context of interaction and social action. They are no more 'authentic' (a favourite word of narrative researchers), he claims, than other forms of research. Readers of narratives need 'thick description' of socio-cultural settings in which the narratives are embedded. Atkinson and Delamont (2006) add that overuse and uncritical acceptance is a recurrent problem in narrative inquiry. The research suffers from a lack of analysis and attention to social context and culture. Researchers, they suggest, should approach narrative research with 'a degree of caution and methodological scepticism, (p.18). Narrative research is not merely a re-telling or re-storying of narratives of personal experience that help participants to have their voice heard and represented but also detailed scholarly analysis and evaluation.

Frank (2000) answers Atkinson by presenting his own ideas on some of the issues important in narrative. He makes five major points:

1. He suggests that, although narrative and story are used interchangeably, people tell stories, they are not telling narratives. Narratives contain structures on which stories are based. Storytellers use these but are not fully aware of them.
2. People share their stories with the listener, and through this sharing of the story the listener becomes part of a relationship in which the story is told.
3. Stories create distance between storytellers and the threats they experience. They do perform the 'recuperative role' that Atkinson attributes to them.
4. Stories are not just the data for analysis to be transformed into text. They affirm the purpose of the story, namely forming relationships.
5. The stories of illness need to be heard. Frank (2000: 355) refutes 'Atkinson's dichotomy' between storytelling and story analysis; he maintains that 'any good story analysis accepts its place in relations of storytelling' and researchers can only listen inside a relationship with ethical and intellectual responsibilities.

Ultimately Frank sees storytelling in a different way from Atkinson. Frank (2000: 355) states emphatically: 'Storytellers do not call for their narratives to be analysed; they call for other stories in which experiences are shared, commonalities discovered and relationships built'.

The discussion about the purpose of narrative and storytelling is ongoing. Regardless of the stance of individual health researchers, they should be aware of the ongoing debate.

Conclusion

The writer, the participants and the reader together 'create' the final story. The researcher interprets the participants, stories in the research account, and the readers in turn read through the lenses of their own understanding. Although researchers interpret and edit the thoughts and ideas of the participants, 'even edited stories remain true' (Frank, 1995: 22). The 'good' research report entails collaboration between researcher and participant. The social and cultural world of narrators or researchers is not simple but complex; it always influences the story.

Summary

- Narratives are tales of experience or imagination and come naturally to human beings.
- Narratives are rarely simple or linear, and they often consist of many different stories rather than of a clearly defined tale.
- Illness narratives are expressions of illness, suffering and pain.
- Narratives are often tales of identity.
- Health professionals gain knowledge of the illness experience from their patients which assists in understanding the condition and the person.
- There are a number of different ways of analysing narrative data, and all are legitimate.
- In narrative inquiry the final story is constructed by participant, researcher and reader.
- Illness and professional narratives are always located in the socio-cultural context as well as in the individual.

References

Atkinson, P.A. (1997) Narrative turn or blind alley? *Qualitative Health Research*, 7 (3), 325–44.

Atkinson, P. & Delamont, S. (2006) Rescuing narrative from qualitative research. *Narrative Inquiry*, 16 (1), 164–72.

Brody, H. (2003) *Stories of Sickness*, 2nd edn. New York, NY, Oxford University Press.

Brown, L. (2008) *The Adjustment Journey of International Postgraduate Students at a University in England: An Ethnography*. Unpublished PhD thesis, Bournemouth University.

Brown, J. & Addington-Hall, J. (2008) How people with motor neurone disease talk about their illness: a narrative study. *Journal of Advanced Nursing*, **62** (2), 200–8.

Bruner, J. (1991) The narrative construction of reality. *Critical Inquiry*, **18** (1), 1–21.

Bruner, J. (2004) Life as narrative. *Social Research*, **71** (3), 691–710.

Carter, B. (2004) Pain narratives and narrative practitioners: a way of working 'in relation' with children experiencing pain. *Journal of Nursing Management*, **12** (3), 210–16.

Charon, R. (2006) The self-telling body. *Narrative Inquiry*, **16** (1), 191–200.

Elliott, J. (2005) *Using Narrative in Social Research: Qualitative and Quantitative Approaches*. London, Sage.

Frank, A.W. (1995) *The Wounded Storyteller: Body, Illness, and Ethics*. Chicago, IL, University of Chicago Press.

Frank, A.W. (2000) The standpoint of storyteller. *Qualitative Health Research*, **10** (3), 354–65.

Frid, I., Öhlen, J. & Bergbom, I. (2000) On the use of narratives in nursing research. *Journal of Advanced Nursing*, **32** (3), 695–703.

Gorman, D., Buikstra, E., Hegney, D. *et al.* (2007) Rural men and mental health: their experience and how they managed. *International Journal of Mental Health Nursing*, **16** (5), 298–306.

Greenhalgh, T. & Hurwitz, B. (1998) Why study narrative? In *Narrative Based Medicine* (eds T. Greenhalgh & B. Hurwitz), pp. 3–16. London, BMJ Books.

Holloway, I. & Freshwater, D. (2007) *Narrative Research in Nursing*. Oxford, Blackwell.

Holloway, I., Sofaer, B. & Walker, J. (2007) The stigmatisation of people with chronic pain. *Disability and Rehabilitation*, **29** (18), 1456–64.

Josselson, R. (1995) Imagining the real: empathy, narrative and the dialogic self. In *Interpreting Experience: The Narrative Study of Lives* (eds R. Josselson & A. Lieblich), pp. 27–44. Thousand Oaks, CA, Sage.

Jovchelovitch, S. & Bauer, M.W. (2000) Narrative interviewing. In *Qualitative Interviewing with Text, Image and Sound* (eds M.W. Bauer & G. Gaskell), pp. 57–74. London, Sage.

Kellas, J.K. & Manusov, V. (2003) What's in a story? The relationship between narrative completeness and adjustment to relationship dissolution. *Journal of Social and Personal Relationships*, **20** (3), 285–307.

Kleinman, A. (1988) *The Illness Narratives: Suffering, Healing and the Human Condition*. New York, NY, Basic Books.

Labov, W. (1972) *Sociolinguistic Patterns*. Philadelphia, PA, University of Pennsylvania Press.

Labov, W. & Waletzky, J. (1967) Oral versions of personal experience. In *Essays on the Verbal and Visual Arts* (ed. J. Helm). Seattle, WA, University of Washington Press.

Lieblich, A., Tuval-Mashiach, R. & Zilber, T. (eds). (1998) *Narrative Research: Reading, Analysis and Interpretation*. Thousand Oaks, CA, Sage.

Lorenz, L. S. (2007) *Living with traumatic brain injury: Narrative analysis of a survivor's photographs and interview*. Poster Presentation, 26th Annual Conference, Brain Injury Association of Massachusetts, Marlborough, MA, March 22.

McCance, T.V., McKenna, H.P. & Boore, J.R.P. (2001) Exploring caring using narrative methodology: an analysis of the approach. *Journal of Advanced Nursing*, **33** (3), 350–6.

McIlfrick, S., Sullivan, K., McKenna, H. & Parahoo, K. (2007) Patients' experience of having chemotherapy in a day hospital setting. *Journal of Advanced Nursing*, **59** (3), 264–74.

Ochs, E. & Capps, L. (2002) Narrative authenticity. In *Qualitative Research Methods* (ed. D. Weinberg), pp. 127–32. Malden, MA, Blackwell.

Paley, J. & Eva, G. (2005) Narrative vigilance: the analysis of stories in health care. *Nursing Philosophy*, **6** (2), 83–97.

Parsons, T. (1951) *The Social System*. New York, NY, Free Press.

Pennebaker, J.W. (2000) Telling stories: the healing benefits of narrative. *Literature and Medicine*, **19** (1), 3–18.

Polkinghorne, D.E. (1995) Narrative configuration in qualitative analysis. In *Life History and Narrative* (eds J.A. Hatch & R. Wisniewski), pp. 5–23. London, The Falmer Press.

Richardson, L. (1990) Narrative and sociology. *Journal of Contemporary Ethnography*, **19** (1), 116–35.

Ricoeur, P. (1984) *Time and Narrative*, Vol. 1. Chicago, IL, Chicago University Press.

Ricoeur, P. (1991) *Time and Narrative*, Vol. 2. Chicago, IL, Chicago University Press.

Riessman, C.K. (1993) *Narrative Analysis*. Newbury Park, CA, Sage.

Riessman, C.K. (2008) *Narrative Methods in the Human Sciences*. Thousand Oaks, CA, Sage.

Riley, T. & Hawe, P. (2005) Researching practice: the methodological case for narrative inquiry. *Health Education Research*, **20** (2), 226–36.

Sakalys, J.A. (2000) The political role of illness narratives. *Journal of Advanced Nursing*, **31** (6), 1469–75.

Sandelowski, M. (1996) Truth/storytelling in nursing inquiry. In *Truth in Nursing Inquiry* (eds J.F. Kikuchi, H. Simmons & D. Romyn), pp. 111–24. Thousand Oaks, CA, Sage.

Skultans, V. (1998) Anthropology and narrative. In *Narrative Based Medicine* (eds T. Greenhalgh & B. Hurwitz), pp. 225–33. London, BMJ Books.

Sparkes, A. (1996) The fatal flaw: a narrative of the fragile body-self. *Qualitative Inquiry*, **2** (4), 463–94.

Thomas-MacLean, R. (2004) Understanding breast cancer stories via Frank's narrative types. *Social Science and Medicine*, **48** (9), 1647–57.

Whitehead, L. (2006) Quest, chaos and restitution: living with chronic fatigue syndrome/myalgic encephalomyelitis. *Social Science and Medicine*, **62** (9), 2236–45.

Further reading

Adams, M., Squire, C. & Tamboukou, M. (eds). (2008) *Doing Narrative Research*. Los Angeles, CA, Sage.

Atkinson, P.A. & Delamont, S. (eds). (2006) *Narrative Methods*, 4 Volumes. London, Sage.

Charon, R. (2006) *Narrative Medicine: Honoring the Stories of Illness*. New York, NY, Oxford University Press.

Clandinin, D.J. (ed). (2007) *Handbook of Qualitative Inquiry: Mapping a Methodology*. Thousand Oaks, CA, Sage.

Harter, L.M., Japp, P.M. & Becker, C.S. (eds). (2005) *Narratives, Health and Healing: Communication Theory, Research and Practice*. Mahwah, NJ, Lawrence Erlbaum.

Hatch, J.A. & Wisniewski, R. (eds). (1995) *Life History and Narrative*. London, The Falmer Press.

Hydén, L. & Brockmeyer, J. (2008) *Health, Illness and Culture: Broken Narratives*. New York, NY, Routledge.

Josselson, R. & Lieblich, A. (eds). (1999) *Making Meaning of Narratives*. Thousand Oaks, CA, Sage.

CHAPTER 13

Phenomenology

Phenomenology is an approach to philosophy and not specifically a method of inquiry; this has often been misunderstood. Indeed, Caelli (2001: 275–6) argues: 'Because phenomenology is first and foremost philosophy, the approach employed to pursue a particular study should emerge from the philosophical implications inherent in the question'. To give a basis to phenomenological research, we have traced the complex history of the philosophy of phenomenology and then discussed its adaptation as a qualitative research approach in nursing, midwifery and other health professions. This might set the scene for the phenomenological research approach. As a method of inquiry, phenomenological research has not often been carried out at undergraduate level in the past but has recently been much more popular particularly in postgraduate health studies. Unfortunately, some phenomenological researchers, especially novices, neglect the philosophical origin of the method.

Various ways of 'doing' phenomenology exist. They all have similar aims however; their data gathering and analytic procedures overlap. The major aim of a descriptive phenomenological research approach is to generate a description of a phenomenon of everyday experience to achieve an understanding of its essential structure while hermeneutic inquiry emphasises understanding more than description and relies on interpretation (see Giorgi, 1992).

Descriptive phenomenologists, such as Giorgi and Todres in particular, mainly use the philosophy of Husserl and his followers, others incorporate the ideas of Heidegger and his colleagues who believe that phenomenology is interpretive, for instance Van Manen (1990, 1998) or Rapport (2005). Either approach can be used; researchers have overlapping though not congruent ideas on the way of doing phenomenological research (see later in this chapter).

Essentially, phenomenology has three major streams: the *descriptive* phenomenology of Edmund Husserl (1859–1938); the *hermeneutic* phenomenology of Martin Heidegger (1889–1976); and the *existentialist* phenomenology of Merleau-Ponty (1908–1961) and Jean-Paul Sartre (1905–1980). There are ongoing philosophical debates about the distinctions and overlaps between these streams, but the differing emphases indicated in this chapter generally remain.

The term 'phenomenology' derives from the Greek word *phainomenon* meaning 'appearance' (the concept was first developed by the philosopher Kant). Phenomenological philosophy is partly about the epistemological question – about the theory of knowledge – of 'how we know', the relationship of the person who knows and what can be known (McLeod, 2001). It is also connected to the ontological question: 'what is *being*'. The ontological question is concerned with the nature of reality and our knowledge about it, 'how things really are'. Giorgi and Giorgi (2003) suggest that phenomenology is 'a study of consciousness.'

As philosophy in general, the study of phenomenology is not immediately understandable. It has, however, informed the human sciences and in particular phenomenological psychology where it is used within qualitative research.

It is useful to trace the history of phenomenology. The following section will outline the background of phenomenology from so-called 'continental philosophy', the subsequent ideas Edmund Husserl (initially based on Brentano), as well as the later development of the phenomenological movement and schools of phenomenology.

Intentionality and the early stages of phenomenology

Phenomenology begins with Husserl who was the core figure in the development of phenomenology as a modern movement. It is important, however, to trace the earlier history of phenomenology in the influence of Franz Brentano (1838–1917) on the work of Husserl. Brentano was part of the preparatory phase of this movement (Cohen *et al.*, 2000).

One of the main themes of phenomenology is the concept of *intentionality*. Husserl takes this term from Brentano though he does not use it in the same way. Giorgi (1997: 237) describes the notion of intentionality as Husserl sees it. In Husserl's work, intentionality is 'the essential feature of consciousness' which is directed towards an object. When human beings are conscious, they are always conscious of something. Consciousness in phenomenology relates to the person's consciousness of the world (Langridge, 2007)

This critical statement concerning the notion of intentionality shows the complexity of any attempt to define the act of conscious thought. In the human sciences, according to Giorgi, consciousness overcomes the dilemma of the subject–object debate, the mind–body relationship which is understood holistically and structurally. Philosophers, psychologists and natural scientists, including doctors and psychiatrists, neither agree nor have firmly established what exactly consciousness is, or what is the true relationship between mind and body. The ideas presented in this chapter cannot resolve the mind–body problem. However, it is useful to note that phenomenology is, in fact, one approach that attempts to do this. Priest places phenomenology within mind–body theories arising from the following:

- Descartes' dualism which separates mind and body.
- So called logical behaviourism: this is a belief that everything concerns behaviour.
- Notions of idealism: all that exists can be explained in terms of the mind.
- Materialism: everything in the universe can be explained in terms of matter.
- Functionalism: everything is a kind of cause and effect. The mind is given a stimulus and responds physically or behaviourally.
- So-called 'double aspect theory': the physical and mental are, in fact, merely aspects of something else, another reality, outside notions of the mental and the physical.
- The phenomenological view: this is an attempt to describe lived experiences, without making previous assumptions about the objective reality of those experiences.

Whilst these ideas are presented as theories within philosophy, phenomenology is, in fact, also a practice. It is this practice that is so exciting for nursing, health and social care alike, because it offers the possibility of '...characterizing the contents of experience just as they appear to consciousness with a view to capturing their essential features' (Priest, 1991: 183).

Phases and history of the movement

As has already been stated, phenomenology has philosophical origins. In 1960, the first edition of Spiegelberg's review of the history of the phenomenological movement was published. He described what he termed three phases in the movement, the preparatory, the German and the French phases. Cohen (1987) summarises these in a paper giving her account of the history and importance of phenomenological research for nursing and stated that Brentano influenced this preparatory phase.

The German phase

The German phase involved primarily Husserl and later Heidegger. Cohen *et al.* (2000) discuss Husserl's contribution to the movement and highlight his centrality for phenomenology, his search for rigour, his criticism of positivism (all knowledge is derived from the senses – linked to scientific inquiry of observation and experiment) and his concepts of *Anschauung* (phenomenological intuition) and phenomenological reduction. In the former, a different kind of experience is apparent, closely involved with the imagination. Experience suggests a relationship with something real, such as an event, while *Anschauung* can also occur in imagination or memory. The latter is a process to suspend attitudes, beliefs and suppositions in order to properly examine what is present. Husserl termed this part of phenomenological reduction *epoché* (from the Greek, meaning 'suspension of belief'). Bracketing (a mathematical term) is the name given by Husserl to this process of suspending beliefs and prior assumptions about a phenomenon. Bracketing and phenomenological reduction are important features of the method, the actual 'doing' of phenomenology. The complex approach of various forms of phenomenology and the idea of bracketing in Husserl's and Heidegger's work has been debated in many books and articles explaining phenomenology to and for nurses both by well-known and new researchers, such as, for instance, Jasper (1994), Crotty (1996), Paley (1997), Berg *et al.* (2006), Streubert Speziale and Rinaldi Carpenter (2007).

Husserl's major contribution to phenomenology consisted of three elements in particular: intentionality, essences and phenomenological reduction (bracketing).

Several important elements of phenomenology were developed by colleagues and students of Husserl. The major concepts are intersubjectivity and the idea of 'lifeworld' (*Lebenswelt*). Intersubjectivity is about the existence of a number of subjectivities which are shared by a community, that is, by individual persons who share a common world. The intersubjective world is accessible because humans have empathy for others. The way of making sense of experience is essentially intersubjective (Schwandt, 2007).

The concept of lifeworld (*Lebenswelt*) is about the lived experience that is central to modern phenomenology. Human beings do not often take into account the commonplace and ordinary; indeed, they do not even notice it. Phenomenological inquiry is the approach needed to help examine and recognise the lived experience that is commonly taken for granted.

The next stage in the German phase of phenomenology involved Heidegger who was an assistant to Husserl for a while. Due to the upsurge of interest (particularly in North America) in using the phenomenological framework for nursing and midwifery research, Heidegger is often mentioned in the work of a number of health researchers over the years. Benner's (1984) phenomenological research uncovered excellence and power in clinical nursing practice, and she references, amongst others, Heidegger. Her well-known study had a profound influence, particularly on nursing research. Heidegger's changed direction from Husserlian phenomenology and his break with it occurred in the way he developed the notion of *Dasein* which is explained fully in his work *Being and Time* in 1927 and translated into English in 1962. Heidegger's concern was to ask questions about the nature of being and about temporality (being is temporal). In this sense, he was interested in ontological ideas. Heidegger's notion of *Dasein* is an explanation of the nature of being and existence and, as such, a concept of personhood. Leonard (1994) makes five main points concerning a Heideggerian phenomenological view of the person. These are as follows.

1. The person has a world, which comes from culture, history and language. Often this world is so inclusive that it is overlooked and taken for granted until we reflect and analyse.

2. The person has a being in which things have value and significance. In this sense, persons can only be understood by a study of the context of their lives.
3. The person is self-interpreting. A person has the ability to make interpretations about knowledge. The understanding gained becomes part of the self.
4. The person is embodied. This is a different view from the Cartesian, which is about possessing a body. The notion of embodiment is the view that the body is the way we can potentially experience the action of ourselves in the world.
5. The person 'is' in time. This requires a little more elaboration as outlined below.

Heidegger had a different notion from the one of traditional time, which is perceived to flow in a linear fashion, with an awareness of 'now'. According to Leonard (1994) he used the word 'temporality' which denotes a new way of perceiving time in terms of including the *now*, the *no longer* and the *not yet*.

As well as these ideas, Heidegger developed phenomenology into interpretive philosophy that became the basis for hermeneutical methods of inquiry (in classical Greek mythology Hermes was the transmitter of the messages from the Gods to the mortals). This often involved interpreting the messages for the recipients to aid understanding. Hermeneutics developed as a result of translating literature from different languages, or where direct access to authoritative texts, such as the Bible, was difficult. Hermeneutics became the theory of interpretation and developed into its present form as the theory of the interpretation of meaning. Text means language. Gadamer (1975) suggests that human beings' experience of the world is connected with language.

Linking the ideas of hermeneutics with phenomenology, Koch (1995: 831) states:

'Heidegger (1962) declares nothing can be encountered without reference to the person's background understanding, and every encounter entails an interpretation based on the person's background, in its 'historicality'. The framework of interpretation that we use is the foreconception in which we grasp something in advance.'

Heidegger's goes beyond mere description to interpretation. Heideggerian interpretive phenomenology is a popular research approach in nursing. This form of research explores the meaning of being a person in the world. Rather than suspending presuppositions, researchers examine them and make them explicit.

The French phase

Cohen (1987) argues that Heidegger's major contribution to the phenomenological movement was his influence on French philosophy. She points out that the main figures in this phase were Gabriel Marcel (1889–1973), Jean-Paul Sartre (1905–1980) and Maurice Merleau-Ponty (1908–1961). Marcel did not call himself a phenomenologist but viewed phenomenology as an introduction to analysing the notion of *being*.

Jean-Paul Sartre was the most influential figure in the movement but again did not want the label phenomenologist; rather he was termed as an *existentialist*. Phenomenological concepts and terms are difficult to grasp and it is often difficult to find a starting point. Understanding of terminology can be obviously further enhanced in progression from general to specific.

The idea of existence and essence are from Sartre; his famous and often quoted phrase is 'existence precedes essence'. This is Sartre's idea that a person's actual consciousness and behaviour (existence) comes before character (essence) (Cohen, 1987). In this sense, research would focus on real and concrete thoughts and behaviour before imaginary or idealised qualities or essences. The notion of intentionality features also in Sartre's work.

Merleau-Ponty's interest in phenomenology focused on perception and the creation of a science of human beings (for the purpose of this chapter it is not necessary to develop this further).

Another major figure in French phenomenology is Paul Ricoeur. Spiegelberg (1984) argues that Ricoeur's phenomenology is primarily descriptive and based on a Husserlian eidetic concern with essential structures. Ricoeur, like Gadamer, focuses on the intersubjective and on issues of language and communication.

There are then different approaches within phenomenology. Indeed most researchers acknowledge that phenomenology is not a single and integrated philosophical direction. In the next stage of this chapter, we will examine the schools of phenomenology outlined by Cohen and Omery (1994).

Schools of phenomenology

It has been shown thus far that phenomenology is an approach within continental philosophy. For purposes of qualitative research however, phenomenology has also been adapted and used as a framework within the so-called interpretive tradition that broadly includes grounded theory and ethnography as Lowenberg (1993) points out. She states: 'Basic to all these approaches is the recognition of the interpretive and constitutive cognitive processes inherent in all social life' (p. 58) and shows that there are many 'quandaries in terminology' which lead to misinterpretations in the nursing and education research literature, and sometimes in social research. She argues that there is a problem with phenomenology, the distinctions between the assumptions that lie behind the theories (e.g. Husserl and Heidegger) and the actual method, the 'doing' of phenomenology. Part of the purpose of this chapter is to try to unravel these perplexities.

A useful outline of phenomenological philosophy, guiding research and describing the development of schools with different approaches, is presented by Cohen and Omery (1994). The broad goal in each school remains the same, that is, to gain knowledge and insight about a phenomenon.

Three major schools can be found, but there is overlap and linkage between them. The first is the *Duquesne* School, guided by Husserl's ideas about eidetic structure (so called because its followers worked at one stage in time at Duquesne University). The second school is about the *interpretation* of phenomena (Heideggerian hermeneutics). The combination of both is found in the *Dutch* School of phenomenology.

The Duquesne School focuses mostly on the notion of description. Giorgi (1985) states that social scientists should describe what presents itself to them without adding or subtracting from it. His advice is to acknowledge the evidence and not go beyond the data although he believes that description cannot ever be complete. The 'interpretation of phenomena' approach concentrates on taken-for-granted practices and common meanings, whilst the Dutch School aims to combine both description and interpretation.

The phenomenological research process: doing phenomenology

Giorgi has always recognised the problem in applying a philosophical approach to a practice discipline. This means that new researchers are often uncertain of how to proceed when wishing to use phenomenological research. While developing ideas about complementarities of different phenomenological approaches as a philosophical basis for nursing research, Todres and Wheeler (2001: 2) discuss some philosophical distinctions in the approach to human experience that need to be included when carrying out practical research. They approach three areas in which they show that phenomenology, hermeneutics and existentialism have a contribution to make to health research: *grounding, reflexivity* and *humanisation*.

Grounding

Grounding means taking the lifeworld as a starting point. It includes the everyday world of common experiences. The lifeworld is more complex than that which can be said about it and contains inherent tensions. Lived experience for Husserl is the *ground* of inquiry. There is also a *need* for inquiry. The commonplace, taken for granted, becomes a phenomenon when it becomes questionable. The understanding of the lifeworld demands an open-minded attitude in which prior assumptions are bracketed so that descriptions can clarify meanings and relationships.

Reflexivity and positional knowledge

Hermeneutics has added certain dimensions to phenomenological research. Gadamer (1975) developed Heidegger's ideas about interpretation as integral to human existence. Human beings are self-reflective persons who are based in everyday life. Their personal relationships and experience happen in a temporal and historical context and depend on their position in the world. Preconceptions and provisional knowledge are always revised in the light of experience and reflection. The text is always open to multiple interpretations because researchers or reflective persons are involved in their own relationships with the world and others.

Humanisation and the language of experience

Human beings cannot be separated from their relationships in the world. Heidegger's notion of *Dasein*, being-in-the-world, entails a relationship between being human and being-in-the-world. Researchers search for fundamental and general categories of human existence that illuminate experiences that reveal a world. Heidegger (Todres and Wheeler, 2001: 5) reflects on fundamental structures that characterise the essential qualities of being-in-the-world such as

- the way in which the body occurs;
- the way the co-constituting of temporal structures occurs;
- the way the meaningful word of place and things occurs;
- the way the quality of interpersonal relationships occurs.

This is how Heidegger shows that body, time and space reflect the qualities of human presence rather than being notions of quantitative measurement.

From these ideas Todres and Wheeler (2001) conclude that phenomenology *grounds* research and stays away from theoretical abstraction. They also claim that hermeneutics adds the notion of *reflexivity*, which makes researchers ask questions meaningful and relevant in cultural, temporal and historical contexts. Lastly, these writers state that the ontological existential dimension *humanises* the research so it is not merely technical and utilitarian.

Phenomenological research focuses on the lifeworld, lived experiences which are described by the participants who reflect on them. These experiences might include 'the experience of diabetes', 'being a first-time father', 'living with epilepsy', and similar phenomena. From these experiences phenomenologists gain insight and extract common themes – essential structures or essences – which human beings have in common and that go beyond individual cases (Todres and Holloway, 2006). Thus, a phenomenological study presents the essential structure of a phenomenon. Here the concept of bracketing becomes useful for the researcher who, as said before, must exclude (bracket) prior assumptions gained through experience or literature to see the phenomenon with an open mind. It is, however, not sufficient to confirm that bracketing has occurred; the researcher also has to show how and where this took place. This is important for the early stages of the inquiry, while later on the researcher has a dialogue with the literature about the phenomenon that is being illuminated. Bracketing means that the researchers can experience things as fresh and new as they do not prejudge. Husserl uses the term epoché (from the Greek for cessation) to characterise this suspension of judgement or bracketing. This phenomenological reduction is necessary to gain the essence of a phenomenon.

Van Manen (1990: 5) outlines some of the important features that characterise phenomenological research.

- Phenomenological research is the study of lived experience.
- Phenomenological research is the explication of phenomena as they present themselves to consciousness.
- Phenomenological research is the study of essences or meaning (depending on the specific approach).
- Phenomenological research is the description of the experiential meanings we live as we live them.
- Phenomenological research is the human scientific study of phenomena.
- Phenomenological research is the attentive practice of thoughtfulness.
- Phenomenological research is a search for what it means to be human.
- Phenomenological research is a poetizing activity.

The latter means that reflexive writing and aesthetic presentation is an essential and integral element in phenomenological research. Indeed, it is crucial. Giorgi and Giorgi remind the researcher that phenomenological inquiry should stay as close as possible to the phenomenon to be illuminated. To begin the process of phenomenological inquiry, researchers obviously need an area of interest, puzzlement, concern or a gap in general or specific knowledge about a phenomenon. 'Practising science', as Giorgi (2000) calls it, is distinctly different from 'doing philosophy'. Indeed he criticises researchers who write on nursing research, such as Crotty (1996) or Paley (1997) for not distinguishing between the two. Giorgi sees value in the use of phenomenological research in nursing but suggests that this means scientific work rather than doing philosophy. (Giorgi's engagement with the ideas of Crotty and Paley is important but cannot be followed up here.)

In all approaches the researcher has a responsibility to justify the type of theoretical framework (e.g. symbolic interactionism, phenomenology or any other) and specify and outline the approach to data analysis (e.g. grounded theory for the former, or Colaizzi's (1978) and other writers' approaches as regards the latter). Holloway and Todres (2003) argue that there is a need to avoid 'method-slurring' and preserve the integrity of the approach. This is particularly important in phenomenology because of its distinctive underlying philosophy.

In data analysis for phenomenological inquiry, the researcher aims to uncover and produce a description of the lived experience. The procedural steps to achieve this aim vary with the approach taken by the researcher in terms of the three main types of phenomenology previously outlined. Various researchers have developed approaches to data analysis that follow the requirements of bracketing, intuition and reflection. One of these, Colaizzi (1978), outlined a seven-stage process of analysis. Although there has been criticism of pioneering work such as this (Hycner, 1985), this particular process of analysis for the eidetic approach of phenomenology is both logical and credible. Hycner (1985: 279) states, however, that 'there is an appropriate reluctance on the part of phenomenologists to focus too much on specific steps in research methods for fear that they will become verified as they have in the natural sciences'. There are, however, several interpretations of the data analysis process depending on the school of phenomenology chosen. For example Streubert Speziale and Rinaldi Carpenter (2007: 83) outline the different procedural steps from other, earlier, authors, such as Van Kaam (1959), Paterson and Zderad (1976), Colaizzi (1978), Van Manen (1990) and Giorgi (1985).

Procedures for data collection and analysis

The data collection starts with the specific and proceeds to the general. For instance in their search for the description of a phenomenon, researchers attempt to ask for a concrete example of their everyday experience of this phenomenon within its context. For instance, a first-time father might be asked: 'What was this experience like for you?' A study of the phenomenon of backpain might start with the researcher's question: 'Describe a situation in which your backpain occurred.' While asking these questions, the researcher brackets prior assumptions and presuppositions. During the rest of the interview the researcher will focus on clarifying the phenomenon. Many such interviews will uncover the essential structure or essence of the phenomenon which is common to all participants.

Many phenomenological research studies originate in the Duquesne School and use the approaches from one of the following authors, Colaizzi (1978), Giorgi (1985) or Van Kaam (1966). Although these authors are still popular – especially Giorgi – who made this his life's work – other approaches, in particularly interpretive phenomenology, have also flourished, though analysis is often similar to that of the following authors. Colaizzi advocates seven steps, Giorgi four and Van Kaam six but many of these steps are similar or overlap, and they are never rigidly applied.

In selecting a school of phenomenology, the researcher will be guided by the approach to the most appropriate procedural steps in data analysis. For the purposes of this chapter, we outline and discuss those developed by Giorgi (1985, 2000) and Colaizzi (1978). It is, however, a decision for student and supervisor (novice or expert researcher) to select the approach best suited for the phenomenon under investigation and to utilise the appropriate literature to guide the research methodology and analysis.

Both Giorgi (1985, 2000, 2008) and Colaizzi (1978) argue for a descriptive approach and provide a method for data analysis, for instance from transcribed tapes of interviews with participants. These are just examples of qualitative data analyses.

Giorgi's steps for analysis are as follows.

1. The entire description is read to get a sense of the whole. This is important as phenomenology is holistic and focuses initially on the 'Gestalt', that is the whole.
2. Once the Gestalt has been grasped, researchers attempt to constitute the parts of the description, make and differentiate between 'meaning units' – as the parts are labelled (these parts have to be relevant) – and centre on the phenomenon under study. It is important that these units are not theory-laden but the language of everyday life is used.
3. When the meaning units have been illuminated, the researcher actively transforms the original data and expresses the insight that is contained in them and highlights common themes which are illustrated by quotes from participants.
4. Giorgi suggests making the implicit explicit and to go from a concrete situation as an example to demonstrate of what this situation is an example. The researcher integrates the transformed meaning units into a consistent statement about the participants' experience across individual sources. This is called the *structure* of experience. In other words, it is the essence of the experience.

Although the researchers uncover structures of experience, finding it from the themes generated by individuals, they look at the phenomenon rather than focusing on individual narratives. This does not mean that there is no interest in individuals, but the search is for the overall structure of experience.

Colaizzi's seven-stage process is another approach to data analysis for the researcher but similar to that of Giorgi. The seven-stage process of analysis occurs as follows.

1. Read all of the subject's [sic] descriptions (conventionally termed *protocols*) in order to acquire a feeling for them, and to make sense out of them.

2. Return to each description and extract from them phrases or sentences which directly pertain to the investigated phenomenon; this is known as *extracting significant statements*.
3. Try to spell out the meaning of each significant statement; these are known as *formulated meanings*.
4. Repeat the above for each description and organise the aggregate formulated meanings into *clusters of themes*.
   (a) Refer these clusters of themes back to the original protocols in order to *validate* them.
   (b) At this point, discrepancies may be noted among and/or between the various clusters; some themes may flatly contradict others, or may appear to be totally unrelated to others. (The researcher is advised by Colaizzi to refuse the temptation to ignore data or themes which do not fit).
5. The results of everything so far are integrated into an *exhaustive description* of the investigated topic.
6. An effort is made to formulate the exhaustive description of the investigated phenomenon in as unequivocal a statement of *identification of its fundamental structure* as possible. This has often been termed as an essential structure of the phenomenon.
7. A final validating step can be achieved by returning to each participant, and, in either a single interview session or a series of interviews, asking the subject about the findings thus far.

These are descriptions of procedural steps adapted from Colaizzi (1978: 59–61).

Colaizzi encourages researchers to be flexible with these stages, and we have found this to be useful. For example, we have encouraged students to take the exhaustive description back to informants, rather than the final, essential structure, because it appears to be more recognisable for them for comment. This ensures rigour. A formal member check is not useful for phenomenologists as they translate the research to a more theoretical level, that of the researcher. It can be seen that many of the steps overlap in the analysis process of different writers on phenomenological research. However, many writers, including van Manen, have a less structured approach and focus on the general insight that phenomenological research offers. In any case, all inquiry goes beyond the formal steps. When Todres (2000: 43) discusses a specific example of phenomenological research, he lists some signposts that go beyond mechanical stages, and they could gain major importance for other researchers.

The presentation of his discoveries involves the following:

- It will go beyond a definition or a series of statements; it will reflect a narrative coherence.
- It will tell us something that connects with universal human qualities so that the reader can relate personally to the themes.

- It will tell a story with which readers can empathise in imaginative ways.
- It contributes to new understanding.
- It will clarify and illuminate the topic to help the reader make sense of it without wholly possessing it.

These signposts are significant for phenomenological studies. They show that the search for the essence of a phenomenon and its meaning within a defined context is not merely a technique or a series of mechanical steps but an exploration of meaning.

Phenomenology and health research

Streubert Speziale and Rinaldi Carpenter (2007) suggest that professional nursing orientation towards holistic care provides the background for deciding whether to undertake phenomenological research. This should also be so for other health researchers. The holistic perspective, coupled with the study of lived experience, provides the foundation for phenomenological research. These authors like others advise the researcher to ask several questions about the intended topic. For example: is there some need for clarity concerning a phenomenon? Has there been anything published in relation to this, or is there a need for further inquiry? If there is, the health researcher should question whether inquiry concerning the lived experience is the most appropriate approach to collecting data. As the accounts of those experiencing the phenomenon are the primary data, the researcher needs to consider that this will yield both rich and descriptive data. Streubert Speziale and Rinaldi Carpenter argue that researchers examine their own style, preference and ability to engage with this approach to research. Further considerations for the research process concern completion and presentation of the study to relevant audiences.

Todres and Holloway (2006) see that this research approach yields very rich data, gives deep insight into the lifeworld of participants and does not stay on the surface. The findings resonate with researchers and readers alike because they concern essential perspectives of human beings. This is one of the reasons why participant observation is problematic as that is seen from the perspective of the researcher, an 'outsider' to the research, while interviews give the ideas of the 'insider'. Researchers need very varied skills, both scientific and communicative; they should be able to do 'good' and rigorous research as well as communicate the findings and meanings in a language that captures the richness of the lifeworld of the participants. It is also stated by Dowling (2007) that phenomenological research is complex and not easy although it can be successful in exploring the 'human condition' if attempted in a rigorous way and if health researchers place it within its philosophical base. It would be difficult for novice researchers to carry out phenomenological research.

Topics for phenomenological approaches

Wojnar and Swanson (2007) suggest that healing and caring are important phenomena to be illuminated, discussed and understood by health researchers.

Appropriate areas for phenomenological research include topics that are important to life experience such as happiness, fear and anxiety or what it means to be a physiotherapist, a doctor or a community midwife. There are other health and illness-related topics such as the experience of having a myocardial infarction, an acute illness or chronic pain.

Recently, phenomenological research in healthcare has become very popular. It covers a range of topic areas including caring, the lived experience of patients, meaningful life experiences and the elderly, the phenomenon of living with breast cancer, infertility, first-time motherhood, chronic illness and relationships in healthcare, action learning, addiction, violence and therapeutic touch. The phenomenological approach can also be used in professional education. The following are other examples of phenomenological research.

Example of descriptive phenomenological research in nursing

Billhult *et al.* (2007) aimed to describe the feelings of ten participants about their lived experience of treatment with massage in a study which examined this type of care after breast cancer surgery. The treatment with massage was the phenomenon to be explored. First, individual variations in meaning were examined, and then researchers searched for the essential invariant meaning. The researchers used Giorgi's methods of analysis and found that participants took a retreat from the feeling of uneasiness about chemotherapy which massage offered them.

Examples of hermeneutic research
Example 1

My research investigated factors influencing clinical decisionmaking by cardiopulmonary physiotherapists in acute care settings. I was interested in why physiotherapists make the decisions they do. I recruited 14 participants from across a range of clinical experience – novice, intermediate and experienced. I chose to use qualitative methods as I wanted to deeply understand the nature of their decisionmaking. The philosophical and methodological framework that I used was hermeneutics as I aimed to interpret the descriptions of decisionmaking that I collected. I also liked the recognition that hermeneutics pays to prior understanding. I had practised as a cardiopulmonary physiotherapist and rather than bracket this I wanted to be able to deal with this in the research process. My data collection methods were observation and semi-structured interviews. The outcomes of my research were an understanding of the factors that influence decisionmaking but also the decision-making process itself and also the effects of experience.

Megan Smith

Charles Sturt University, Albury Australia

(Dr Megan Smith sent this example from physiotherapy by email on October 2008)

Example 2

In a study on nurse practitioners' experience of role transition and professional autonomy, Mercer (2008) explored the phenomenon of autonomy and its relationship to professional practice. He used the phenomenological hermeneutical approach which placed emphasis on the meaning of the participants' lived experience and through hermeneutic analysis developed an understanding of the phenomenon.

Example of existentialist phenomenological research

Thomas and Johnson (2000) published their research which was based on the ideas of Merleau-Ponty who focuses on the existential world as it is lived and experienced and on the body as 'a fundamental category of human existence'. They involved 13 female and male participants who were asked to share their experience of chronic pain. These participants showed – unlike individuals in many other chronic pain studies – that they saw chronic pain as a major burden and often experienced hopelessness focusing on bodily experiences which became the centre of their existence.

These examples illustrate the breadth of phenomenological research and the potential of this method of inquiry. For health professionals, phenomenological research is a rewarding enterprise. It is not easy because researchers have to understand the underlying philosophies before carrying out a study and decide which type of phenomenological approach to use.

Choice of approach: descriptive or interpretive phenomenology

Researchers usually choose one of these phenomenological approaches. They are similar and many of the ideas overlap as they both have their roots in Husserl's philosophy. Both start with the lifeworld, 'the lived experience' of the participants and focus initially on individual and unique everyday experiences and concrete examples of the phenomenon to be researched. After reflection and analysis, more general ideas about the phenomenon emerge. As stated before,

Giorgi, his many students and followers who are descriptive phenomenologists (such as, for instance, Les Todres, Barbro Giorgi and Karin Dahlberg) stay close to Husserl while hermeneutic phenomenologists, such as Frances Rapport, make use of the philosophies of Heidegger, Gadamer and Ricoeur. Van Manen is one of the present-day hermeneutic researchers whose work is particularly known in the field of education.

These approaches differ in their details. For instance, while descriptive phenomenological researchers find and describe essential and universal structures, researchers who take the hermeneutic approach attempt to interpret the meaning of the phenomenon in context. Bracketing prior assumptions and preconceptions is important for descriptive phenomenologists, but hermeneutic researchers believe that these prior experiences might become sources of knowledge and sensitise the researcher to the meanings that might be presented in the narratives of participants. Interpretive phenomenology uses the term 'fusion of horizons' which has its origin in Gadamer's work on intersubjectivity, one horizon being that of the 'text' and the other that of the interpreter of the text. In the research approach it indicates the intersection of the researcher's and the participants' ideas. Both have individual perspectives on the phenomenon but they also live in a shared world where they have common perceptions. The term 'hermeneutic circle' also has its origin in the philosophy of Heidegger. In research it means that interpretation of text (participant narratives) looks at parts of the lived experience, then at the whole, and then back again in a spiralling process, the end of which is achieved when the researcher has gained a reasonable understanding and meaning of the text.

Summary

- Phenomenology is primarily a philosophy but is sometimes applied as a research approach.
- There are three main phases in the phenomenological philosophical movement: preparatory, German and French. There is overlap and interaction of ideas between the phases.
- Writers developed different conceptual formulations, (very broadly) descriptive (Husserl), interpretive (Heidegger) and ontological-existential (Sartre) which have been adapted as methods of inquiry by researchers.
- Researchers who use phenomenological methods have formulated various methods of data analysis.
- The approach should not be mechanical but insightful and illuminate the phenomenon under study and capture its essence.

References

Benner, P. (1984) *From Novice to Expert: Excellence and Power in Clinical Nursing.* Menlo Park, CA, Addison-Wesley.

Berg, L., Scott, C. & Danielson, E. (2006) An interpretive phenomenological method for illuminating the meaning of caring relationship. *Scandinavian Journal of Caring Sciences*, **20** (1), 42–50.

Billhult, A., Stener-Victorin, E. & Bergbom, I. (2007) The experience of massage during chemotherapy in breast cancer treatment. *Clinical Nursing Research*, **16** (2), 85–99.

Caelli, K. (2001) Engaging with phenomenology: is it more of a challenge than it needs to be? *Qualitative Health Research*, **11** (2), 273–81.

Cohen, M.Z. (1987) A historical overview of the phenomenologic movement. *Image: Journal of Nursing Scholarship*, **19** (1), 31–4.

Cohen, M.Z. & Omery, A. (1994) Schools of phenomenology: implications for research. In *Critical Issues in Qualitative Research Methods* (ed. J.M. Morse), pp. 136–56. Thousand Oaks, CA, Sage.

Cohen, M.Z., Kahn, D.L. & Steeves, R.H. (2000) *Hermeneutic Phenomenological Research: A Practical Guide for Nurse Researchers.* Thousand Oaks, CA, Sage.

Colaizzi, P. (1978) Psychological research as a phenomenologist views it. In *Existential Phenomenological Alternatives for Psychology* (eds R. Vallé & M. King), pp. 48–71. New York, NY, Oxford University Press.

Crotty, M. (1996) *Phenomenology and Nursing Research.* Melbourne, Churchill Livingstone.

Dowling, M. (2007) From Husserl to Van Manen. A review of different phenomenological approaches. *International Journal of Nursing Studies*, **44** (1), 131–42.

Gadamer, H. (1975) *Truth and Method.* New York, Seabury Press (Originally published in 1960. Translated by G. Barden & J. Cumming; 2nd edn. 1989).

Giorgi, A. (ed.) (1985) *Phenomenology and Psychological Research.* Pittsburgh, PA, Duquesne University Press.

Giorgi, A. (1992) Description versus interpretation: competing strategies for qualitative research. *Journal of Phenomenological Psychology*, **23** (2), 119–35.

Giorgi, A. (1997) The theory, practice and evaluation of the phenomenological method as a qualitative procedure. *Journal of Phenomenological Psychology*, **28** (2), 235–60.

Giorgi, A. (2000) Concerning the application of phenomenology to caring research. *Scandinavian Journal of Caring Science*, **14** (1), 11–15.

Giorgi, A. (2008) Workshop on Phenomenology, Bournemouth University.

Giorgi, A. & Giorgi, B. (2003) Phenomenology. In *Qualitative Psychology: A Practical Guide to Research Methods.* (ed. J. Smith), pp. 25–50. London, Sage.

Heidegger, M. (1962) *Being and Time.* New York, Harper and Row (Translated from the original 1927 publication by J. Maquarrie and E. Robinson).

Holloway, I. & Todres, L. (2003) The status of method: flexibility, consistency and coherence. *Qualitative Research*, **3** (3), 345–57.

Hycner, R.H. (1985) Some guidelines for the phenomenological analysis of interview data. *Human Studies*, **8** (3), 279–303.

Jasper, M.A. (1994) Issues in phenomenology for researchers of nursing. *Journal of Advanced Nursing*, **19** (2), 309–14.

Koch, T. (1995) Interpretive approaches in nursing research: the influence of Husserl and Heidegger. *Journal of Advanced Nursing*, **21** (5), 827–36.

Langridge, D. (2007) *Phenomenological Psychology*. Edinburgh, Pearson Education.

Leonard, V.W. (1994) A Heideggerian phenomenological perspective on the concept of person. In *Interpretive Phenomenology: Embodiment, Caring and Ethics in Health and Illness* (ed. P. Benner), pp. 43–63. Thousand Oaks, CA, Sage.

Lowenberg, J.S. (1993) Interpretive research methodology: broadening the dialogue. *Advances in Nursing Science*, **16** (2), 57–69.

McLeod, J. (2001) *Qualitative Methods in Counselling and Psychotherapy*. London, Sage.

Mercer, A. (2008) Role transition and the nurse practitioner: An investigation into the experience of professional autonomy. Unpublished PhD thesis, Bournemouth University.

Paley, J. (1997) Husserl, phenomenology and nursing. *Journal of Advanced Nursing*, **26**, 187–93.

Paterson, J.G. & Zderad, L.T. (1976) *Humanistic Nursing*. New York, NY, Wiley.

Priest, S. (1991) *Theories of Mind*. London, Penguin Books.

Rapport, F. (2005) Hermeneutic phenomenology: The science of interpretation of text. In *Qualitative Research in Health Care* (ed. I. Holloway), pp. 125–46. Maidenhead, Open University Press.

Schwandt, T.A. (2007) *Dictionary of Qualitative Inquiry*, 3rd edn. Newbury Park, CA, Sage.

Spiegelberg, H. (1984) *The Phenomenological Movement: A Historical Introduction*, 3rd edn (1st edn 1960). The Hague, Martinus Nijhoff.

Streubert Speziale, H.J. & Rinaldi Carpenter, D.R. (2007) *Qualitative Research in Nursing: Advancing the Human Imperative*, 4th edn. Philadelphia, PA, J.B. Lippincott & Co.

Thomas, S.P. & Johnson, M. (2000) A phenomenologic study of chronic pain. *Western Journal of Nursing Research*, **22** (6), 683–705.

Todres, L. (2000) Writing phenomenological psychological descriptions: an illustration to balance texture and structure. *Auto/Biography*, **8** (1/2), 41–48.

Todres, L. & Holloway, I. (2006) Phenomenology. In *The Research Process in Nursing*. (eds K. Gerrish & A. Lacey), pp. 224–38. Oxford, Blackwell.

Todres, L. & Wheeler, S. (2001) The complementarity of phenomenology, hermeneutics and existentialism as a philosophical perspective for nursing research. *International Journal of Nursing Studies*, **38** (1), 1–8.

Van Kaam, A. (1959) A phenomenological analysis exemplified by the feeling of being understood. *Journal of Individual Psychology*, **15** (1), 66–72.

Van Kaam, A. (1966) *Existential Foundations of Psychology*. Pittsburgh, PA, Dusquesne University Press.

Van Manen, M. (1990) *Researching Lived Experience: Human Science for an Action Sensitive Pedagogy*. New York, NY, State University of New York Press.
Van Manen, M. (1998) *Researching Lived Experience: Human Science for an Action Sensitive Pedagogy*, 2nd edn. New York, NY, State University of New York Press.
Wojnar, D.M. & Swanson, K.M. (2007) Phenomenology: an exploration. *Journal of Holistic Nursing*, **25** (3), 172–80.

Further reading

Dahlberg, K., Dahlberg, H. & Nyström, M. (2008) *Reflective Lifeworld Research*, 2nd edn. Lund, Studentlitteratur.
Todres, L. (2007) *Embodied Enquiry: Phenomenological Touchstones for Research, Psychotherapy and Spirituality*. Basingstoke, Palgrave Macmillan.

CHAPTER 14

Action Research

What is action research?

Action research (AR) is a type of inquiry generally undertaken by practitioners who become researchers, or who work in partnership with university researchers, to examine issues and problems in their own settings; it is carried out through a cyclical process in which each cycle depends on the one before. The aim is to solve practical problems in a specific location and improve the situation. It is a useful approach to organisational or professional change and improvement; it has been increasingly applied to professional and organisational settings in education since the early 1990s and in nursing and other forms of healthcare in the late 90s. Community development is another area in which AR is often carried out. Researchers can use both qualitative and quantitative methods, but many see it as 'the antithesis of experimental research' (see Hart and Bond, 1995: 39) and hence as essentially qualitative. Indeed AR is not a 'pure' research approach but a particular style and development, and researchers can use many of the well-known methods and strategies. AR is not distinguished from other types of research by the use of different research procedures but it differs in some of its aims and processes (see later in this chapter); any of the conventional approaches may be carried out in its research phase. As the name implies, AR includes both research and action. It should fulfil a number of criteria, which will be discussed in this chapter. Other terms often used instead of AR are co-operative inquiry or collaborative research. Badger (2000) claims that AR stands within a continuum of definitions and philosophies; it is not a single unitary approach.

Reason and Bradbury (2006) speak of a variety or 'a family' of approaches in the introduction to their book; these derive from various philosophical and psychological assumptions and have their basis in different traditions. Usually, action researchers use qualitative methods, as this type of inquiry is a reaction against positivist approaches.

Although some agreement exists about the nature and features of AR, there are a number of definitions, some of which are quoted here. All involve the concepts of change, participation and action. In one of the definitions (Carr and Kemmis, 1986: 162) it is claimed that AR is 'a form of self-reflective inquiry undertaken by participants in social situations in order to improve the rationality and justice of their own practices, their understanding of these practices, and the situations in which practices are carried out'. (Carr and Kemmis are educationists, and in the past AR has most often been used in education.)

Action research is more than mere production of knowledge about a problem, a topic or an area of study and involves situations where change is necessary or desirable, and researchers employ interventions to improve practice. Action researchers claim that AR differs from other research mainly because

- it has different aims, one of them being evaluation;
- researchers collaborate with practitioners, or are themselves participants in the setting to be studied;
- the process integrates action as an essential element;
- as well as research, it includes intervention and change in the situation under study;
- it is research in the setting where the changes take place;
- the findings can be of immediate benefit as solutions to problems can be implemented and assessed straight away.

Because of its complexity and time consumption, AR is more appropriate for small rather than large studies. Language use also differs from that of other approaches as it must be understood by all the participants and not be full of academic terminology or researcher jargon. Newman (2000) suggests that there is no 'right' way of carrying out AR, but that action researchers should modify their approach as they go through the process of planning, acting and evaluating.

Example 1

Davies *et al.* (2008) developed an AR project in which a research partnership was established between members of local communities in Wales and a professional researcher. The intentions were to improve health and well-being of over-50s individuals. The aim of the research was to work for positive change concerning disadvantaged groups. Free exercise classes were set up in local communities. This was achieved through people deciding on their own agenda. Programmes were set up, evaluated and discussed over a period of time to improve through 'feedback, reflection and adjustment'. (Although this study is not wholly qualitative, it incorporates the main features of AR)

Example 2

As hospital mealtimes tend to be problematic in many institutions, Dickinson *et al.* (2005) carried out an AR study which focused on the needs of patients in a unit for elderly people rather than fulfilling the agenda of the hospital. The research aimed ultimately to improve mealtimes and help to make them patient-centred. The first phase consisted of observations and interviews with staff and patients about mealtimes. The data from the first stage were presented to the staff who, in the second phase, developed an action plan to improve the situation. Phase three consisted of the evaluation of the implementation of the plan. At all stages, practitioners and research facilitator worked together. Dickinson *et al.* noted the necessity to educate and train the research team in the appropriate skills.

The origins of action research

AR does not have a very long history but started in the 1940s. It is becoming popular and interdisciplinary, but in education it has been used often and for a long time. Lewin (1946), the social psychologist, was one of the early pioneers to develop AR although he used it differently from more recent action researchers. The concept of change, however, was already present in this type of research, and he wanted to employ AR to bring about change in behaviour. Lewin adopted a number of stages, which consisted of

- planning an initial step to change a setting or individuals' behaviour;
- implementing the change;
- evaluating the results of the change;
- modifying the actions in the light of the evaluation;
- starting the process all over again.

Although modern action researchers still use the stage approach, much has changed; in particular AR has become more democratic and participatory. Action researchers now take account of the power relationships inherent in a setting.

The Tavistock Institute of Human Relations set up organisational AR from the late 1940s onwards – although at this stage the type of research was not called AR. The members of the Institute, in general psychologists, developed a problem-solving approach. At a later stage, this problem-solving approach was also used to help deprived communities to solve social and educational problems and ameliorate the 'cycle of deprivation'. Since the work of the Tavistock Institute, AR has been carried out in many disciplines including management, sociology, healthcare and other disciplines. Often it is interdisciplinary and interprofessional.

Critical social theory

Many ideas of modern AR have their basis in critical social theory and critical social science. Carr and Kemmis (1986) give an overview of these, and some of their ideas are summarised here.

Critical theory is critical of positivist and complementary to interpretive research. Critical theorists of the 1950s, such as Horkheimer, Adorno, Marcuse and others, criticised the dominance of positivist social science in the twentieth century which conformed to rigid rules and stifled critical and creative thinking although they did agree with the scientific aim of generating rigorous knowledge about social life. While retrieving for social science those elements that are connected with values and human interests, they also tried to integrate these into a new framework that included ethical and critical thought. Like positivists however, they still considered rigorous knowledge about social life as a requirement of social science.

Habermas (1974) discusses human behaviour in terms of interests and needs. He argues that knowledge consists of three constitutive interests, which he calls the *technical*, the *practical* and the *emancipatory*. The technical interest helps people to gain knowledge in order to achieve technical control over nature. This instrumental knowledge requires scientific explanations. Habermas suggests that, although this form of knowledge is necessary, not everything can be reduced to scientific explanations, and people need to grasp the social meanings of life to understand others. Generating knowledge through interpretive methods can serve 'practical' interests, but this still does not suffice. Human beings need 'emancipatory' knowledge in order to achieve freedom and autonomy, overcome social problems and change power relationships. This will diminish alienation. Habermas's (1972, 1974) thinking (developed in his books) is based in Marxist philosophy. (His theories cannot be developed here; this section merely gives a flavour of the thinking behind modern AR. Habermas also discusses the relationship between theory and practice.)

Educationists in the 1970s and 1980s developed ideas for AR, because they pressed for change in educational settings and society within a critical theory framework. The concept of 'conscientization' discussed by Freire (1970), the Marxist educationist, is also connected to critical social science. Freire believed that people become increasingly aware of the social and historical reality that influences their lives and are able to take action in order to change it. McTaggart and Kemmis (1982) developed guidelines in an AR planner. Although educational and community development studies are not directly connected to AR in nursing and healthcare, the underlying ideas are important as health researchers too desire the empowerment of patients who will be able to take control of their own lives and change their situation. AR has, however, lost much of the ideas of its Marxist antecedents, while valuing democracy and equality in action.

Action research in healthcare

As AR focused on improving education and society, it was also seen as useful in nursing and other healthcare arenas. In the words of Hart and Bond (1995:3), 'it represents a counter to positivism and can develop reflexive practice and general theory from this practice'. It is, in their view, a tool for practitioners, as knowledge is vital for improving healthcare practice; only those involved in the setting are fully able to apply this knowledge. AR generates practical knowledge intended to assist in raising standards of care and delivery of service in general. It is not 'blue skies research'. Health workers now use it frequently but do not always go back to its base and develop it merely on a practical level rather than taking into account its added importance in developing theory.

One of the aims of AR is bridging the theory–practice gap as this gap has been seen as detrimental to professional and clinical work. Rolfe (1996) argues that engaging practitioners from the clinical setting to carry out research in their own practice area would help to overcome this gap and generate direct improvement in practice and generate nursing knowledge. This, after all, is one of the justifications for doing health research. In the health professions, AR is also a useful way of attempting and evaluating change in order to improve settings and care in the clinical arena. Professionals are able, through AR, to undertake research into their own practices. Earlier deeply held assumptions might be questioned. This is linked to the reasons McNiff (1988) gives for engaging in AR, and these can be applied to nursing and health research. She suggests that the aims are political, professional and personal. Through AR, health professionals are able to make sense of the clinical situation and become aware of the impact of policies and practices imposed on them through the system. They will also recognise more clearly that the health services and guidelines for care and treatment should exist initially for the good of the patients and ultimately for the health of society.

As professionals, health researchers make independent decisions while adopting procedures based on theory and research rather than being controlled by outside forces. AR helps professionals to make decisions in the interest of their clients (Carr and Kemmis, 1986). Rather than accepting unsatisfactory decisions imposed on them, they observe and diagnose problems as well as plan and implement changes that are based on the knowledge gained through the research. In AR, professionals need to adopt a thinking and self-critical stance towards their practice which enables them to justify what they do.

On a personal level, AR not only improves the situation for clients and patients, but also enlightens the practitioners themselves and enhances their lives through reflection and engagement in the situation. The clinical setting provides the opportunity for active involvement and personal satisfaction and hence for personal growth.

The main features of action research

Action research is more than just the generation or production of knowledge about an area of interest in which change is seen as necessary or desirable to improve practice. Researchers carry out interventions in the setting to be investigated. The main features of good AR include the following:

- AR draws data and information from a range of sources.
- AR is cyclical and dynamic.
- AR is collaborative and participatory.
- The aim of AR is to devise solutions to practical problems and to develop theory.
- Researchers and practitioners are critical, self-critical and reflective.

AR draws data from a range of sources and perspectives: for instance, data sources might be interviews and observation, documents or diaries. AR is cyclical in the sense that it represents an action cycle consisting of planning, implementing action, observing and reflecting. Then the process starts again. Lewin (1946) already demanded these four stages which he developed into a 'spiral'. The difference between his and modern AR is that present-day research is not imposed from outside the organisation or setting but planned and carried out by insiders, namely participants in the setting.

Lewin's (1946) stages still form the basis for AR, and Parahoo (2006) describes the use of this process in nursing where the stages are similar, though the aims and character of AR are different in some ways in clinical and educational nursing from those of earlier AR:

- Researchers identify a problem in practice.
- They carry out research to assess the problem.
- They plan and implement the change.
- They evaluate the outcome.
- After this, the cycle starts again.

These stages will be developed further in the section on practical considerations Waterman *et al.* (2001) demonstrated the cyclical process and the research partnership as 'fundamental' for AR.

Example of AR in nursing

Researchers from the Netherlands reported on a study of AR to enhance care of people who used heroin before attending methadone substitute outpatient clinics. The participatory action research (PAR) approach involved innovative care strategies and their evaluation. Its ultimate purpose was to improve the quality of nursing care, and it was – to a large extent – successful. Loth *et al.* (2007), the researchers, demonstrated that enhanced nursing knowledge can lead to enhanced nursing practice and better care for clients.

> ## Example of AR in midwifery
>
> Choucri (2005) chose an AR project to evaluate the work of the education and development group of the maternity services in a British hospital trust with the midwives involved in this, focusing in particular on women's needs. This happened in the context of the National Health Service modernisation agenda and was intended to develop innovations in practice. The work and its effect on practice was evaluated and re-planned for improvement. The steps the researchers took were those of AR, namely: preliminary exploration, choosing the research question, planning action, collecting and analysing data, re-planning in the light of findings, taking action and re-evaluating and re-planning (each step dependent on the previous stage). Throughout, the researchers reflected on the processes employed.

AR is collaborative. It involves individuals who choose this approach in the design, data collection and analysis and evaluation of the research as well as in its dissemination. This fulfils the criterion of empowerment and assists emancipation. Because the research influences and intervenes in the participants' working lives, they should be included in decisionmaking.

Once a problem or an important issue has been highlighted and the need for change and improvement is clearly observed, participants develop the focus for the research as co-researchers. The research centres on the problem or issue in the situation in which they work or learn and on a specific location. Modern day AR is always collaborative and participatory. The researchers are often themselves involved in the system they study, but even when they are not, they work with practitioners and professionals to carry out the research.

The methodological continuum

There are different types of AR as suggested before and many of these are used depending on the intentions of the co-researchers. The most common in nursing are identified by Hart and Bond (1995) and Holter and Schwartz-Barcott (1993), but the differences between them are not vast, and they overlap. Because the typology of the latter is inclusive, it will be discussed here.

Holter and Schwartz-Barcott distinguish between three approaches:

1. Technical collaborative
2. Mutual collaborative
3. Enhancement

In the *technical collaborative* approach, the researcher acts as a professional expert who pre-plans the research, carries out the research with practitioners, advises on action and acts as facilitator. It has a pre-specified framework and theory and is rarely qualitative.

The *mutual collaborative* approach entails a more democratic process. The researcher(s) as facilitator and the practitioners collaborate to identify a problem. They plan intervention and change together, and they work as equal partners. Theory is developed rather than predetermined. This mode of AR is more flexible than the technical approach. It is designed to solve immediate and practical problems and needs quick decisionmaking. There is the danger, however, that the practitioners will not continue when the facilitator leaves the clinical area.

The goals of the *enhancement approach* are first, to bridge the theory and practice to solve problems and explain them and second, to raise awareness so that practitioners can identify problems and make them explicit. While the mutual collaboration approach fosters mutual understanding, the enhancement approach leads to emancipation of all participants. Some suggest that one of the aims of this approach is the creation of action-oriented policy which means that this type of AR continues after the facilitator leaves (Berg, 2006). The link between theory and practice generates empowerment because practitioners gain deeper understanding and are therefore able to apply it in different settings, not just in one location at a particular time.

Hart and Bond (1995) maintain that AR is not linked to just one approach but can involve a progression through the typology. Lax and Galvin (2002) describe the differences between AR and PAR, two terms that are often used interchangeably. The focus in their research was the development of a working group for 'families and young children'. The AR approach was adopted to support the development of improved childcare. Although often used in community development, PAR has not often been used in nursing. Kemmis and McTaggart (2000) stress the significance of participation in PAR which has a stronger element of participation than other types of AR. They state that it usually has three main features of importance:

- *Shared ownership*: the projects are owned by all who take part in them
- *Community based analysis*: the collaborators investigate social problems that occur in a community
- *Orientation towards community action*: the findings will be acted upon among the participating group

Example of PAR

A PAR project on diabetes in a primary care setting was carried out in the United States by Mendenhall and Doherty (2007). Patients and their relatives as well as health professionals were involved over three years. A partnership in diabetes was established where support partners were trained 'to reach out' to those with diabetes and their relatives. The partnership was created to overcome the hierarchical relationship between patients and physicians and other providers of care. The study had all the features of PAR such as a challenge to existing modes of care, community collaboration, a cyclical approach that highlights the problem, develops solutions and interventions, and evaluates outcomes. The researchers acknowledge that community-based participatory research can be a slow and rather chaotic process (a general problem with AR) but is worthwhile.

Early developers of PAR include Reason (1988), Heron (1996) and Fals Borda (2001) who claim that it is a way by which participants can take power and control in the research. Its aim is empowerment, emancipation and the generation of knowledge that benefits them directly. The researchers in this type of AR are much more aware of the elements of power and control.

Practical steps

We will now describe the practical steps which researcher-practitioners take while going through an AR cycle in clinical or educational practice. Meyer (2006) calls these phases the exploration, intervention and evaluation phase.

1. Researchers and practitioners carefully observe what is happening in the setting. Before starting the AR, all participants should agree on their participation in the project. Usually they formulate the question together and take decisions. This entails a number of meetings in which procedures will be discussed. These meetings include managers and policy makers who need to give permission for the project to proceed and for access to all the participants. Initially there is a critical assessment of all the aspects of current practice and a review of its effectiveness, quality and cost-effectiveness. In this early stage, much negotiation between different factions takes place.
2. Researcher-practitioners identify problem areas that they want to improve and thoroughly examine the practices that seem to need change and intervention. They 'explore the nature of the problem' (Meyer, 2006: 282) and then discuss this with their colleagues and others interested in the project, including clients, and ask for their ideas and confirmation of the areas in need of improvement. Observations, interviews and brainstorming and focus group sessions take place to ascertain the problem.
   At this stage, researchers plan changes and interventions and implement them in the practice setting. Planning includes drawing up a budget, suggesting a timescale and giving the details of procedures happening.
3. During the implementation of change or intervention, an evaluation process takes place which carefully monitors all the steps and procedures. This is done through a number of meetings with the people in the setting as well as observation and interviewing.

4. In the light of this careful evaluation, practitioners modify their practices to improve on the intervention or change. Meyer states that there is no tidy end to AR; processes are often ongoing beyond the formal project, or they are sometimes disrupted because of new managers and colleagues that enter the setting.

The action and monitoring process continues until practitioners are satisfied with the level of improvement. Throughout the whole process there will be meetings and discussions. The number of meetings depends on the size and duration of the project. Record keeping too, is of major importance, and participants write progress reports and give account of their actions to each other and to their managers. One can use both focus groups, individual interviews, meetings and discussions about the research and the outcomes of actions but groups are more fruitful as these can generate quicker results and stimulate ideas (Stringer, 2007).

Example

Dowswell *et al.* (1999) report on their participatory process in developing a collaborative stroke training programme. Physiotherapists, nursing staff and managers were asked to identify training needs. They observed and interviewed practitioners and gave an account of what needed to be done. At the end of the research phase their reports were used to inform the content of the training course and its structure. The professionals interviewed were also involved in the development, implementation and evaluation of the training course.

Much useful AR can be carried out with patients, users of the services and lay carers. Dowswell *et al.* (1999: 751) advise researchers on the stages of AR while describing their own project. The following are some excerpts from their account and demonstrate what needs to be done by other researchers.

- *Preliminary stage*: All participants are involved in the proposal and understand the reasons for the project. It is important that they all agree and willingly take part in it.
- *Assessment phase*: Ethical issues are clarified and anonymity ensured. Aims and limitations are truthfully described.
- *Planning phase*: Participants find innovative ways of solving problems and carry out agreed tasks and reflect on decision making.
- *Implementation phase*: All participants, regardless of ability, must be comfortable with the materials and incorporate both theory and practice.
- *Evaluation phase*: Interviews, observations and written reviews are used to evaluate the project.

The processes of data collection and analysis are those of other qualitative research.

Learning the skills of action research

It is advisable that all collaborators are trained in research skills to carry out observation and interviews as well as acquiring skills to analyse the data. They also learn to reflect on their own beliefs and assumptions and to make them explicit as well as on the situation. This also means identifying the audit trail of the research process, explaining in detail what they have done and thought. The ongoing documentation of what goes on also helps planning and avoids chaos.

Trustworthiness in AR

The criteria for validity or its equivalent are often discussed and developed by qualitative researchers (see Chapter 18). Waterman claims that an unquestioning acceptance of general criteria for qualitative research does not suffice for AR and describes three types of validity:

1. *Dialectical validity:* tensions and processes
2. *Critical validity:* moral responsibilities
3. *Reflexive validity:* valuing ourselves

First, Waterman (1998) points to the importance of examining the inherent tensions of an AR project. It implies attention to and description of details in the ongoing process as well as the conflicts and tensions between practice, theory and research. Second, she describes the moral responsibility of researchers who have to be aware and take account of the problems of people in the setting. Decisionmaking not only includes action but also knowing when not to take action. Waterman goes on to say that researchers have the responsibility to give reasons for their decisions and argue their cause, as the ultimate aim is 'to improve people's lives'. Third, the reflexive nature of AR is acknowledged. The final report of an AR project should reflect the variety of perspectives that were examined. There is the important dilemma of the multiple roles of researchers who are, in the same study, research participants, change agents and evaluators of change. This position needs a reflexive stance by researchers on their own practices and assumptions. Whilst 'valuing themselves', researchers must also be aware of their own biases and limitations. Another important aspect for judging AR is the existence of more than one cycle. Some researchers who maintain they have used AR do not go further than a single cycle.

Whatever the criteria for trustworthiness might be, all the collaborators involved in an AR study must agree on the issues. For a project to be truly based on AR, they should reflect together on data collection, analysis and other methodological and procedural issues, because reflection on action is inherent in this approach. In AR, researchers need perhaps more reflection and reflectivity than in other research projects. Evaluation of a programme or action needs careful consideration, particularly when further actions are based on it. Meyer (2006: 284) asks the questions that can identify whether an AR project had 'quality'. This includes questions about the usefulness of the research and whether it led to major improvement, the involvement of all people in the setting, and the appropriateness of research methods. AR depends on active collaboration.

Guidance on assessment of the quality of AR projects and proposals can be found in Waterman *et al.* (2001: 43).

Problems and critique

Of course, AR can be problematic for a number of reasons. First, it is obvious that not everybody may wish to be involved. It takes diplomacy and persuasion to recruit reluctant participants. While undertaking the research, practitioners may be in conflict with each other. Managers too, may make objections especially if the process takes too much time or is expensive.

AR is not always appropriate, and it can be a-theoretical. Morton-Cooper (2000: 25) suggests certain situations in which it should not be used:

- If the policy or service to be implemented is forced on the people in the setting, especially when managers have already made their own decisions about this
- If the procedures and methodology used have not met the same quality criteria as other clinically based studies
- If the members of the team giving care, treatment or service do not work well together
- If the researchers want to enhance their own status and reputation

We would have to add that AR takes time and is complex because of its cyclical nature.

Meyer (1993) also notes some problems and limitations of AR. She identifies the problem of defining stages in AR when it is difficult to describe them before the start of the research as they develop during its process. This also means that informed consent is problematic because the stages are unknown beforehand. She warns researchers that the members of the participating team – which may consist of practitioners and facilitators as experts in research – have to be able to collaborate willingly and with a common aim rather than by edict and selection of management. Power relationships may also have inherent problems: research experts from outside have to negotiate rather than using their expertise as control. Waterman *et al.* (2001) suggest, among other problems, that the familiarity of co-researchers with the setting might 'cloud understanding'. Again, this means that they have to become 'professional strangers' or naïve observers of their own situation.

While researchers in other types of inquiry are advised to avoid research in their own setting, AR is carried out in their own location and thus situationally specific and unique. This of course, makes it more difficult and ethically complex. When undertaking research in one's own setting, issues of anonymity and confidentiality might become problematic; because of the different personalities and backgrounds of the people involved, it is not always easy to gain consent. Indeed, often tensions and conflicts between individuals occur which have to be resolved. All must be consulted and agree to the steps that will be undertaken and the decisions that are being made. As in all health research, participation should be voluntary.

Some health professions still do not see AR as a respectable, scientific type of research because it is not generalisable. It is, however, increasingly used in healthcare because it can offer practical solutions to problems and enhancement of theory. Morrison and Lilford (2001) describe the dilemma inherent in AR. Action researchers have developed innovative and imaginative ways of developing practice and theory that could be applied in all research approaches. In their enthusiasm, however, they maintain that a major difference from traditional research (or mainstream research) exists. In fact, so Morrison and Lilford argue, many of the tenets of AR could be applied to mainstream research. There is only one major difference: AR takes account of its unique social context. However, one might argue that this is true for much of qualitative research which is context-bound, meaning that the specific context in which it takes place has to be taken into account. This does not necessarily indicate that the findings of one specific context cannot be applied in other contexts, or that the theoretical advances are not useful in other settings. The researcher should also be able to apply what is learnt from one situation to another setting. AR is, nevertheless, of most use in a specific context in which a local problem needs a solution or where actions and thinking need improvement. This supports the claim by Waterman et al. (2001) about AR as 'real world research'.

This chapter does not tell researchers how to carry out the research, as the research strategies may include many types of qualitative (and indeed, occasionally quantitative) approach. Data collection and analytic procedures can be found in the other chapters of this book.

Summary

- Inherent in AR is the wish for empowerment, collaborative working.
- The outcome of AR is improvement in a specific situation.
- AR draws data from a range of sources.
- Researchers can apply a number of different approaches.
- AR bridges the theory–practice gap and is 'real world' research.
- AR includes planning, action or intervention and evaluation.
- It is cyclical, reflective and dynamic.

References

Badger, T.G. (2000) Action research: change and methodological rigour. *Journal of Nursing Management*, **8** (4), 201–7.

Berg, B.L. (2006) *Qualitative Research for the Social Sciences*, 6th edn. Boston, MA, Allyn and Bacon.

Carr, W. & Kemmis, S. (1986) *Becoming Critical: Education, Knowledge and Action Research*. London, The Falmer Press.

Choucri, L. (2005) Creating change: developing a midwifery action research project. *British Journal of Midwifery*, **13** (10), 629–32.

Davies, J., Lester, C., O'Neill, M. & Williams, G. (2008) Sustainable participation in regular exercise among older people: developing an action research approach. *Health Education Journal*, **67** (1), 45–55.

Dickinson, A., Welch, C., Ager, L. & Costar, A. (2005) Hospital mealtimes: action research for change? *Proceedings of the Nutrition Society*, **64**, 269–75.

Dowswell, G., Forster, A., Young, J., Sheard, J., Wright, P. & Bagley, P. (1999) The development of a collaborative stroke training programme for nurses. *Journal of Clinical Nursing*, **8**, 743–52.

Fals Borda, O. (2001) Participatory (action) research in social theory. In *Handbook of Action Research: Participatory Inquiry and Practice* (eds P. Reason & H. Bradbury), pp. 27–37. London, Sage.

Freire, P. (1970) *Cultural Action for Freedom*. Cambridge, MA, Centre for the Study of Change.

Habermas, J. (1972) *Knowledge and Human Interest* (translated by J. Shapiro). London, Heinemann.

Habermas, J. (1974) *Theory and Practice* (translated by J. Viertel). London, Heinemann.

Hart, E. & Bond, M. (1995) *Action Research for Health and Social Care: A Guide to Practice*. Buckingham, Open University Press.

Heron, J. (1996) *Co-operative Inquiry*. London, Sage.

Holter, I.M. & Schwartz-Barcott, D. (1993) Action research: what is it? How has it been used and how can it be used in nursing? *Journal of Advanced Nursing*, **18** (2), 298–304.

Kemmis, S. & McTaggart, R. (2000) Participatory action research. In *Handbook of Qualitative Research* (eds N.K. Denzin & Y.S. Lincoln), pp. 567–605. Thousand Oaks, CA, Sage.

Lax, W. & Galvin, K. (2002) Reflections on a community action research project: interprofessional issues and methodological problems. *Journal of Clinical Nursing*, **11**, 1–11.

Lewin, K. (1946) Action research and minority problems. *Journal of Social Issues*, **2**, 34–46.

Loth, C., Schippers, G.M., Hart, H. & Van de Wijngaart, G. (2007) Enhancing the quality of nursing care in methadone substitute clinics using action research: a process evaluation. *Journal of Advanced Nursing*, **57** (4), 422–31.

McNiff, J. (1988) *Action Research: Principles and Practice*. London, Routledge.

McTaggart, R. & Kemmis, S. (1982) *The Action Research Planner*. Geelong, Victoria, Australia, Deakin University Press.

Mendenhall, T.J. & Doherty, W.J. (2007) Partners in diabetes: action research in a primary care setting. *Action Research*, **5** (4), 378–406.

Meyer, J.E. (1993) New paradigm research in practice: the trials and tribulations of action research. *Journal of Advanced Nursing*, **18** (7), 1066–72.

Meyer, J.E. (2006) Action research. In *The Research Process in Nursing* (eds K. Gerrish & A. Lacey), 5th edn, pp. 274–88. Oxford, Blackwell Science.

Morrison, B. & Lilford, R. (2001) How can action research apply to health services? *Qualitative Health Research*, **11** (4), 436–49.

Morton-Cooper, A. (2000) *Action Research in Health Care*. Oxford, Blackwell Science.

Newman, J.M. (2000) Action research: a brief overview. *Forum Qualitative Sozialforschung/Forum Qualitative Research* **1** (1), On-line journal. Available at http://www.qualitative-research.net/fqs

Parahoo, K. (2006) *Nursing Research: Principles, Process and Issues*, 2nd edn. Basingstoke, Palgrave, Macmillan.

Reason, P. (ed.) (1988) *Human Inquiry in Action: Developments in New Paradigm Research*. London, Sage.

Reason, P. & Bradbury, H. (eds). (2006) *Handbook of Action Research: Participatory Inquiry and Practice*, 2nd edn. London, Sage.

Rolfe, G. (1996) Going to extremes: action research, grounded practice and the theory–practice gap in nursing. *Journal of Advanced Nursing*, **24**, 1315–20.

Stringer, E.T. (2007) *Action Research: A Handbook for Practitioners*, 3rd edn. Thousand Oaks, CA, Sage.

Waterman, H. (1998) Embracing ambiguities and valuing ourselves: issues of validity in action research. *Journal of Advanced Nursing*, **28** (1), 101–5.

Waterman, H., Tillen, D., Dickson, R. & de Koning, K. (2001) Action research: a systematic review and guidance for assessment. *Health Technology Assessment*, **5** (23), iii-157.

Further reading

Koch, T. & Kralik, D. (2006) *Participatory Action Research in Health and Social Care*. Oxford, Blackwell Science.

McNiff, J. & Whitehead, J. (2005) *All You Need to Know about Action Research*. London, Sage.

McNiff, J. & Whitehead, J. (2009) *Doing and Writing Action Research*. London, Sage.

Winter, R. & Munn-Giddings, C. (2001) *A Handbook for Action Research in Health and Social Care*. London, Routledge.

Whitehead, J. & McNiff, J. (2006) *Action Research: Living Theory*. London, Sage.

CHAPTER 15

Additional Approaches

Case study research

The term 'case study' is used for a research approach with specific boundaries and can be both qualitative and quantitative. Stake (2000) states that much qualitative research is called case study research but argues that it is very specific, 'a bounded system' and both a process as well as a product of the inquiry. Thus some researchers call anything that has boundedness and specificity a case study, but in this chapter it is referred to as research in a unit, a location, a community or an organisation (Bryman, 2008: 53). It can be the study of a single individual though it need not be. A case study is an entity studied as a single unit, and it has clear confines and a specific focus and is bound to context. The boundaries of the case should be clarified in terms of the questions asked, the data sources used and the setting and person(s) involved.

Case studies can be quantitative, qualitative or both, but we shall here summarise the main features of the qualitative case study which tends to be more common in health research. It is often combined with a specific approach to research.

Example of early case study 1

One of the most famous early case studies is that of Whyte (1943) in which he studied a neighbourhood gang in Chicago. Other researchers who used ideas from this study found that it was a 'typical case', meaning that theories emerging from this work could be applied to their own research on groups of young people. This case was studied within an ethnographic research approach.

Overview

The case study is used in a number of disciplines such as anthropology, sociology or geography, though not all studies of limited cases are case studies. It has been most popular in business studies, but is also used in social work and nursing.

The best-known writer on this type of research, Robert Yin, has discussed case studies in various editions of his books (for example, Yin, 2003, 2009). Although his writing, on the whole, focuses on the quantitative framework, he sees the qualitative approach as valid. Case study research is not to be confused with other types of case work, case history or case study as sometimes used in student education to give examples and flavour of cases in clinical settings.

Features and purpose of case study research

Generally researchers who develop case studies are familiar with the case they explore and its context before the start of the research. Health professionals study cases because they may be interested in it for professional reasons or because they need the knowledge about the particular case.

As in other types of qualitative research, the case study is a way of exploring a phenomenon or several phenomena in context. The researchers therefore use a number of sources in their data collection, such as observation, documentary sources and interviews so that the case can be illuminated from all sides. Observation, interviewing and documentary research are the most common strategies used in case study inquiry. The case study is neither a method nor a methodology as neither data collection nor analysis occurs through case study but through specific research approaches, but it can make use of a variety of methods (VanWynsburghe and Khan, 2007). It is something that the researcher chooses to study. Travers (2001) gives a range of qualitative approaches which can be applied to case study research which can be used; for instance, ethnography, grounded theory, narrative analysis or other ways of inquiry can be useful in doing case study research.

Example 2

The aim of the case study research by Walshe *et al.* (2008) was to examine the impact of referral decisions in community palliate care service. The case in point was the community care service in three specific settings within a primary care trust. Interviews took place with patients and health professionals in these settings. The researchers illuminated the influences on referral services.

The case study is determined by the individual case or cases, not by the approach to it that is taken by the researcher. The analysis of qualitative case studies involves the same techniques as that of other qualitative methods: the researcher codes and categorises, provides exhaustive descriptions, develops typologies or generates theoretical ideas.

Studies focus on individuals such as a patient or a group which might consist of individuals with common experiences or characteristics, a ward or a hospital. Life histories of individuals would also be interesting examples of cases. A process or procedure might also constitute a case.

> **Example 3**
>
> Walton *et al.* (2007) explored priority-setting in cardiac surgery at three cardiac centres of the University of Toronto. Data sources consisted of documents, observations and interviews with surgeons, cardiologists and triage nurses. The case is the process of priority-setting itself.

In health research with a psychological emphasis, cases often focus on individuals and an aspect of their behaviour, while the sociologist is more interested in groups. In any health organisation, single or multiple cases can be examined. The local 'case' focuses on both the physical and social elements in the setting.

As in other qualitative research, case studies explore the phenomenon or phenomena under study in their context, and indeed contextualisation is an important feature of all case studies. The lines of division between the phenomenon under study and the context, however, are not always clear (Yin, 2003).

Case studies can be exploratory devices, for instance as a pilot for a larger study or for other, more quantitative research, or they could illustrate the specific elements of a research project. One of our students demonstrated all the ideas she obtained from informants by writing up the case of one single participant. Usually the case study stands on its own and involves intensive observation. The description of specific cases can make a study more lively and interesting.

Case study research is used mainly to investigate cases that are tied to a specific situation and locality, and hence this type of inquiry is even less readily generalisable than other qualitative research (a debate can be found in Gomm *et al.* 2000). Therefore researchers are often advised to study 'typical' and multiple cases (Stake, 1995). Atypical cases, however, may sometimes be interesting because their very difference might illustrate the typical case. It is important, though, that the researcher does not make unwarranted assertions on the basis of a single case. Although there can be no generalisability of the findings from a single case, there might be some transferability of ideas if the researcher has given a detailed audit trail and used 'thick description' so that this case can illuminate other, similar cases.

Conversation analysis

Within the great variety of qualitative methods, some emphasise language and language use. Any professional–client interaction relies on language as a major communication device. Conversation(al) analysis (CA) is a type of discourse analysis (DA) that examines the use of language and asks the question of how everyday conversation works; in its basic form it is the study of talk in everyday interaction (Hutchby and Wooffitt, 2008). This type of inquiry focuses on ordinary conversations and on the way in which talk is organised and ordered in speech exchanges. While researchers primarily examine speech patterns, they also analyse non-verbal behaviour in interaction such as mime, gesture and other body language. As Nofsinger (1991:2) explains: 'If we are to understand interpersonal communication, we need to learn how this is accomplished so successfully'.

The origins of conversation analysis

Harold Garfinkel, Harvey Sacks, Emmanuel Schegloff and others initially developed CA in the 1960s and 1970s in the United States within the ethnomethodological movement. While other types of DA have their roots in the field of linguistics, CA originates in ethnomethodology, a specialist direction of sociology and phenomenology. Ethnomethodology focuses in particular on the world of social practices, interactions and rules (see Turner, 1974). Garfinkel attempted to uncover the ways in which members of society construct social reality. Ethnomethodologists focus on the 'practical accomplishments' of members of society, seeking to demonstrate that these make sense of their actions on the basis of 'tacit knowledge', their shared understanding of the rules of interaction.

The use of conversation analysis

CA focuses on what individuals say in their everyday talk, but also on what they do (Nofsinger, 1991). Through conversation, movement and gesture, we learn of people's intentions and ideas. The sequencing and turn taking in conversations demonstrate the meaning individuals give to situations and show how they inhabit a shared world. Body movements too, are the focus of analysis. Conversation analysts do not use interviewing to collect data but analyse ordinary talk, 'naturally occurring' conversations. Most sections of talk analysed are relatively small, and the analysis is detailed. According to Heritage (1988: 130), CA makes the assumptions that talk is structurally organised, and each turn of talk is influenced by the context of what has gone on before and establishes a context towards which the next turn will be oriented. There are two other fundamental tenets of CA according to Heritage: sequential organisation and empirical grounding of analysis. Talk happens in organised patterns; the action of the member who takes part in the conversation is dependent on and makes reference to the context, and researchers should avoid generalities and premature theory building (Silverman, 2006).

CA is more often used in sociological or education studies than in nursing or other disciplines within the healthcare arena. Indeed, Jones (2003) found few in nursing journals. We think, however, that it can contribute a valuable research approach in nursing and healthcare and lead to changes in the interaction between health professionals and patients. Researchers generally audio- or videotape these interactions and transcribe the conversations in a particular way (see transcription techniques in detail, in Button and Lee (1987)) largely developed by Gail Jefferson.

There are examples in health research of doctor–patient or nurse–patient interaction, particularly in consultations which show how talk is generated and organised by the participants and follows an orderly process in which a turn-taking system exists (Sharrock and Anderson, 1987; Bergstrom *et al.*, 1992). All the recent examples we discovered were in the area of medical consultations (see for instance Campion and Langdon, 2004). These interactions are usually taped and the tapes show what actually takes place in a setting.

> **Example**
>
> Maynard and Heritage (2005) use CA in medical education to demonstrate its value to the understanding of the interaction between doctors and patients. As these interactions are occurring in natural settings and are spontaneous, nothing has to be set up especially for the research. Maynard and Heritage show that CA is systematic and analytic in examining the structure of medical interviews. They give examples of how this method of research can be used for medical education.

Jones (2003) investigated the communication and interaction between nurses and patients in healthcare consultations and found that CA was a useful way to undertake this. He regrets that this way of studying talk is not often used in the field. Sequences of talk can be studied, and he suggests that they illuminate processes such as treatment, advice and assessment. The disadvantages of CA he sees as the length of time that is needed for this research approach, and the potential lack of context as the focus on direct interaction and communication might become isolated from the social context.

The analysis of CA includes the discovery of regularities in speech or body movement, the search for deviant cases and the integration with other findings without over-generalisation (Heritage, 1988). One of the disadvantages is the way in which conversation analysts emphasise the formal characteristics of interaction at the expense of content, however, much can be discerned from the way the communication and interaction proceeds. ten Have (2007) describes ways of analysing CA data, and researchers might find his book useful.

CA is difficult, highly complex and very detailed. Researchers may not find it easy, and we do not recommend it to novice researchers.

Critical incident technique

The critical incident technique (CIT) is a procedure designed to solve problems in clinical practice or educational settings. In the past, it was not often used in the health arena, but it has been applied in this field, and although neglected for a number of years, it has become more often used in the recent decade. It is not a specific method or methodology but a means of developing questions, whilst focusing on people's behaviour in critical situations in order to solve problems in task performance. A critical incident is an observed event that is perceived as particularly important or critical. Researchers examine those events that are significant for a particular process. They collect examples of critical incidents in the situation under study by observation of behaviour and by asking participants to give an account of the way in which they deal in critical situations or times of crisis.

Flanagan (1954) who first developed this technique, suggests that in this approach, an incident has to occur in a situation with definite consequences and effects. CIT was initially developed as a result of the Aviation Psychology Program in the United States to collect information from pilots about their behaviour when flying a mission. In particular, psychologists asked for reports about critical incidents that helped or hindered the successful outcome of the mission. Through analysis of these reports, a list of components for successful performance was generated from the data. Flanagan refined the procedure for industrial psychology to assess the outcomes of task performance, and it was used also in other fields such as personnel selection. Although the method was neglected after the 1950s, it can be a useful, effective and qualitative approach to studying critical events in order to improve task performance and is thus very useful for the health professions. Flanagan (1954: 335) states that the technique is 'a procedure for gathering certain important facts concerning behaviour in defined situations'.

Critical incidents might occur in clinical practice, make visible problems in care and are noticed by health professionals who then decide to examine these, as well as the reasons for their occurrence. They then develop the specific plan and aim of their research and start collecting and analysing data. It can be seen that this type of inquiry follows the traditional path of data collection and analysis in qualitative research.

Researchers examine those events that are significant for a particular process. They collect examples of critical incidents in the situation under study, and participants give an account of the way in which they act in critical situations or times of crisis. Direct observation is the most important part of the data collection. Generally the researchers ask about the critical event and gain a perspective about effective and ineffective behaviour in specific decisive and important situations.

Example of CIT in clinical practice

Broström *et al.* (2003) developed a study in the area of congestive heart failure (CHF) breathing disorders which aimed to explore situations in which spouse influence and support was crucial in the sleep situation. Participants, the partners of individuals with CHF, were asked through semi-structured interviewing to provide specific situations in which they gave support or where their influence and support was inhibited. The implications of this study meant that health professionals could gain insight into the problems of the sleep situation and increase understanding, as well as learn how to facilitate support in practical ways.

The process of critical incident technique

Schluter *et al.* (2007) in a short guide to CIT (p.108) describe the five steps which Flanagan suggests:

1. Identification of the research question and aim
2. Identification of the specific types of incidents to be observed
3. Collection of data by observation and recording
4. Analysis and interpretation of the observed and recorded data
5. Writing the report and disseminating the data

The aim of the technique is to obtain information about each specific incident. This will include choosing the type of events on which researchers wish to focus, generally critical events or incidents in care or educational settings. The second stage involves selecting a purposive sample of incidents and people from which to collect data. The sample size depends on the number of critical incidents, not on the number of people interviewed or observed (Kemppainen, 2000). Initially, health researchers find out about critical incidents through incidental and casual observation, but when they decide to do the research, they observe and ask questions more purposefully. The data are analysed in a similar way as in other approaches. There is, however, a slight difference: Researchers choose a more defined frame of reference in this type of research as they wish to focus on particular events. It is also important that the terminology used is clear and appropriate for CIT; indeed, Butterfield *et al.* (2005) deplore the lack of consistency in studies which use this technique.

The goal of the researcher is to investigate a recurring problem and to find a solution to it. To examine the critical incidents, the health researcher has to be familiar with the setting and the nursing or midwifery tasks that are performed. Kemppainen (2000) advises that the responses of the participants to the researcher's questions should be specific and accurate, and not vague or unclear. We feel that this way of researching is under-explored and could be specifically useful in the healthcare field.

Discourse analysis

Cheek (2004) suggests that CA and DA are complex concepts and that confusion exists about this area of research. DA cannot be easily identified, as people use it in different ways; it is more a framework or holistic theoretical stance. Discourse in general is applied to talk and text, such as conversations, interviews or documents. Traynor (2006) re-emphasises that it is an analysis of naturally occurring talk, one of the most important sources of data, although talk is not the only discourse that might be analysed.

DA in psychology is an analysis of text and language drawing on 'accounts' of experiences and thoughts that participants present. This type of DA has been carried out mainly by psychologists. Accounts consist of forms of ordinary talk and reasoning of people, as well as other sources of text, such as historical documents, diaries, letters or reports and even images such as photographs, drawings or paintings. DA is not a method but a specific approach to the social world and research (Potter, 1996; Cheek, 2004). It focuses on the construction of talk and text in social action and interaction. In common with other types of qualitative inquiry, discourse analysts initially use an inductionist approach by collecting and reviewing data before arriving at theories and general principles as do other qualitative researchers. The way people use language and text is taken for granted within a culture (Gill, 1996) and this shows that discourse is context-bound. DA as the structural analysis of discourse, is often used in media and communication research to analyse data. An example would be an analysis of the speech messages of politicians.

Language itself and reality are socially constructed. The vocabularies which individuals and groups use are located in interpretive 'repertoires' that are coherent and related sets of terms. Crowe (2005: 55) adds to this that discourses show how 'social relations, identities, knowledge and power are constructed in spoken and written text.'

It is important to read the documents and transcripts carefully before interpreting them. The first step in the analysis is a close look at and detailed description of other, less language-based sources. The relevant documents are read and re-read until researchers have become familiar with the data, be they textual or visual. Immersion in the data, after all, is a trait of all qualitative research. Important issues and themes can then be highlighted. The analysis proceeds like other qualitative research: analysts code the data, look for relationships and search for patterns and regularities that generate tentative propositions. Through the process, they always take the context into account and generate analytical notes as in other forms of qualitative inquiry.

Also, like for other qualitative research, the findings from DA are not instantly generalisable; indeed researchers are not overly concerned with generalisability, because the analysis is based on language and text in a specific social context. There are a number of similarities between CA and DA: both CA and DA focus on language and text. While DA generally considers the broader context, CA emphasises turn-taking and explains the deeper sense of interaction in which people are engaged, particularly 'naturally occurring' talk, while discourse analysts look at the material more holistically, and they can also use records, newspaper articles or reports of meetings, etc.

Discourse analysts are interested in the ways through which social reality is constructed in interaction and action. DA is based on the belief that language (and presentation of images) does not just mirror the world of social members and cultures but also helps to construct it.

> **Example 1**
>
> DA is demonstrated by Fealy (2004) who analysed the way in which nurses were presented and the changes in their status in images to the Irish public over time. They pointed to the fact that the image of the nurse is both culture and time specific. Class, economic position, power and gender relationships were all important in the process of presenting images of the nurse to the public. (Fealy does draw parallel to images of nursing in other countries too.)

Potter and Wetherell (1987) developed the notion of 'interpretative repertoires' which they saw as a set of related concepts organised around one or several important metaphors. These provide researchers with common sense concepts of a group or a culture. Language is 'action oriented': it is used so people can 'do' and shaped by the cultural and social context in which it occurs. Social groups possess a variety of repertoires and use them appropriately in different situations. The discourses or narratives of people about various specific areas in their lives generate a text. Discourse analysts must therefore be aware of the context in which action takes place so that the context can be analysed as well. The same text can be interpreted in different ways: different versions of reality exist in different contexts. The DA of psychologists and linguists focuses on language and text. Readers can make judgements about this type of research because they themselves possess knowledge of everyday discourse and its construction. Wetherell *et al.* (2001) and Potter and Wetherell (2007) have since updated their work.

McHoul and Grace (1995) differentiate between Foucauldian and non-Foucauldian discourse (although these are not really separate). Michel Foucault, the French historian and philosopher, made the concept of discourse famous while describing the links of language with disciplines and institutions. For him, discourses are bodies of knowledge, by which he means both academic scholarship and institutions, which exist in disciplines. Indeed, he claims that discourse reproduces institutions. Social phenomena are constructed through language. Specific language is connected with specialist fields, for instance 'professional discourse', 'scientific discourse' or 'medical discourse'; for instance, Rayner *et al.* (2006) examine the values of the National Health Service Framework for coronary heart disease and identify three different discourses, the managerial, the clinical and the political, all with different messages and overtones.

In Foucault's works, discourses as specialist languages are linked to power.

Example 2

Hui and Stickley (2007) analysed the discourses of the literature and health policies of the government and those of service users in the mental health arena in a Foucauldian DA. These two types of discourse were distinct and competing. Different concepts had different meanings among these two perspectives. 'Power' in particular had varied connotations.

DA discovers the language that operates within the particular discourse under study and which has almost moral connotations. For instance, professionals use particular types of discourse to impose their own or the official version of reality on their clients. Traynor (2006) stresses that people persuade others, present themselves to others, and act in particular ways; how this occurs is important and involves power relationships. This can be shown in speech, text or image.

Feminist research

Feminist inquiry is research that focuses on the experience, ideas and feelings of women in their social and historical context. Researchers adopt a gender perspective to the phenomenon under investigation. Feminist approaches do not prescribe methods of analysing research but instead suggest ways of thinking about it. The intention is to make women visible, raise their consciousness and empower them. As Oleson (2000) states: 'It is research for rather than about women'. Because qualitative research has affinity with the ideas of feminists, it is used more often than quantitative approaches (although feminist researchers also see the latter as valid).

Feminist research is important for health researchers which are still female professions, and their members are well aware of gender and power issues. Some feminists believe in a separate and distinctive feminist research methodology, and that this type of inquiry is not merely a variation or branch of qualitative research (Stanley and Wise, 1993). Many early feminist researchers maintained (for instance Harding, 1987) that a distinctive feminist method does not exist, but that feminist authors address certain epistemological and methodological issues related to gender. They show in particular that structural and policy issues are as important as personal or individual factors. One major element of feminist research is critical theory. Feminist researchers often see women as an oppressed group controlled by the media, the political and economic systems and ultimately by men. Structural and political forces, so they believe, work against equality for women. Feminists believe that women are economically exploited and suffer social discrimination. Hearing the voices of women and raising their consciousness through research may therefore assist in overcoming inequalities.

The most common form of feminist inquiry is narrative or life history research, because it gives women the chance to tell their own stories in their own way, 'letting the women speak'. Feminist research and cooperative inquiry share many of their most important features such as complete equality between researcher and participant and a democratic non-judgemental stance (though one might say this about all qualitative research).

The feminist approach to research gives women the opportunity to voice their concerns and interests and is not merely concerned with the technical details of data analysis. The latter depends on the field in which researchers work and on the specific research question, although methods, too, reflect the feminist principles of equality between researcher and participant and focus on women's experiences and their empowerment. Taking into account the requirements of feminist research, researchers use grounded theory, ethnography and other types of data analysis. The focus on the 'lived experience' and the affective elements in the participants' lives mean that phenomenological approaches are often taken in feminist qualitative research.

The term 'feminist standpoint research' is used. It is a less specific term than feminist methodology and carries with it the implication that feminist research uses a specific type of analysis. Feminist standpoint researchers recognise that their view of the world is distinctive and different. There should be a fit, they suggest, between the world view of feminism and the methods adopted for research.

The origins of feminist methodology

Feminist methodology has its roots in feminist theory. Writers such as Millett (1969), Mitchell (1971) and Oakley (1972) as well as others, particularly in the United States and Britain, were the pioneers who helped to direct the focus on women's interests and ideas. Early feminist writers in the professions in Britain include Stanley and Wise (1993) in social work and Webb (1984) in nursing.

A number of major issues emerge in thinking and doing research within a feminist methodological framework. Initially, feminist research was a reaction against positivist research and traditional strategies, which were seen as male-dominated and androcentric. Feminist approaches take up the issues of power, oppression and subordination although they are not only about women but also about the interests of men (Peters *et al.*, 2008). Feminist writers used consciousness-raising as a methodological tool to empower women. It also becomes a tool for narrowing the distance between researchers and participants by generating reciprocity and collaboration. This affects all participants and gives individuals – including researchers – a sense of their identity. Women, so feminists believe, become aware of their position through the research process and relationships and aim to change their situation and become more powerful.

Feminist researchers emphasise an alternative social reality and value women's lives and experience. Researchers intend to contribute to the improvement of the state of women who will learn to control their own lives through this. Feminists are concerned with the importance of women's lives and their position in the social structure. They claim that unequal relations are not only embedded in the structure of society but have taken part in the construction of social relationships.

Travers (2001) claims that feminism has been one of the most important movements in the late twentieth century. The aversion to main stream research which was often seen as embodied in positivism has helped feminist researchers to value qualitative research though they do not use it exclusively; indeed Oakley (2000) stresses the importance of 'scientific' quantitative research.

Feminist thought and methodology

Even before feminism, disenchantment with natural scientific methods had emerged, which led to a critique of positivism. Researchers who took the approach of natural science believed that objectivity was possible, and that to use the scientific method was the best way to examine social reality as it would be neutral and objective. Feminists question the notion of value-neutral research and agree with other qualitative researchers who react against the positivist and neopositivist approach.

Traditional research was often male dominated. Feminist critics of this approach maintain that it is often stripped of its context while questions and answers are predefined and controlled by researchers who, whilst claiming objectivity, impose their own subjective framework. Feminists believe that researchers cannot achieve complete objectivity. They can only state their bias or assumptions and demonstrate the value bases from which they come; that is, they are reflexive. They criticise the differentiation between the objective and subjective and put an emphasis on the relationships and realities of everyday life through which social structures can be understood.

Women explain their social reality in personal accounts of their lives, and these accounts emerge from their shared experiences. The researcher listens to these accounts and, while interpreting them, gives a faithful picture of the personal histories and biographies of women. Feminist research aims to raise the consciousness of people in general and of the women participants specifically. Consciousness of their reality can guide women to an understanding, and helps them to change their lives and empower them. Research makes emotions, personal values and the participants' thoughts legitimate topics of research.

The relationship between researchers and women participants

The research relationship follows that of other types of qualitative research but collaboration and equality between the researcher and women participants is stressed even more. Empathy with women may be easier to achieve by female researchers because of their gender (though feminists do not claim that men cannot have empathy, nor that research supports a woman's perspective just because it is done by a woman). The personal experience and values of the researcher become important in feminist research. Feminists often describe and integrate their own feelings while recounting and analysing women's experiences, pains and passions. Sometimes they study women's conditions or problems that they have experienced in their own lives. Feminist qualitative research allows for interactive interviewing where participants can ask professional as well as personal questions.

There are considerable variations in feminist research that we do not intend to discuss here. New books on feminist research appear quite often. We believe, however, that this can be a useful perspective in nursing, midwifery and physiotherapy, where women are still presently in the majority. We refrain from giving a great deal of space to the feminist standpoint because it is not a specific approach to qualitative research, although it more often adopts qualitative than quantitative methods. This does not detract from its importance. It is a way of seeing rather than a method or methodology, although some writers such as Ramazanoglu and Holland (2002) for instance would take issue with this statement.

It must be stated, however, that some feminist research neglects the issue of men's oppression and submission to economic and structural forces, particular of those in unskilled occupations. Everybody is influenced by political and structural forces (Peters *et al.*, 2008), not women alone.

Performative social science

Performative (or performance-based) social science (PSS) is an innovative and unconventional approach to collecting, presenting or disseminating data through images, poetry and performances such as theatre or dance. It is becoming increasingly used in qualitative health research. The researcher thus uses tools borrowed from the arts and humanities (Jones, 2006) and seeks alternative ways to generate and present research. This type of approach is employed in auto/biographical and narrative inquiry. PSS is being used across a variety of disciplines and uses a wide range of techniques, media and creative processes. In research, it indicates a change from text to performance and it has become increasingly popular, though text is still the preferred way of presenting qualitative data. Guiney Yallop *et al.* (2008) claim that performative data presentation could reach a wider audience as it might be easier to understand than traditional ways of researching and presenting. A lay audience in particular will find it easier to grasp complex issues this way because of its greater accessibility, but it can also have an impact on academic peers and funding agencies. Performance is, however, not suitable in all studies.

The concept of performance in research emerged in the 1970s. It is linked to the enactment of research in various ways. Austin, the philosopher, for instance, uses the term 'performative' in relation to utterances in text or speech which perform and enact (Schwandt, 2007). A text itself might be a performative production. The concept of PSS relates, however, mostly to the visual and audible. In the last two decades, qualitative researchers have often translated their data, findings and presentations into performances. Indeed, Denzin (2001: 26) states that we 'inhabit a performance-based dramaturgical culture'. Film, poetry and video for instance, open up new ways for qualitative inquiry and are often appropriate to evoke emotion and response in the audience; hence, they help listeners and viewers to grasp human concerns more fully.

Drama, dance and music and other tools also are performance-based modes of presenting research; it is not all image-based. Saldaña (2003) speaks of 'dramatizing data' where the participants play roles and are characters in a play. Some of our students, for instance, showed a fictional film about old people in a care home which presented the findings from their research. Rossiter *et al.* (2008) show how and why findings can be usefully communicated, through theatre for instance.

New and innovative technology is often the medium through which performative events can happen and films or dramatic presentations are obvious choices. Jones ties performativity to post-modernity and social constructionism, because of its multi-voiced and interdisciplinary character and for its diversity and lack of linearity. Roberts (2008: 1), however, warns against the collapsing of artistic or social science or activity into mere performance or simply transferring it, as this needs careful examination of 'skills, purpose, tradition and context'.

The Gergens (Gergen and Gergen, 2000) have used performances in their work for decades. They declare that in research, writing is only one way of expression. Films, drama and other modes of presentation can be used to this end, while in the past they were merely complementary to scientific writing. They also believe that in this genre boundaries between data collection and report become blurred in the process of research. Collecting data through images, poems and other means empowers the participants and centres on their perspectives.

Example of data collection

Spiers (2004) used an innovative, observational approach to the study about teenagers with diabetes to whom he gave cameras so they could film what it was like living with diabetes and the processes needed to care for themselves and to be cared for. He states as an advantage the control of events by the participants. Spiers also filmed interactions of these teenagers with nurses.

Keen and Todres (2007) give several examples of dissemination through performance methods and discuss the value of this type of presentation of findings.

The data collected by these techniques need of course to be analysed in detail to be used by health professionals. Indeed, vigorous and rigorous analysis is essential to make performance-based collection and presentation of data acceptable, particularly in academic settings. Nevertheless, through presentation in a storytelling or image-based way, the audience, particularly an audience of patients or users of services, is able to grasp the experience of pain and joy, stigma and other problems which are made more visible and concrete.

PSS is useful in health research as it can present vividly the voices of the participants – be it in film, theatre or other media. It is more immediate than reading a text produced by researchers, and assists the audience in understanding the experience of patients or health professionals. The producer of a performance, whether it is in a play, a film or any other form, becomes a recorder of experiences. His or her observations evoke a response in audiences who bring their own interpretations to the situation in interaction with the data or their presentation.

Performance cannot be used as a 'gimmick' where the dramatic is all important. Curtin (2008) suggests that drama and other performances need to have the same academic credentials such as rigour and analytic quality.

(Much of this material for this section is based directly on Holloway, 2008)

Conclusion

This chapter is aimed to give an overview of some qualitative research approaches that are either embedded in other methods, such as case study research and CIT, or those that are more (DA, PSS) or less (conservation analysis) frequently used in health research. All qualitative researchers need to have at least some knowledge about these methods. We have focused mainly on main stream approaches in the preceding sections.

References

Case studies

Bryman, A. (2008) *Social Research Methods*. Oxford, Oxford University Press.
Gomm, R., Hammersley, M. & Foster, P. (2000) *Case Study Method*. London, Sage.
Stake, R.E. (1995) *The Art of Case Study Research*. Thousand Oaks, CA, Sage.
Stake, R.E. (2000) The case study method in social inquiry. In *Case Study Method* (eds R. Gomm, M. Hammersley & P. Foster), pp. 19–26. London, Sage.
Travers, M. (2001) *Qualitative Research through Case Studies*. London, Sage.
VanWynsburghe, R. & Khan, S. (2007) Redefining case study. *International Journal of Qualitative Methods*, **6** (2), Article 6. Retrieved January 2009 from http://www.ualberta.ca/iiqm/backissues/6_2/vanwynsberghe.pdf

Walshe, C., Chew-Graham, C., Todd, C. & Caress, A. (2008) What influences referrals within community palliative care services: a qualitative case study. *Social Science and Medicine*, **67** (1), 137–46.

Walton, N.A., Martin, D.K. & Peter, E.H., *et al.* (2007) Priority setting and cardiac surgery: a qualitative case study. *Health Policy*, **80** (3), 444–58.

Whyte, W.F. (1943) *Street Corner Society: The Social Structure of an Italian Slum*. Chicago, IL, University of Chicago Press.

Yin, R.K. (2003, 2009) *Case Study Research*, 3rd and 4th edn. Thousand Oaks, CA, Sage.

Conversation analysis

Bergstrom, L., Roberts, J., Skillman, L. & Seidel, J. (1992) You'll feel me touching you, sweetie: vaginal examination during the second stage of labour. *Birth*, **19**, 11–18.

Button, G. & Lee, J.R.E. (eds). (1987) *Talk and Social Organisation*. Clevedon, Multilingual Matters.

Campion, P. & Langdon, M. (2004) Achieving multiple topic shifts in primary care medical consultations: a conversation analysis study in UK general practice. *Sociology of Health and Illness*, **26** (1), 81–101.

ten Have, P. (2007) *Doing Conversation Analysis*, 2nd edn. London, Sage.

Heritage, J. (1988) Explanations as accounts: a conversation analytic perspective. In *Analysing Everyday Explanation: A Casebook of Methods*, pp. 127–44. London, Sage.

Hutchby, I. & Wooffitt, R. (2008) *Conversation Analysis*. Cambridge, Polity Press.

Jones, A. (2003) Nurses talking to patients: exploring conversation analysis as a means of researching nurse-patient communication. *International Journal of Nursing Studies*, **40** (6), 609–18.

Maynard, D. & Heritage, J. (2005) Conversation analysis, doctor-patient interaction and medical communication. *Medical Education* **39** (4), 428–35.

Nofsinger, R.E. (1991) *Everyday Conversation*. Newbury Park, CA, Sage.

Sharrock, W. & Anderson, R. (1987) Work flow in a paediatric clinic. In *Talk and Social Organisation* (eds G. Button & J.R.E. Lee). Clevedon, Multilingual Matters.

Silverman, D. (ed.) (2006) *Interpreting Qualitative Data: Methods for Analysing Talk, Text and Interaction*, 3rd edn. London, Sage.

Turner, R. (ed.) (1974) *Ethnomethodology*. Harmondsworth, Penguin Books.

Critical incident technique

Broström, A., Strömberg, A., Dahlström, U. & Fridlund, B. (2003) Congestive heart failure, spouse support and the couple's sleep situation. *Journal of Clinical Nursing*, **12** (2), 223–33.

Butterfield, L.D., Borgen, W.A., Amundson, N.E. & Asa-Sophia, T.M. (2005) Fifty years of the critical incident technique: 1954–2004 and beyond. *Qualitative Research*, **5** (4), 475–97.

Flanagan, J. (1954) The critical incident technique. *Psychological Bulletin*, **51**, 327–58.

Kemppainen, J.K. (2000) The critical incident technique and nursing care quality research. *Journal of Advanced Nursing*, **32** (5), 1264–71.

Schluter, J., Seaton, P. & Chaboyer, W. (2007) Critical incident technique: a user's guide for nurse researchers. *Journal of Advanced Nursing*, **61** (1), 107–14.

Discourse analysis

Cheek, J. (2004) At the margins? Discourse analysis and qualitative research. *Qualitative Health Research*, **14** (8), 1140–50.

Crowe, M. (2005) Discourse analysis: towards an understanding of its use in nursing. *Journal of Advanced Nursing*, **51** (1), 55–63.

Fealy, G. (2004) 'The good nurse': visions and values in images of the nurse. *Journal of Advanced Nursing*, **46** (6), 649–56.

Gill, R. (1996) Discourse analysis: practical implementation. In *Handbook of Qualitative Research in Psychology and the Social Sciences* (ed. J.T.A. Richardson), pp. 141–56. Leicester, BPS Books.

Hui, A. & Stickley, T. (2007) Mental health policy and mental health service user perspectives on involvement: a discourse analysis. *Journal of Advanced Nursing*, **59** (4), 416–26.

McHoul, A. & Grace, W. (1995) *A Foucault Primer: Discourse, Power and the Subject*. Melbourne, Melbourne University Press.

Potter, J. (1996) *Representing Reality: Discourse, Rhetoric, and Social Construction*. London, Sage.

Potter, J. & Wetherell, M. (1987) *Discourse and Social Psychology: Beyond Attitudes and Behaviour*. London, Sage.

Potter, J. & Wetherell, M. (2007) *Discourse and Social Psychology*, 3rd edn. London, Sage.

Rayner, M., Scarborough, P. & Allender, S. (2006) Values underlying the National Service Framework for coronary heart disease. *Journal of Health Services Research and Policy*, **11** (2), 67–73.

Traynor, M. (2006) Discourse analysis: theoretical and historical overview and review of papers in the Journal of Advanced Nursing. *Journal of Advanced Nursing*, **54** (1), 62–72.

Wetherell, M., Taylor, S., Yates, S.J. (eds). (2001) *Discourse as Data: A Guide for Analysis*. Milton Keynes, The Open University.

Feminist research

Harding, S. (ed.) (1987) Introduction. In *Feminism and Methodology*, pp. 1–14. Bloomington, IN, Indiana Press.

Millett, K. (1969) *Sexual Politics*. London, Abacus.

Mitchell, J. (1971) *Women's Estate*. Harmondsworth, Penguin.

Oakley, A. (1972) *Sex, Gender and Society*. London, Temple Smith.

Oakley, A. (2000) *Experiments in Knowing: Gender and Method in the Social Sciences*. Cambridge, Polity Press.

Oleson, V. (2000) Feminisms and qualitative research at and into the millennium. In *Handbook of Qualitative Research* (eds N.K. Denzin & Y.S. Lincoln), 2nd edn, pp. 215–55. Thousand Oaks, CA, Sage.

Peters, K., Jackson, D. & Rudge, D. (2008) Research on couples: are feminist approaches useful? *Journal of Advanced Nursing*, **62** (3), 373–80.

Ramazanoglu, C. & Holland, J. (2002) *Feminist Methodology: Challenges and Choices*. London, Sage.

Stanley, L. & Wise, S. (1993) *Breaking Out Again*. London, Routledge.

Travers, M. (2001) *Qualitative Research through Case Studies*. London, Sage.

Webb, C. (1984) Feminist methodology in nursing research. *Journal of Advanced Nursing*, **9** (3), 249–56.

Performative Social Science

Curtin, A. (2008) How dramatic techniques can aid the presentation of qualitative research. *Qualitative Researcher* (8), pp. 8–10.

Denzin, N.K. (2001) The reflexive interview and a performative social science. *Qualitative Research*, **1** (1), 23–46.

Gergen, M.M. & Gergen, K.J. (2000) Qualitative inquiry: tensions and transformations. In *Handbook of Qualitative Research* (eds N.K. Denzin & Y.S. Lincoln), pp. 1025–46. Thousand Oaks, CA, Sage.

Guiney Yallop, J.J., Lopez de Vallejo, I. & Wright, P.R. (2008). Editorial: overview of the performative social science special issue [20 paragraphs]. *Forum Qualitative Sozialforschung(Forum: Qualitative Social Research)*, **9** (2), Article 64. Retrieved July 2008 from http://nbn-resolving.de/urn:nbn:de:0114-fqs0802649

Holloway, I. (2008) *A-Z of Qualitative Research in Healthcare*. Oxford, Blackwell Science.

Jones, K. (2006) A biographic researcher in pursuit of an aesthetic: the use of arts-based (re) presentations in 'performative' dissemination of life stories. *Qualitative Sociology Review*, **2** (1), 66–85.

Keen, S. & Todres, L. (2007) Strategies for disseminating qualitative research findings: three exemplars [36 paragraphs]. *Forum Qualitative Sozialforschung(Forum: Qualitative Social Research)*, **8** (3), Article 17. Retrieved July 2008 from http://nbn-resolving.de/urn:nbn:de:0114-fqs0703174

Roberts, B. (2008) Performative social science: a consideration of skills, purpose and context [122 paragraphs]. *Forum Qualitative Sozialforschung(Forum: Qualitative Social Research)*, **9** (2), 1, Article 58. Retrieved July 2008 from http://nbn-resolving.de/urn:nbn:de:0114-fqs0802588

Rossiter, K., Kontos, P., Colantonio, A., Gray, J. & Keightley, M. (2008) Staging data: theatre as a tool for analysis and knowledge transfer in health research. *Social Science and Medicine*, **66** (1), 130–46.

Saldaña, J. (2003) Dramatizing data: a primer. *Qualitative Inquiry*, **9** (2), 218–36.

Schwandt, T. (2007) *A Dictionary of Qualitative Inquiry*. Thousand Oaks, CA, Sage.

Spiers, J.A. (2004) Tech tips: using video management/ analysis technology in qualitative research. *International Journal of Qualitative Methods*, **3** (1), Article 5. Retrieved July 2008 from http://www.ualberta.ca/iiqm/backissues/3_1/pdf/spiersvideo.pdf

Further reading

Hessebiber, S.N. & Leavy, P.L. (2007) *Feminist Research: A Primer*. Thousand Oaks, CA, Sage.

McHoul, A. & Grace, W. (1997) *A Foulcault Primer: Discourse, Power and Subject*. New York, NY, NYU Press.

Rose, G. (2007) *Visual Methodologies: An Introduction to the Interpretation of Visual Materials*, 2nd edn. London, Sage.

The special issue of *Forum Qualitative Research*, Vol. 9, No 2, a free on-line journal, contains a number of important and explanatory articles.

CHAPTER 16

Mixed Methods: Combining Qualitative and Quantitative Research

The nature of mixed methods studies

Mixed methods research (MMR) means the use of both qualitative and quantitative approaches in one empirical study. (It must be noted, however, that mixed methods (MM) can also be conducted *within* qualitative research itself when several approaches are employed. See later in this chapter.) MMR has become fashionable – O'Cathain *et al.* (2007) state that some writers even call it a fad. MMR is more difficult than mono-method research for several reasons: First, traditionally writers proposed that qualitative and quantitative research come from different world views and each has a distinct epistemological stance and conceptual framework (the debate is discussed in the introduction of this book). While Punch (2005: 3) claims that not all research questions are 'driven by paradigm considerations', others, such as some of the authors in the text edited by Tashakkori and Teddlie (2003) see it as a third paradigm (see also Johnson and Onwuegbuzie, 2004). Secondly, some authors maintain that technically and operationally it might be difficult to use both approaches in one single study (for instance Sandelowski, 2000). In spite of its complexity, MMR in nursing and healthcare has been frequently carried out in a pragmatic and practical way throughout the last decade. Researchers who pursue this type of inquiry need an understanding of both qualitative and quantitative research and realisation that this type of inquiry is more time-consuming.

Qualitative and quantitative methods are often used together in one single study for practical purposes only, or to satisfy members of grant-making bodies who believe that a research study can be strengthened through using both methods. MMR is used to illustrate different aspects of a phenomenon or to illuminate a problem from different angles, gaining a variety of different types of information. Many approaches used in nursing and healthcare researches employ MM occasionally, for instance ethnography and – mainly in the early days – grounded theory.

Mason (2006) gives two main reasons for MMR:

1. Social reality has many dimensions and MM illustrate this complexity of the social world.
2. People's lives and life experience happens on both macro and micro levels. MM demonstrate these levels of people's lives.

MMR is particularly useful for translational research (where basic research and scientific discoveries are applied to clinical or practice settings). Tripp-Reimer and Doebbeling (2004) state that the use of qualitative research in a quantitative study adds 'human dimensions' to the care of patients; policy changes too might be more easily put into place as a result of this strategy.

Mixed methods and pragmatism

Mixed methods (mixed methodologies) research has its roots in pragmatism, a direction in philosophy with its origin in the work of Charles Peirce (1839–1914), William James (1842–1910) and John Dewey (1859–1952) in the nineteenth and early twentieth century. Seeing the world as a reality of diverse experiences, they considered mainly the practical consequences and effects of actions and their expedience. In the view of pragmatists, theory and practice are not only related, but theory is just an abstraction from reality (this is a very simplistic description of some elements of pragmatism, but there is no place for discussing the whole of pragmatism here. Researchers who are interested can pursue this themselves). Johnson and Onwuegbuzie (2004: 16) stress 'workable solutions' to problems and hence pragmatism as the 'philosophical partner' for MM which are seen as instrumental in achieving the research aims. The practical consequences of actions are seen as important and the research should be meaningful. The 'paradigm wars' and the dichotomy or dualism of qualitative and quantitative research have no place here. Clinical and applied research often gain from the practical and instrumental approach. Practice has priority over theory in pragmatism, although pragmatists are by no means a-theoretical. It is interesting however, that Giddings and Grant (2007) suggest that pragmatism is not the preserve of MMR alone but can play a part in any type of research. Pragmatists, so these writers observe (p. 53): 'rather than focusing on epistemological integrity, emphasise the importance of getting "the job done".'

Many researchers see MM as a way of improving, enhancing or extending a research study. In the words of Johnson et al. (2007: 113):

'Mixed methods research is generally speaking an approach to knowledge (theory and practice) that attempts to consider multiple viewpoints, perspectives, positions and standpoints (always including the standpoints of qualitative and quantitative research).'

Flemming (2007) defends MMR in nursing specifically, by stating that many nursing questions need input from both quantitative and qualitative perspectives to provide the broad knowledge in the field. These types of knowledge, she maintains, are neither incompatible nor mutually exclusive. The effectiveness of care or interventions can be measured by a randomised controlled trial (RCT) while patient perceptions and experience are more likely to be elicited by qualitative methods. Both contribute to practical use in clinical practice regardless of their ontological and epistemological base.

Doing mixed methods research

To design a piece of multimethod or MMR is a complex process because several approaches are involved which have different epistemologies and strategies as explained earlier, and hence clarity is of major importance. As in all research, the research question and the following proposal must address the issue of design, and this in turn should fit the problem. The research question(s) need to be robust; Tashakkori and Creswell (2007) state that they include the 'what and how' and 'what and why'.

Researchers need to be clear from the beginning about the type of MMR they wish to adopt and the strategies to be used. The important issues focus on the sequencing of the methods, the priority one might have over another, the question of combination of the two, including integration or non-integration. As MMR includes both qualitative and quantitative elements the aims of each approach should be made explicit. This might be challenging researchers but would enable them to make a more robust case for MMR

Types of mixed methods research

Methods in MMR can be used either sequentially, concurrently or transformatively according to Creswell (2009). When researchers use sequential procedures, one method follows the other and expands or enhances the findings from the first. For instance, a health professional might start a study with participant observation and conduct a survey about a particular issue that arose during observing the setting. On the other hand, the researcher might have been involved in an RCT and wish to deepen knowledge about the feelings or thoughts of the participants.

When concurrent procedures are carried out, quantitative and qualitative data converge as they are both gathered at the same time. The researcher also integrates and interprets qualitative and quantitative information concurrently. When using transformative procedures, a 'theoretical lens' (Creswell, p. 62) is used which provides a framework for the study. This is the most complex approach.

Creswell makes further distinctions by identifying several types or strategies of MMR.

1. Sequential explanatory
2. Sequential exploratory
3. Sequential transformative
4. Concurrent triangulation
5. Concurrent nested
6. Concurrent transformative

(we shall only give examples for the most commonly used studies)

Sequential explanatory design is the least controversial form of these types. The researcher collects and analyses quantitative data and, based on the results, uses a qualitative approach to gain more depth and interpretive possibilities for the study. Quantitative method has priority and therefore the results of the study can be generalised. In this and other types of sequential design, separate questions are asked and answers emerge sequentially; this means that the findings from the quantitative research form the basis for questions in qualitative research or vice versa.

Example of sequential explanatory strategy

Ivankova *et al.* (2006) developed a sequential explanatory mixed method design to research doctoral students' persistence in taking part in the distance-learning programme and identify the factors which contribute to this perseverance. They established and used a complex survey, including Likert-type scales and other instruments using statistical analysis for the data. The quantitative sample consisted of almost 300 students. The analysis showed that five main variables contributed to the discriminating function linked to students' persistence in the programme. Thus the in-depth explanation of the quantitative study was the study's major aim.

The qualitative part of the study had a sample of only four participants. Various in-depth interview techniques were used and the data thematically analysed. The qualitative findings showed that quality of the programme, the infrastructure and student commitment were elements in the persistence of students.

Sequential exploratory design seems another logical and useful way of MMR. In this, primacy is usually given to qualitative research methods of data collection and analysis which are used at the start of the study to illuminate a phenomenon. Quantitative strategies follow these to help interpret the findings, show generalisability or test the propositions developed in the qualitative part. It can also illustrate the distribution of the phenomenon within a particular population.

> ## Example of sequential exploratory design
>
> Murphy (2007) reports on a sequential exploratory design in which the qualitative phase preceded the quantitative. Interviews were the basis of the qualitative research which was then used to design a questionnaire; factor analysis was employed to analyse the questionnaire. This study was, however, undertaken in two completely separate phases which together formed MMR. The focus was on the phenomenon of quality of care and the factors contributing to this.

Sequential transformative or *concurrent transformative* strategies can develop approaches sequentially or concurrently. They do have, however, as Creswell states, an overarching perspective which is provided by looking at the topic through a 'theoretical lens'. Depending on which type of strategy is used, the researcher again collects data either sequentially or at the same time. We could find little about these two strategies and no examples in the healthcare research literature.

Concurrent triangulation strategies are the best known and are also undertaken within some of the other MMR designs. One distinct method is used to validate or confirm the other type selected. Each is employed to overcome the weaknesses of the other and they are integrated. It is obviously better when the methods have equal importance.

The *concurrent nested strategy* is often employed when one approach is strongly dominant and the embedded method is used merely to ask a somewhat different question. The main framework is the dominant approach. Many studies where qualitative research has priority use a nested strategy. The answer to the research question might also be broader and enhance the study. According to Creswell, this procedure could also be undertaken when different groups or levels are being examined.

> ## Example of a nested design
>
> Day (2008), a nurse researcher, has started a concurrent nested study aimed to explore the phenomenon of the meaning of pain – in this case chronic low back pain – through examining Focusing (a technique and process in psychotherapy, developed by the philosopher Gendlin). It explores the phenomenon of self-care through descriptive phenomenology in which a quantitative strategy is embedded to examine pain scores and quality of life. The qualitative element of the study will have primacy. Day states that as a clinician she needs both qualitative and quantitative data to make decisions.

In concurrent MMR, parallel questions are asked from the very beginning. It is important to note, however, that both qualitative and quantitative ways of researching are valid.

The process of MMR

The approach to designing and doing a mixed method study is very similar, though more complex than undertaking mono-method research. Wilkins and Woodgate (2008) propose a nine-step approach to MMR whose steps do not necessarily all need to be used sequentially:

1. *Researchers reflect on the appropriateness of MMR* which means that both qualitative and quantitative aims need to be considered. Of course, if only one researcher is involved, he or she should be knowledgeable about both qualitative and quantitative approaches.
2. *The rationale of employing MM is developed*. A number of questions are asked about this, for instance whether the methods are used as complementary approaches or for triangulation.
3. *The researcher chooses a specific design*, concurrent or sequential, and decides on the priority of qualitative or quantitative procedures or whether they should have equal weight. The research question influences the data collection and analysis.
4. *The sample is selected* according to the methods used, probability sampling in quantitative research, and purposeful sampling for the qualitative section
5. *Data are collected*, and the type of collection depends on the design of the study, whether it is concurrent or sequential.
6. *The researcher analyses the data* according to the specific analysis needed for both the qualitative and quantitative procedures.
7. *Data need interpretation*. This, of course depends on the particular combination or integration of the research. The interpretation of qualitative and quantitative data can be combined. The findings from each might be compared or might be used for enrichment or expansion.
8. *The validity and trustworthiness of the findings are established*. This includes the audit trail, member check (if appropriate), and reflexivity for qualitative findings and procedures such as probability sampling and inclusion of a control group for quantitative findings.
9. *The researcher gives an account of the findings* which have to be reported in writing through a formal report or thesis, and disseminated through journal articles, books or conference papers.

Wilkins and Woodgate do not mention ethical considerations and the step to gain ethical approval which is important soon after deciding on the research design.

The place and purpose of the literature

The literature review in a MM design depends on the way in which these methods are used in the particular study. Where quantitative method has priority in a sequential approach, the initial review is usually lengthy as the gap in knowledge demonstrated by the literature has to be established. On the basis of this, the rationale for the study can be developed. In a sequential type where qualitative research has primacy, there is merely an overview to show that the specific topic has not been researched in the way in which the researcher wants to study it. Of course the dialogue with the literature is ongoing in the qualitative section and closely linked to the findings and developing ideas. In a concurrent study, the researcher has choice, but ultimately, the literature review depends on the topic under study.

Triangulation

A long debate has arisen about the use of triangulation, and many MMR studies have included an attempt at this. Triangulation is the process by which several methods (data sources, theories or researchers) are used in the study of one phenomenon in order to ensure validity in a study. The concept has its origin in ancient Greek mathematics; in modern times it is employed in topographic surveying as a checking system. Denzin (1989) differentiates between four different types of triangulation: triangulation of *data*, *investigators*, *theories* and *method/ologies*. The triangulation of methods is most often used, and the discussion in this chapter centres on this type of triangulation. (The other forms are explained in Chapter 18).

Usually researchers use *methodological triangulation* in its two main forms: Within-method (intra-method) triangulation and between-method (across method or inter-method) triangulation. Within-method triangulation adopts different strategies but stays within a single paradigm; for instance, participant observation and open-ended interviews are often used together in one qualitative study. In this chapter we are discussing the triangulation between methods.

Researchers use between-method triangulation to confirm the findings generated through one particular method by another. It is suggested that triangulation can improve validity and overcome the biases inherent in one perspective.

Critique of MMR

MM studies are not always seen as the solution to the problems of mono-method research.

Lipscomb (2008) considers pragmatism and its place in MM studies and points out some caveats on the interpretation of data from this research. He tells health researchers that MMR should be neither naïve, nor should it lack theory; indeed he intimates that many studies suffer from serious flaws and cautions against 'unreflective pragmatism and theoretical indifference'

(p. 35), and suggests that MMR should be truly mixed and not contain two separate studies in one. Adding that qualitative, quantitative, and even different qualitative approaches, cannot be seen as having the same underlying beliefs and diverge from each other and hence are not always suited to be built into a MM study (*our comment*: for instance, grounded theory which develops theories and hypotheses might be useful for sequential explorative inquiry but not for another type of MMR). In Lipscomb's words (p. 37):'... it is unlikely that all combinations of qualitative and quantitative methodologies can be blended'.

The often-mentioned claim that MMR is a 'third paradigm' is contested by Giddings and Grant (2007) who see this belief as problematic. Much MMR fits into the positivist paradigm or has its basis in a post-positivist stance. Often quantitative methods have dominance over the qualitative and many MMR studies add the qualitative at some stage to enhance or deepen the findings from the quantitative approach. The vocabulary of MMR also shows that there is no clarity between the mixing of methods or methodologies; most MM researchers would advocate the mixing of methods rather than that of methodologies as the latter is linked to underlying philosophical bases of methods while the former are mainly techniques for data collection and analysis. Giddings and Grant see in MMR a distancing of researchers from philosophical and theoretical issues.

Conclusion

Freshwater (2007: 140) calls MM inquiry 'an unfinished story', and indeed new discussions and developments are being processed. We suggest that undergraduate students use a single method/ology in their research because of the limited time frame; they might also find difficulty reconciling the distinct world views of qualitative and quantitative research; they need to know of its existence however. MA/MSc students might attempt a simple MM approach if it is appropriate for the research question. For doctoral students this approach can be useful as they learn to use a variety of research methods when carrying out MMR. They can then engage with the philosophical and theoretical tensions within it. Experienced researchers might or might not employ a mixed methodology and take a pragmatic approach. This type of research is highly regarded by funding bodies and agencies because they wish researchers to take a pragmatic and practical route. Many qualitative and quantitative researchers appreciate MMR especially when they are carrying out interprofessional or interdisciplinary research. Members of different health professions and disciplines are able to work together in one study in which each is using their own expertise in one study. MMR can change clinical practice and provide new insights.

Summary

- MMR as understood in this chapter uses both qualitative and quantitative methods within a single research project.
- MMR is intended to illuminate all sides of a problem or phenomenon.
- MMR has its basis in pragmatism and takes a practical empirical approach.
- There are a number of types of MMR.
- The complexity of this research needs expert researchers and a considerable time span.

References

Creswell, J.W. (2009) *Research Design: Qualitative, Quantitative and Mixed Methods Approaches*. Los Angeles, CA, Sage.

Day, R. (2008) *An Exploration of the Meaning and Experiences of Pain when Journeying with 'focusing' in One's Life*. Bournemouth University, Research Study.

Denzin, N.K. (1989) *The Research Act: A Theoretical Introduction to Sociological Methods*, 3rd edn. Englewood Cliffs, NJ, Prentice Hall.

Flemming, K. (2007) The knowledge base for evidence-based nursing: a role for mixed methods research. *Advances in Nursing Science*, 30 (1), 41–51.

Freshwater, D. (2007) Reading mixed methods research. *Journal of Mixed Methods Research*, 1 (2), 134–146.

Giddings, L.S. & Grant, B.M. (2007) A Trojan horse for positivism? A critique of mixed methods research. *Advances in Nursing Science*, 30 (1), 52–60.

Ivankova, N.V., Creswell, J.W. & Stick, S.L. (2006) Using mixed methods sequential explanatory design: from theory to practice. *Field Methods* 18 (1), 3–20.

Johnson, R. & Onwuegbuzie, A.J. (2004) Mixed methods research: a paradigm whose time has come. *Educational Researcher*, 33 (7), 14–26.

Johnson, R.B., Onwuegbuzie, A.J. & Turner, L.A. (2007) Towards a definition of mixed methods research. *Journal of Mixed Methods Research*, 1 (2), 112–33.

Lipscomb, M. (2008) Mixed method nursing studies: a critical realist technique. *Nursing Philosophy*, 9 (1), 32–5.

Mason, J. (2006) Mixing methods in a qualitatively driven way. *Qualitative Research*, 6 (1), 9–25.

Murphy, K. (2007) Nurses' perceptions of quality and the factors that affect quality care for older people living in long-term care in Ireland. *Journal of Clinical Nursing*, 16 (5), 873–84.

O'Cathain, A., Murphy, E. & Nicholl, J. (2007) Why, and how, mixed methods research is undertaken in health services research in England: a mixed methods study. *BMC Health Services Research* 7, 85. Open access journal. Retrieved July 2008 from http://www.pubmedcentral.nih.gov/articlerender.fcgi?artid=1906856

Punch, K.F. (2005) *Introduction to Social Research: Qualitative and Quantitative Approaches*, 2nd edn. London, Sage.

Sandelowski, M. (2000) Focus on research methods: combining qualitative and quantitative sampling, data collection and analysis techniques in mixed methods studies. *Research in Nursing and Health*, **23** (3), 246–55.

Tashakkori, A. & Creswell, J.W. (2007) Exploring the nature of mixed methods research. *Journal of Mixed Methods Research*, **1** (3), 207–11.

Tashakkori, A. & Teddlie, C.B. (eds). (2003) *Handbook of Mixed Methods in Social and Behavioral Research*. Thousand Oaks, CA, Sage.

Tripp-Reimer, T. & Doebbeling, B. (2004) Qualitative perspectives in translational research. *Worldviews on Evidence-Based Nursing*, **1** (Suppl 1), S65–S72.

Wilkins, K. & Woodgate, R. (2008) Designing a mixed methods study in pediatric oncology research. *Journal of Pediatric Oncology*, **25** (1), 24–33.

Further reading

Bryman, A. (2006) Integrating qualitative and qualitative research: how is it done? *Qualitative Research*, **6** (1), 97–113.

Bryman, A. (2006) (ed.) *Mixed Methods*, 4 vol. set. London: Sage

Creswell, J.W. & Plano Clark, V.L. (2006) *Designing and Conducting Mixed Methods Research*. Thousand Oaks, CA, Sage.

Gilbert, T. (2006) Mixed methods and mixed methodologies: the practical, the technical and the political. *Journal of Research in Nursing*, **11** (3), 205–17.

Greene, J. (2008) Is mixed methods social inquiry a distinctive methodology? *Journal of Mixed Methods Research*, **2** (7), 7–22.

PART FOUR

Data Analysis and Completion

CHAPTER 17

Data Analysis: Procedures, Practices and Computers

The process of data analysis

Qualitative data analysis (QDA) is a complex, non-linear process but also systematic, orderly and structured. Not all qualitative forms of inquiry take the same approach to analysis, as can be seen in the chapters on specific approaches. Indeed, grounded theory (GT) and phenomenology in particular have very distinct ways of analysing data (and also a different approach to data collection). Data reduction or collapsing, description and/or interpretation, however, are common to many types of QDA although the approach to these procedures is flexible and creative. There is no rigid prescription as long as the eventual research account has its roots directly in the data generated by the participants. In this chapter we shall only attempt an overview of generic data analysis in qualitative research. For complete beginners an examination of relevant chapters in clearly written introductory texts might be useful, such as that of Hansen (2006).

Data analysis is an iterative activity. Iteration means that researchers move back and forth from collection to analysis and back again, refining the questions they ask from the data. Knowledge of this process means that researchers will be able to allocate and segment their time appropriately. Health researchers often lack time at the end of their study to carry out the appropriate data analysis, because they do not foresee the complexity of the data and the length of time needed for analysing them. The iterative character of qualitative research also makes it more time consuming.

Qualitative researchers usually collect and analyse the data simultaneously, unlike those involved in quantitative inquiry who complete collection before starting analysis. Indeed in GT, data collection and analysis interact (see Chapter 11), and in several other approaches researchers often use data collection and analysis in parallel and interactively (for instance in ethnography). Even when recording and transcribing initial data, researchers reflect upon them and so start the process of analysis at an early stage.

The process of analysis goes through certain stages common to many approaches:

- Transcribing interviews and sorting fieldnotes
- Organising, ordering and storing the data
- Listening to and reading or viewing the material collected repeatedly

All this means immersion in and engagement with the data.
Other stages depend on the approach taken by the qualitative researcher:

- Coding and categorising (this is particularly appropriate in interpretive methods)
- Building themes
- Describing a cultural group (in ethnography)
- Describing a phenomenon (this is appropriate in phenomenology)

These steps also involve storing ideas, interpretations and theoretical thought which is carried out through memoing and writing fieldnotes (see Chapters 10 and 11 on fieldnotes and memos respectively)

Silverman (2006) discusses the status of interview data in particular, which must be taken into account before the process of data analysis can start. These data are rarely raw but have been processed through the mind of the interviewer and can only be seen in context. In observations too, fieldnotes do not always show how the environment might shape the interaction, in particular elements such as the presence or absence of certain people, the work climate and other factors.

Transcribing and sorting

Transcription of interviews is one of the initial steps in preparing the data for analysis. The fullest and richest data can be gained from transcribing verbatim. We advise that if possible, novice researchers transcribe their own tapes because this way they immerse themselves in the data and become sensitive to the issues of importance. Transcription takes a long time: one hour of interviewing takes between four and six hours to transcribe. For those who are not used to audio-typing, it can be much longer. Transcription is very frustrating and can take time that researchers often lack. A typist using a transcription machine could do it more quickly, but this would be expensive. On the other hand, it would give more time to the researcher to listen and analyse. The decision about this depends on the researcher. Any outsider who transcribes must, of course, be advised on the confidentiality relating to the data.

Initial interviews and fieldnotes should be fully transcribed so that the researcher becomes aware of the important issues in the data. Novice researchers should transcribe all interviews verbatim, while more experienced individuals can be more selective in their transcriptions and transcribe that which is linked to their developing theoretical ideas. It is always better that the interviews or fieldnotes are fully transcribed by the researchers themselves if they have the time. There is danger that researchers who fail to record the interviews will overlook significant issues, which they would uncover on reflection when listening to the tape or considering the transcript. Pages are numbered, and the front sheet should contain date, location and time of interview as well as the code number or pseudonym for the informant and important biographical data (but no identifier). Many researchers number each line of the interview transcript so that they can retrieve the data quickly when revisiting the transcript. Transcription pages are most useful when put into a column which takes half the sheet while the other half is left for coding and comments.

A minimum of three copies (usually more) should be made of the transcripts and a clean copy without comments for locking away in a safe place in case other copies are lost or destroyed.

Occasionally researchers use formal transcription systems (some invent their own systems); the best known of these is Gail Jefferson's which uses symbols for non-verbal actions such as coughing, pausing, emphasising. These systems are more often applied to 'naturally occurring data' such as those from conversation or discourse analysis. However, for some approaches the type of transcribing Jefferson developed would be an anathema; Langridge (2007) reminds researchers that phenomenology in particular does not need a micro-level of transcription, and we would suggest the inappropriateness of this for ethnography and GT too. Silverman (2006) gives a list of simplified transcription symbols which could be helpful in conversation analysis and some forms of discourse analysis.

Of course, researchers transcribe in detail, and as accurately as possible, often more than they analyse as they choose sections from the data which answer their research questions. There is however the danger that they select according to their own assumptions about the importance of data rather than focusing on the participants' words, hence careful reading and listening is advised.

Taking notes and writing analytic memos

Some researchers use the tape-recorder and also take notes during the interview so that participants' facial expression, gestures and interviewers' reactions and comments can be recorded. Making notes might disturb the participant. We would suggest this only when taping is not feasible or if interviewees do not wish to be tape-recorded. Notes can also be taken immediately after the interview.

When participants deny permission for recording or when it seems inappropriate – for instance in very sensitive situations – interviewers generally take notes throughout the interview, and these notes reflect the words of the participants as accurately as possible. As interviewers can only write down a fraction of the sentences, they select the most important words or phrases and summarise the rest, and this might distort meaning. Patton (2002) advises on conventions in the use of quotation marks while writing notes. Researchers use them only for full, direct quotations from informants. Patton suggests that researchers adopt a mechanism for differentiating between their own thoughts and informants' words. When reading transcripts and writing memos, researchers should also collect a series of pithy quotes, which are representative of the thoughts of the participants and the phenomenon or phenomena under study.

Another method of recording is to take notes after the interview is finished. This should be done as soon as possible after the interview to capture the flavour, behaviour and words of the informants and the concomitant thoughts of the researcher. It should not be done in the presence of the participants.

The process of listening to the tapes will sensitise researchers to the data and uncover ambiguities or problems within them. At this time, any theoretical or other ideas that emerge should be written down in the field diary. The process of writing fieldnotes and memos is in itself an analytic process and not just data recording. It helps the researcher to reflect on the data and engage with them.

During the process of analysis researchers write analytical memos or notes containing ideas and thoughts about the data as well the reasons for grouping them in a particular way. Sometimes researchers draw diagrams to demonstrate this, and these diagrams can be taken directly into the report when they discuss the methods and the decision trail. Researchers might develop concepts in the memos, ask analytic questions of the data, or elaborate ideas from the literature that link directly with the data. There are different ways of keeping memos: in field journals or diaries, or on a computer. This all helps 'tacking', that is, going back and forth between the data and theoretical ideas, between codes and themes. This is called 'iteration'.

Some researchers do not code or categorise because they wish to perceive the essence of the phenomenon as a whole, a *Gestalt*. Breaking the data into codes may lose this holistic view of the phenomenon and fragment the ideas contained in the data. Memoing goes on throughout the research process but is of particular importance in assisting analysis. (Specific types of analysis are discussed in the chapters on the various approaches.)

Ordering and organising the data

Qualitative researchers generate large amounts of data consisting of narratives from interviews, fieldnotes and documents, as well as a variety of memos about the phenomenon under study (Bryman, 2008). Many use the literature linked to the research as data.

Through organisation and management, the researcher brings structure and order to the unwieldy mass of data. This will help eventual retrieval and final analysis. All transcripts, fieldnotes and other data should have details of time, location and specific comments attached. The use of pseudonyms or numbers for participants prevents identification during the long process of analysis when the data might fall into the hands of individuals other than the researcher. Everything has to be recorded, cross-checked and labelled. Then the material has to be stored in the appropriate files for later retrieval.

From the very beginning of the study, nurses and other health professionals will recognise significant ideas and themes in the material they generated. On listening to tapes, reading transcriptions and other documents or looking at visual data common themes and patterns will begin to emerge and become crystallised.

Borkan (1999) discusses the initial process of analysis and describes two strategies from which researchers can choose depending on their approach, namely *horizontal* and *vertical* 'passes' of the data. The horizontal pass involves

- reading the data and looking at themes, emotions and surprises, taking in the overall picture;
- reflective and in-depth reading of the data to find supporting evidence for these themes;
- re-reading for elements that might have been overlooked;
- searching for possible alternative meanings;
- attempting to link discrepancies together.

Vertical passes involve

- concentrating on one section of the data and analysing it before moving on;
- reflecting on and reviewing the data in the section;
- looking for insights and feeding them back into the data collection process.

The horizontal is more holistic than the vertical pass. However, researchers not only analyse according to the methods they adopt, but they also have different personal styles, which demand different ways of looking at the data.

Analytical styles

Different approaches to research have different types of data analysis. Even within one approach, researchers adopt a variety of analyses. Phenomenologists, ethnographers or grounded theorists for instance, use a variety of analytic strategies. They all involve the steps of listening to, viewing and gaining a holistic view of the data as well as dividing them into units or segments of meaning. Dahlberg *et al.* (2008) ask that each part of the transcribed text, analysed for meaning, should be understood in relation to the whole of the text and the whole understood in terms of its parts.

Moustakas (1994), a hermeneutic phenomenologist, gives a general overview of analysis styles and comes up with overlapping steps in which researchers carry out the following:

- They reflect on each transcript and search for significant statements.
- They record all relevant statements.
- They delete repetitive and overlapping statements, leaving only invariant constituents of the phenomenon, and organise them.
- They link and relate these into themes.
- Including verbatim quotes from the data, they integrate the themes into a description of the texture of the experience as told by the participants.
- They reflect on this and their own experiences.
- They develop a description of the meanings of the experience.

At all times, researchers search for links and relationships between sections of data, categories or themes.

There are more detailed discussions of analytic procedures in the chapters on specific approaches.

Coding and categorising

Coding means marking sections of data and giving them labels or names. It is an early stage in analysis and proceeds towards the development of categories, themes or major constructs (the nomenclature depends on the language of the specific approach). It breaks the data into manageable sections.

Line-by-line coding identifies information which both participant and researcher consider important. In their initial coding, many researchers single out words or phrases that are used by participants – these are called *in vivo* codes. This type of coding prevents researchers from imposing their own framework and ideas on the data, because the coding starts with the words of the participants.

> **Example of *in vivo* coding**
>
> A transcript might contain the sentence 'I was really worried when I went to the doctor with my problem; it could have been serious'. The *in vivo* code might be: *worried when going to the doctor*. At a later stage, of course, this would have to be refined by the words of the researcher but still seen from the perspective of the participant. It might become: *Fear of diagnosis*. As the coding process goes on, the codes might become more abstract.

In the beginning, line-by-line and *in vivo* coding can be useful, but it would be difficult to carry out in all transcriptions of the interviews and sets of fieldnotes.

It does, however, help researchers discern important ideas in the data initially until they become used to coding.

Initial or *open* coding gives a name to specific pieces of data. The codes may be words, expressions or other chunks of data. Researchers might start with a mass of codes and reduce them so that each of them represents a concept. These concepts are *units of meaning*. Once simple coding has been completed, researchers group together the codes with similar meanings which are linked to the same phenomenon. If different terms are applied to the same concept, the best label is used as a name for the concept. Rather than coding line by line or sentence by sentence, many researchers code paragraph by paragraph. Others search for meaningful statements in the text. Ziebland and McPherson (2006) remind researchers not only to focus on what they think is important but mainly on the ideas that emerge from the participants and what the latter think significant. This means that the collected data have primacy, and not the researchers' prior assumptions about themes. However, these authors also speak of 'anticipated' and 'emergent' themes (p. 407). When looking at the data, researchers anticipate particular elements which have roots in their experiences and disciplines. The dialogue with the literature takes place at the stage when the findings have been established. The relevant literature will then be related and integrated into the findings.

There are some problems with coding and categorising. One is the loss of the holistic view or *Gestalt* of the phenomenon, which is the aim of phenomenologists. The other, according to Silverman (2005), is the loss of important information, because it does not 'fit' the code or category, hence the importance of the search for discrepant and alternative ideas.

When analysing data from different data sources, for instance from observation, interviews and documents, researchers search for similarities and differences. All the material that has conceptual links is grouped together for later categorisation. Some researchers actually cut up the data and keep them in a file, after pasting them on pages of paper and putting them into a ring binder, others use coloured pencils or pens to identify closely linked material. Researchers need to keep a list of the categories or themes to compare each section of new data with the early-established themes. The new ideas might fit into these, or new themes have to be uncovered. Eventually, a greatly reduced list might be established to form a diagram. Often, researchers generate a hierarchy of themes and codes with more abstract and general themes at the top. They might also establish a typology. Typologies are classification systems. Bluff (2005), for instance, distinguishes between 'flexible' and 'prescriptive' midwives who had different characteristics and acted in different ways in particular situations.

Many researchers go further than merely arriving at an analytic or conceptual description. They take into account conditions under which something occurs, variations in findings according to location and time, the context in which things happen, the strategies that participants adopt to cope with their experiences, causes of actions and events as well as their effects and consequences (See specific approaches such as GT and ethnography).

Problems of QDA

Because of the complexities of QDA, a number of problems might arise. Li and Seale (2007) list several, and one of these relates to not knowing where to start the process. This might be solved by asking novice researchers to analyse short sections of data. Many find the resulting themes or codes ambiguous, and of course, there is sometimes overlap of meaning. Reporting or recording problems can be overcome more easily. These issues are often connected with forgetting to note down the identifier of the participant, or not being able to retrieve ideas that had previously been discovered. Some new researchers over-interpret – everything has meaning for them – or they report inaccurately and give no evidence where ideas have their roots.

Inferential leaps and 'premature closure'

As part of the process of data analysis, researchers should check against inferential leaps. In our early days of research supervision, it became apparent that students would infer conclusions from the data too quickly. In their haste to make sense of the data and develop a picture, students can too readily make inferential leaps. It seems that health researchers remember concepts or frameworks previously learned or discovered as a background to the research, and they try to fit these to the data. The researcher has to return to the data continually, checking and verifying so that inferential leaps are not made. This is closely connected with the warning against premature closure (Glaser, 1978) that is one of the problems of qualitative research. Often novice researchers decide on a theme or category at an early stage of the research process. In GT in particular, the danger exists that once researchers have generated some theoretical ideas, they then sit back and decide that they arrived at full explanations for the phenomenon under study. Sometimes there has been no full investigation of the data; sometimes they close their minds to new ideas. Premature closure and inferential leaps might mean that the research is incomplete or inadequate.

Collaboration in the process of analysis and interpretation

In all types of QDA it is important that researchers stay as close to the data as possible and look at everything connected with the phenomenon under study.

A completed study is never a mere description of the participants' experience. It is important to remember that the final product of research depends on the collaborative effort of participants and researcher. While those observed and interviewed are active agents in their world rather than passive participants and construct their social reality, researcher and participant also construct meaning together. The reader of the study too, will eventually be involved in construction of meaning.

Computer-aided analysis of qualitative data

Computers can of course, carry out the process much more quickly – even when researchers do not use a computer package for the analysis of data. There are, however, arguments both for and against computer use in qualitative research.

Computers have been used in the analysis of qualitative data mainly since the 1980s although they do not seem as popular as they once were. They are most useful for storing or retrieving data, and all researchers use them this way. Computers can be useful and make the process of qualitative research less cumbersome.

The type of approach influences the program for analysis of qualitative data. Managing a large volume of data by hand is boring and tiring because the search for specific ideas, words, incidents or events takes time. The computer is, however, merely a tool, if a useful one for a lengthy study with a large number of participants; it shortens routine and mechanical tasks and can be a device to save labour and time though a novice researcher might spend a lengthy span of time learning to use a particular computer package. In the past, researchers depended for their analysis to a large extent on cutting, sorting and pasting bits of paper. This meant that the researcher was left with a mass of paper cuttings, a great many boxes and envelopes and/or an elaborate card system. Computers have changed these elaborate processes. We do however believe that the researcher is more intimate with the data when the analysis is not computerised.

Several types of computer-aided QDA software (CAQDAS) exist, of which the best known are NUDIST (Non-numerical Unstructured Data Indexing, Searching and Theorising) NVivo, Ethnograph, ATLAS.ti and HyperResearch (for a list and advice for best uses of the various programs see Fielding and Lee, 1998). Ethnograph is one of the earliest packages and NUDIST is one of the most widely used (perhaps because of its name!). The packages have slightly different functions.

Since the early 1980s, when the journal *Qualitative Sociology* (1984, 7 (1) 2) published a special edition on the use of computers in qualitative research, new ideas and packages have been developed. Some programs are more sophisticated than others. Each has its own technical traits depending on the choice of the designer. For researchers who wish to use this software, it is essential to become familiar with it.

For further information and details on particular programs, we advise researchers to look at up-to-date text books such as Bazeley (2007). Older texts such as those by Kelle (1995), Fielding and Lee (1998), and the various writings of Richards (2005) who are advocates of CAQDAS. Lately Lewins and Silver (2007) have written a step-by-step guide. In some of these books, programs and addresses can also be found. Well-known are the courses and books generated by the CAQDAS Network of the University of Surrey (see Caqdas Networking Project in References for website).

The reasons for computer use

Tesch (1993) lists a variety of tasks, formerly done manually, which can now be performed by computers, some of which we list as the most important. Although this book is now quite old, she describes the main tasks for the analyst.

- Storing, annotating and retrieving texts
- Locating words, phrases, and segments of data
- Naming or labelling
- Sorting and organising
- Identifying data units
- Preparing diagrams
- Extracting quotes

Storing, annotating and retrieving texts

Storing and retrieving texts such as interview transcripts, fieldnotes or diaries is the most common use of computer programs in qualitative research. Data are easily accessible – for instance interview transcripts and fieldnotes can be stored in separated files and memos attached to the category to which they belong – and can be called upon when needed. Researchers must always label and date these files to keep order among them. NB: Copies of files should be made on floppy disks and stored safely in different locations.

Locating words, phrases or segments of data

Researchers may want to find particular words or phrases and the context in which they occur as well as their frequency. Sentences, paragraphs and specific key words can be recalled. These can indicate the importance, which informants and researcher attach to particular words or concepts (though it is dangerous to rely on the number of instances rather than an in-depth examination of each instance).

Naming or labelling

These labels are key words that define an idea, or they can be summaries of the content of data. Categorising starts here and is based on this labelling.

Categories are concepts attached to a topic emerging from the data and a step in their interpretation. Researchers give the appropriate label to each segment of data or to instances that belong together. Revision of names in the light of further analysis then becomes less difficult. The creation of categories from the data is a step towards theory building.

Sorting and organising

Sorting and organising the data segments and topic units according to the named categories or key words attached to them is one of the procedures undertaken during the analysis process. Organising data into segments (bits, chunks or strips as they are sometimes called), means dividing them into discrete units (although these can sometimes overlap with each other). All segments with the same inherent themes or categories can be grouped together.

Identifying data units

Researchers identify data units relevant to several categories and discover relationships between them. They always try to see a structure and links between categories. While working with the data these links can be found more easily in and across particular files. This helps in the development of working hypotheses, models or typologies. Of course, the computer does none of these processes; they are based on the researcher's theoretical considerations and decisionmaking but are helped by the machine. Each proposition can be checked out. For instance, a nurse researcher may infer from examining the data that women prefer male to female doctors. This can be checked quickly through viewing the categories and the links between them.

Preparing diagrams

Diagrams illustrate the relationship between themes or categories. The graphic display can enhance the storyline and help to convey its meaning. Many of our students clarify their findings by showing links and connections through diagrams.

Approaches to qualitative computer analysis

Tesch (1991) describes three main approaches to QDA (described below) but acknowledges that these groupings and their subgroups are not neat and discrete; they overlap and do not reflect reality. Both the content of the text and the process of communication are seen as important.

Language oriented

These types of analysis are used by researchers who are primarily interested in language and its meaning – examples are conversation and discourse analysis as well as ethnography. These approaches focus not only on words and verbal interaction but also on the way in which people make sense of their world.

Descriptive/interpretive approaches

These deal with narratives and give descriptions of feelings and actions. Examples are life histories and certain types of ethnography as descriptions and interpretations of a culture. Researchers tell stories and provide interpretations of meanings that participants in the research attach to their experiences.

Theory building

In theory building, the researcher finds patterns and links between ideas and attempts to build theory. From insights generated by the data, general principles often emerge. This is more explanatory than other approaches. GT represents this type of research. The process of theory building is not routine or mechanical but demands engagement, immersion and reflection from the researcher.

The practicalities of using computer-aided analysis

Most students already use word processors for entering and storing data. It is essential for the small minority who do not do so to learn word processing skills because changing a text by correcting, cutting and pasting on the machine takes much less time than rewriting by hand or typewriter. Word processing programs create and revise text and can therefore be helpful to researchers in the transcription of interviews, fieldnotes and in writing the report.

Many researchers would like to learn the use of computers for qualitative analysis, but the practicalities of this must be sorted out before starting a project. The usefulness of computers depends on the researchers' initial knowledge of computers as well as the time span and size of the project. Some of our students started learning to use the computer for data analysis and found it impossible to do so within the allocated time.

We found it difficult to learn the use of computer packages for qualitative analysis from manuals, although some people seem to be able to do so. It is always easier to let expert users teach rather than relying on a manual, but one must be aware that very experienced individuals might be too far advanced to use beginners' terms and explain the skills in a simple way. They take the language and skills needed for computers for granted. It is far better to have a teacher who is just a few steps ahead.

Not only do researchers store and retrieve data, actions that are mechanical and routine, but they also code and categorise. These tasks involve formulating concepts and theory and hence reflection. These two types of activities, procedures and conceptual thinking are always linked to each other and can both be helped by the use of computers.

Advantages of computer use

Researchers use computers as tools for facilitating processes that were done manually in the past; but it is a fallacy to believe that data can be analysed more quickly by computer programs, because it takes time to learn their use. Once learnt though, they can save time and help researchers to be more organised and systematic and facilitate planning. Data are more accessible and fewer hours are spent sorting and coding the data (however, this implies that all approaches use coding and categorising, and that, of course, is not so).

Cutting and pasting is easy when computers are used, and more time can be given to thinking through the analysis. Researchers should remember to back up their data by storing copies on floppy disks or other computers in several locations and update them regularly. Computers can make the process of qualitative research more manageable especially if a great number of participants are involved. They are, however, merely tools to make the analysis easier. While decisions and judgements are still made by the researcher, searching, cutting and pasting is done by machine. Computers cannot formulate categories or interpret the data, but they might make the analysis more accurate and comprehensive. Health researchers who are not familiar with computer analysis when starting research, should not attempt computer analysis unless they are able to extend their project over a lengthy time period.

Problems and critique

Certain problems emerge, however, when using computers. Seidel (1991: 107), one of the major proponents of computer use in qualitative analysis, warns of 'analytic madness' and states that the use of technology may be a problem that can interfere with appropriate qualitative analysis. He discusses a number of issues. Researchers may be tempted to collect and manage more data than necessary, especially when they have mostly used quantitative methods in the past. The overload of data might prevent them from looking for the most interesting and significant ideas. Instead of searching for deeper meaning in the data, they try to make up for the lack of depth by focusing on the volume of data. There is also the issue of the relationship between researchers and data. This might become mechanistic if analysts do not see the need to examine and evaluate the data carefully. The number of instances of a code or category is often seen as more important than a single significant occurrence just because counting is easy. The lack of scrutiny might prevent the researcher from seeing the real meaning of the phenomenon under study. This also happens occasionally when the data are analysed manually, but the danger becomes greater through the use of computers. Morse and Richards (2002) caution against compulsive activity in computing which can interfere with the process of reflection and engagement with the data. They also maintain that researchers sometimes try to fit the research to the computer program and also homogenise the data, rather than seeing the program as a tool which assists them in the analysis.

Some researchers believe that computing skills are not only unnecessary but that their use could make qualitative research mechanistic and rigid, the very characteristics which might change its lively humanistic nature. Even now, there are some who think this. For instance, Becker (1993) warns the grounded theorist about the use of computers; she feels that computers can prevent sensitivity to the data and the discovery of meanings. Computers might distance researchers from the data. In nursing and midwifery research where emotional engagement and sensitivity is necessary, the use of computers could be problematic.

The distancing of the researcher from the data is another problem in the use of computers. The involvement with a file on a computer or a printed sheet of paper, which is coded by machine, seems less personal than coding and categorising by hand. The researchers have to keep close to the data, immerse in them and engage with them.

In spite of these potential problems, many well-known qualitative researchers use computer programs when conducting a major piece of research. Seidel himself is the developer of the much used computer package *Ethnograph* that helps researchers to identify and retrieve text from documents.

Computers have largely been accepted in qualitative research. In our experience, some funding agencies are impressed by computer packages because their members are used to computers in survey research and often worry about the scientific value of qualitative research. (Computer packages do not, of course, confirm or deny the scientific value or quality of qualitative research, as computer-aided analysis is merely an instrument and as good or bad as the thinking and judgement of the researcher who uses it.) The greatest help from computers lies in the management of data especially when there is a large amount. It is important for researchers, however, not to distance themselves from the data.

Depending on their own stance towards the use of computer-aided analysis, or their individual needs and skills, nurses and midwives can, of course, choose whether or not to use computer-aided data analysis.

Summary

There are a number of different ways in which data are analysed depending on the research question and the approach.

- QDA is complex, iterative and time-consuming.
- Many approaches use coding and categorising which proceeds from a basic to a more abstract level, others apply a more holistic approach and focus on the description of a phenomenon.
- Data analysis is not rigid or prescriptive although there are certain commonalities in most approaches.
- Computers may be a useful tool in the analysis of data, especially in some areas of retrieval, organisation and management, but they should be used with caution.

References

Bazeley, P. (2007) *Qualitative Data Analysis with NVivo*. Thousand Oaks, CA, Sage.

Becker, P.H. (1993) Common pitfalls in grounded theory research. *Qualitative Health Research*, **3** (2), 254–60.

Bluff, R. (2005) Grounded theory: the methodology. In *Qualitative Research in Health Care* (ed. I. Holloway), pp. 147–167, Maidenhead, Open University Press.

Borkan, J. (1999) Immersion/crystallisation. In *Doing Qualitative Research* (eds B.F. Crabtree & W.L. Miller), 2nd edn, pp. 179–94. Thousand Oaks, CA, Sage.

Bryman, A. (2008) *Social Research Methods*, 3rd edn. Oxford, Oxford University Press.

Caqdas Networking Project, University of Surrey. http://caqdas.soc.surrey.ac.uk/index.htm

Dahlberg, K., Dahlberg, H. & Nyström, M. (2008) *Reflective Lifeworld Research*, 2nd edn. Lund, Studentlitteratur.

Fielding, N. & Lee, R. (1998) *Computer Analysis and Qualitative Research*. London, Sage.

Glaser, B.G. (1978) *Theoretical Sensitivity*. Mill Valley, CA, Sociology Press.

Hansen, E.C. (2006) *Successful Qualitative Health Research: A Practical Introduction*. Maidenhead, Open University Press.

Kelle, U. (ed.) (1995) *Computer-Aided Qualitative Data Analysis: Theory, Methods and Practice*. London, Sage.

Langridge, D. (2007) *Phenomenological Psychology*. Harlow, Pearson/Prentice Hall.

Lewins, A. & Silver, C. (2007) *Using Software in Qualitative Research: A Step-by-Step Guide*. London, Sage.

Li, S. & Seale, C. (2007) Learning to do qualitative data analysis: an observational study of doctoral work. *Qualitative Health Research*, **17** (10), 1442–52.

Morse, J.M. & Richards, L. (2002) *Readme First: A User's Guide to Qualitative Methods*. Thousand Oaks, CA, Sage.

Moustakas, C. (1994) *Phenomenological Research Methods*. Thousand Oaks, CA, Sage.

Patton, M. (2002) *Qualitative Evaluation and Research Methods*, 3rd edn. Thousand Oaks, CA, Sage.

Richards, L. (2005) *Handling Qualitative Data: A Practical Guide*. London, Sage.

Seidel, J. (1991) Method and madness in the application of computer technology to qualitative data analysis. In *Using Computers in Qualitative Research* (eds N.G. Fielding & R.M. Lee), pp. 107–18. London, Sage.

Silverman, D. (2005) *Doing Qualitative Research: A Practical Handbook*, 2nd edn. London, Sage.

Silverman, D. (2006) *Interpreting Qualitative Data: Methods for Analysing Talk, Text and Interaction*, 3rd edn. London, Sage.

Tesch, R. (1991) Software for qualitative researchers. In *Using Computers in Qualitative Research* (eds N.G. Fielding & R.M. Lee), pp. 16–37. London, Sage.

Tesch, R. (1993) Personal computers in qualitative research. In *Ethnography and Qualitative Design in Educational Research* (eds M.D. LeCompte & J. Preissle, R. Tesch), 2nd edn, pp. 279–314. Chicago, IL, Academic Press.

Ziebland, S. & McPherson, A. (2006) Making sense of qualitative data analysis: an introduction with illustrations from DIPEx (personal experiences of health and illness). *Medical Education*, **40** (5), 405–14.

Further reading

Auerbach, C.F. & Silverstein, L.B. (2004) *Qualitative Data: An Introduction to Coding and Analysing*. New York, NY, New York University Press.

Gibbs, G. (2007) *Analyzing Qualitative Data*. London, Sage (from the Sage Qualitative Research Kit).

Grbich, C. (2007) *Qualitative Data Analysis: An Introduction*. London, Sage

Lacey, A. & Luff, D. (2007) *Qualitative Data Analysis*, Sheffield Trent RDSU, National Institute for Health Research.

Saldaña, J. (2009) *The Coding Manual for Qualitative Researchers*. Thousand Oaks, CA, Sage.

CHAPTER 18

Establishing Quality: Trustworthiness or Validity

Quality

All research is rightly open to scrutiny from its readers. Health researchers too must not only consider the 'truth value' of their studies but also demonstrate that it is credible and valid for professional practice, and that it has quality. Ways of reflecting on validity have reached a variety of conclusions. No single or unitary concept of validity exists in qualitative research which is comparable to its meaning in quantitative inquiry, and as Onwuegbuzie and Leech (2007: 233) state: 'to date, no one definition of validity represents a hegemony in qualitative research'; no one idea of validity dominates.

There are several distinct perspectives on the quality of qualitative research (Murphy *et al.*, 1998), some of which are listed below. Some believe that

- qualitative and quantitative research should be evaluated by the same criteria;
- qualitative research should be evaluated by criteria that have been specially developed for it;
- criteriology should be rejected.

One group, for instance Maxwell (2005) and Silverman (2006) among many others, argues for the retention of the criteria of reliability and validity while arguing, at the same time, that these criteria cannot be directly translated from quantitative to qualitative research because qualitative inquiry has its own criteria by which it can be evaluated. Indeed validity in qualitative research has different implications and applications. Others (see Seale, 1999), reject evaluative criteria as inappropriate for qualitative inquiry and stress that contextualisation is most important. Although qualitative researchers are flexible and open minded, they are also advised to be systematic and well organised and through this the research gains validity.

Proponents of another group follow the ideas. Lincoln and Guba (1985 initially) and Guba and Lincoln (1989) developed the concepts of trustworthiness and authenticity as parallel and alternative criteria. Researchers will come across both groups of terms during their reading and therefore will have to know about them regardless of the terms they themselves apply. However, a simplistic stance is sometimes taken, and concepts developed here are complex. Different qualitative approaches often take a variety of viewpoints on criteria of quality (Whittemore *et al.*, 2001). Sparkes (2001), too claims that there is no shared understanding of 'good' qualitative research. Researchers find difficulty agreeing on how to judge the 'validity' of qualitative research or how to present convincing evidence of its trustworthiness.

Conventional criteria

We will discuss the traditional criteria generally used in quantitative research, their meaning in qualitative inquiry and their alternatives. Trustworthiness and authenticity are more often used than validity and reliability in qualitative healthcare research, and they are discussed in detail later in the chapter.

- Rigour – trustworthiness
- Reliability – dependability
- Validity – credibility
- Generalisability (external validity) – transferability
- Objectivity – confirmability

Porter (2007) claims that standardising and establishing acceptable criteria for evaluating qualitative research enables writers to create mediating tools by which this type of inquiry can be judged by all readers including those who carry out quantitative research. This means that some form of 'criteriology', might be acceptable although criticised by some such as Seale (1999) or Sparkes (2001).

Rigour

The concept of rigour has its origin in science, and quantitative researchers use it because of its particular connotations with measurement and objectivity; hence it has a more appropriate place in quantitative research. In qualitative research rigour indicates thoroughness and competence. Sandelowski (1986, 1993) wrote two classic articles on rigour in qualitative nursing research. Her latter article recognises that the term rigour could imply inflexibility and rigidity and that researchers should not be too preoccupied with it. Instead she advises they should create 'evocative, true-to-life and meaningful portraits, stories and landscapes of human experience...' (p. 1), and she criticises 'the reduction of validity to a set of procedures' (p. 2). Indeed, excessive rigour may hinder creativity and artistry (Bradbury-Jones, 2007).

Reliability

Reliability in quantitative inquiry refers to the consistency of the research instrument. It is also linked to replicability, that is, the extent to which the study is repeatable and produces the same results when the methodology is replicated in similar circumstances and conditions. As the researcher is the main research instrument in qualitative inquiry, the research can never be wholly replicable. Other investigators have different emphases and foci, even when they adopt the same methods and select a similar sample and topic area.

The researcher's characteristics and background will also influence the research.

Validity

Validity in quantitative research is seen as the extent to which an instrument measures what it is supposed to measure. In qualitative research the concept is more complex. Description and interpretation by researchers and truth telling by participants are all important.

One of the threats to validity is posed when collecting incorrect or incomplete data. The field diary must therefore be detailed and extensive. In interpretation, researchers are in danger of imposing their own ideas or distorting the meaning of the participants' accounts. Therefore it is important for the researcher to listen to the participants' voices and let them speak. Researchers hope that the stories of the participants are true; they do occasionally make mistakes or tell deliberately lies, though the latter seems to be rare. However, this does not mean that there is no truth as the participants describe their world as they see it from their own perspective in the context of their time and culture as well as their own biography. Researchers generally trust their participants even if they cannot prove the 'truth' of their tales. The description by the researcher should not only be plausible but also trustworthy. Researchers set aside their own thoughts and preconceptions about the phenomenon under study at some stage. Alternative and rival explanations to the researchers' own initial interpretation should be taken into account. Although researchers can never be fully certain that all threats to validity have been eliminated, awareness of these threats helps produce a valid piece of research.

To the term validity Hammersley (1998) adds that of *relevance* as a criterion for evaluating qualitative research. Relevance means that explanatory factors should have significance related to the purpose of the research and in solving the problems of practitioners in the discipline. The research must not only be meaningful but also useful for those who undertake it.

Internal validity is the extent to which the findings of a study are true, and whether they accurately reflect the aim of the research and the social reality of those participating in it. This can be established to an extent by taking the findings back to the participants (see the section on member check later in this chapter). The researchers can compare their own findings with the perception of the people involved and explore whether they are compatible. Bryman (2008: 376) adds 'the match between the researchers' observations and the theoretical ideas which they develop.' *External validity*, also called generalisability, is described in the next section.

Generalisability or external validity

This is the most contentious concept linked to validity. For some authors generalisability is not an issue to be discussed at length for they believe it is not relevant as they speak of specific situations and cases. For others, however, it is problematic. Most funding agencies and research committees in the UK National Health Service demand that the proposed research be generalisable, and this is understandable. If large amounts of money are given to researchers, funding bodies wish to know whether the outcomes are of general use in clinical practice and not just the results of 'blue skies' research undertaken for its own sake or only applicable to specific situations.

Generalisability exists when the findings and conclusions of a research study can be applied to other similar settings and populations, i.e. when they can be generalised across a variety of settings. The term has its origin in quantitative research with its random statistical sampling procedures. Random sampling ensures that the results of the research are representative of the group from which the sample was drawn. It is clear that this type of generalisability cannot be achieved in qualitative research in which sampling is purposeful or, in grounded theory, theoretical.

Generalisability is difficult to achieve in qualitative research. Positivist and interpretive research differ in the sense that positivists seek law-like generalities while interpretivists focus on unique cases even though they might want to establish patterns. As much quantitative research – though by no means all – is carried out in the positivist tradition and uses deductive methods, it can be more easily generalised. Many qualitative researchers, however, do not aim to achieve generalisability as they focus on specific instances or cases not necessarily representative of other cases or populations. The case(s) may even be atypical. Indeed the concept of generalisability is irrelevant if only a single case or a unique phenomenon is examined. For instance, a nurse or physiotherapist may want to examine a particular phenomenon important for local practice and patients in a particular area rather than of interest to the whole country. However, the study can still be successful, because it highlights specific non-typical features that can be related and compared to those of other, more typical cases.

Many qualitative researchers attempt to achieve some generalisability, however, because they feel that their research should be useful beyond their own studies. Strauss and Corbin (1998) speak of the representativeness of concepts and applicability of theory to other situations. This means that qualitative research can have external validity through 'theory-based generalisation'. Morse (1994) claims that theory contributes to the 'greater body of knowledge' when it is re-contextualised into a variety of settings. It involves the application of theoretical concepts found in one situation to other settings and conditions. If the theory developed from the original data analysis can be verified in other sites and situations, the theoretical ideas are generalisable. The findings from multi-site studies are, of course, more easily generalisable than those from a few unique cases from one setting.

Objectivity

This is a term often used in quantitative research. This means that the research is free of biases and relatively value neutral. Qualitative researchers do not find this concept very useful. Objectivity and neutrality are difficult to achieve; in fact, the values of researchers and participants become an integral part of the research, and they must openly acknowledge their own subjectivity. They do not conceal it but examine and then set it aside. Critical subjectivity, a term originally coined by Carr and Kemmis (1986) and later developed by other writers such as Reason and Heron (1995), is useful here. Although much knowledge is based on subjective experience it should not be accepted in a simplistic way but rooted in critical consciousness. Researchers do not disregard their subjectivity, they are aware of it and attempt to have self-reflexivity, so no prior assumptions can introduce bias in the study.

Validity in various approaches to qualitative research

The concept of validity is used in phenomenological research, but its meaning and the way in which it is ensured is less precise and prescriptive than in other forms of qualitative research. For instance, Dahlberg *et al.* (2001) state that the research report should not contain any internal contradictions if the researcher wants it to be seen as valid.

Research can be valid through intersubjective knowledge. Moustakas (1994) speaks of 'intersubjective truth'. He states (p. 57) that according to Husserl 'each can experience and know the other, not exactly as one experiences and knows oneself but in the sense of empathy and copresence'. Initially truth is based in the unique perspective of unique individuals and their self-knowledge. As individuals inhabit the world of self and others, there is also communication with others. This enhances intersubjective understanding. If the research is to have validity, its readers will have learnt something of the human condition as well as recognise and grasp the essence of the phenomenon under study. This form of 'validity' is similar to, though not the same as the concept of 'ontological authenticity' described by Guba and Lincoln (1989) or that of 'thick description' by Geertz (1973).

In phenomenology and a number of other approaches such as grounded theory, internal validity (being faithful to the ideas of the participants) is a complex concept as the researchers always transform the data and take them to a different level from that of the participants when they describe the phenomenon or interpret the ideas of the participants. The researchers' ideas are more abstract and theoretical than those of the participants, and ultimately the researchers' description and interpretation is presented to the readers of the account, though they are grounded in the participants' thoughts and feelings. Lomberg and Kirkevold develop the ideas about validity in grounded theory, namely those of fit, relevance, and modifiability (see details in Lomberg and Kirkevold, 2003). Hope and Waterman (2003) discuss the re-conceptualisation of validity in action research, stressing the importance of contextualisation and rigorous application of the chosen approach. (It is not possible to develop ideas on validity in each approach, but we hope that researchers might gain more details from the references).

An alternative perspective: trustworthiness

It can be seen that the conventional terms used in quantitative research have different meanings in qualitative inquiry. Guba and Lincoln (1989), as stated before, go further than this and develop alternative terms and criteria. We will show how health researchers can attempt to demonstrate trustworthiness in the last section of this chapter.

Trustworthiness

Trustworthiness in qualitative research means methodological soundness and adequacy. Researchers make judgements of trustworthiness possible through developing dependability, credibility, transferability and confirmability. The most important of these is credibility.

Dependability

Lincoln and Guba (1985; Guba and Lincoln 1989) use the term dependability instead of reliability. If the findings of a study are to be dependable, they should be consistent and accurate. This means that readers will be able to evaluate the adequacy of the analysis through following the decision-making processes of the researcher. The context of the research must also be described in detail. To achieve some measure of dependability an audit trail is necessary. This helps readers follow the path of the researcher and demonstrates how he or she achieved their conclusions. It also guides other researchers wishing to carry out similar research. Although the study cannot be replicated, in similar circumstances with similar participants, it might be repeated.

Credibility

Credibility corresponds to the notion of internal validity (see p. 252). This means that the participants recognise the meaning that they themselves give to a situation or condition and the 'truth' of the findings in their own social context. The researcher's findings are, at least, compatible with the perceptions of the people under study.

Transferability

Lincoln and Guba use transferability instead of generalisability. This means that the findings in one context can be transferred to similar situations or participants. The knowledge acquired in one context will be relevant in another, and those who carry out the same research in another context will be able to apply certain concepts originally developed by other researchers. It seems to us that the concepts of transferability and generalisability are not too different.

Confirmability

Confirmability has taken the place of the term objectivity. As the research is judged by the way in which the findings and conclusions achieve their aim and are not the result of the researcher's prior assumptions and pre-conceptions, Lincoln and Guba demand 'confirmability'. This again needs an audit or decision trail where readers can trace the data to their sources. They follow the path of the researcher and the way he or she arrived at the constructs, themes and their interpretation. For this, details of the research and the background and feelings of the researcher should be open to public scrutiny. When confirmability exists, readers can trace data to their original sources. Dahlberg *et al.* (2001) also demand intellectual honesty and openness from the researcher, as well as sensitivity to the phenomenon under study thus incorporating the idea of the audit trail although they do not explicitly call it this.

Authenticity

Trustworthiness, which relies on the methodological adequacy of the research, does not suffice according to Guba and Lincoln (1989), and therefore they add the concept of authenticity. A study is authentic when the strategies used are appropriate for the true reporting of the participants' ideas. Authenticity consists of the following.

1. *Fairness:* The researcher must be fair to participants and gain their acceptance throughout the whole of the study. Continued informed consent must be obtained. The social context in which the participants work and live also need to be taken into account.
2. *Ontological authenticity:* This means that those involved, readers and participants, will have been helped to understand their social world and their human condition through the research.
3. *Educative authenticity:* Through understanding, participants improve the way in which they understand other people.
4. *Catalytic authenticity:* Decision making by participants should be enhanced by the research.
5. *Tactical authenticity:* The research should empower participants.

A study is authentic when the strategies used are appropriate for the true reporting of the participants' ideas, when the study is fair, and when it helps participants and similar groups to understand their world and improve it. It means that there is new insight into the phenomenon under study.

Trustworthiness and authenticity are achieved by following certain strategies. Indeed Lincoln and Guba developed and systematised these within their writing. The concept of authenticity has not found the same response in qualitative research as the term trustworthiness, which is now popular as an alternative for validity in qualitative research, especially in the United States.

Strategies to ensure trustworthiness

There are a number of ways in which qualitative researchers can check and demonstrate to the reader whether the research is trustworthy. The most common strategies are the following (although not all of these are accepted by all qualitative researchers):

- Member checking
- Searching for negative cases and alternative explanations
- Peer review (also called peer debriefing)
- Triangulation

- The audit or decision trail
- Thick description
- Reflexivity

It is more likely that the study is trustworthy if researchers have been involved in the setting for a lengthy period of time as this may eliminate the reactivity of participants, because they learn to trust and are more likely to tell the truth, and also because their own assumptions can be examined in the process of prolonged engagement, persistent observation and immersion in the setting. This does not seem problematic for health professionals who are deeply involved with clinical practice. However, they occasionally bring preconceptions to the research and it is important to be aware of these.

Member checking

Throughout interviews and observations, a check is needed on the understanding of the data with the people who are studied. Researchers do this by summarising, repeating or paraphrasing the participants' words. They then ask whether the participants feel that the interpretation is a true and fair representation of their perspective. This is called a *member check* (Lincoln and Guba, 1985) or *member validation*. The main reasons for member checking are the feedback of participants, their reaction to the data and findings, and their response to the researcher's interpretation of the data which are obtained from them as individuals.

The specific purposes of member checking are

- to find out whether the reality of the participants is presented;
- to provide opportunities for them to change mistakes which they feel they might have made;
- to assess the researcher's understanding and interpretation of the data;
- to give the participants the opportunity to challenge the ideas of the researcher.

Feedback from others ensures the trustworthiness of the research, and a member check is one of the strategies for achieving this. The procedure will help avoid misinterpretation or misunderstanding of the participants' words or actions. If a member check is carried out, it is more likely that the researcher presents the participant's point of view. After all, the aim of the study is to give a 'convincing account' (a term used by Seale, 1999) of the participants' different perspectives.

There are a number of ways to carry out member checks:

1. The researcher presents participants with a transcript of their interview or fieldnotes of observations and asks them to comment on the contents. This

is a very time-consuming process, and research participants cannot comment on the researcher's interpretations of their perspectives. Although this is an acceptable procedure, we would not advise undergraduates to do this, because of the time it takes.

2. The interviewer can give the participants a summary of their interview, and his or her own interpretation of their words. This is a more useful way of confirming the ideas and the meaning of the account. The interviewers can discuss their own interpretations and discuss the meaning of the participants' words and actions. It is a check on the understanding of the account. Participants may change meaning and correct errors. The check may also add clarity or trigger and extend ideas that go beyond the original interview. The comments can be included in the final report.

3. The researcher might present the final copy or substantial sections of the report and ask the participants to comment on the contents. Again, this is a lengthy process that demands time commitment and thought from participants, which they may not be able or willing to give. Although all or any of these procedures could be employed, we would suggest the second strategy as the most practical. Member checks do not only help in achieving validity in the study, but they also empower participants and give them control to confirm their words and actions and thus some control in the research itself. Member checking demands a large time commitment from both participant and researcher.

However rigorous and detailed the member check, some problems are inherent in it:

- The researcher's and participants' perspectives may be different.
- The reactions of participants may be defensive.
- The close relationship with the researcher may prevent the participant from adopting a critical stance.
- Perceptions may change over time.
- The researcher develops second-order concepts and theories.

Sandelowski (1993) sees member checking as problematic and complex. She points to the fact that participants and researchers have a different agenda. Members are more interested in their own unique experiences. Researchers wish to portray 'multiple realities', while still representing the experience of each participant.

Some of the issues related to member checks pose ethical dilemmas for the researcher. Participants might become aware and anxious that they have disclosed ideas that might be judged as unacceptable by the researcher or a reader of the report. They might hesitate to disagree because they have built up a close relationship with the researcher whom they see as a friend. Also, if the member check does not take place at an early stage after collection or analysis of the data, the participants might have changed their perceptions, and the researcher has to start again. Change over time is, of course, one of the reasons, why several interviews are better than one, and why prolonged engagement in the setting is useful.

Researchers present the participants' perspectives and the meaning they give to their experiences; however, the data are also transformed so that they become uniquely the researcher's who takes them to a more abstract, theoretical level. Bryman (2008) sums up the problematics of member checking. He claims that researchers write for a readership of scholars and peers. This means that they always take the research to the level of developing concepts, an etic view which includes but goes beyond the participants' perspectives. He also suggests that participants may be defensive of their words or reluctant to be critical and change their minds.

Searching for negative cases and alternative explanations

It enhances the validity of the research if the researchers identify data that do not easily fit into the developing theory or their own ideas. There may also be contrary occurrences that do not easily fit into developing patterns. These may provide alternative explanations. In the critical analysis, researchers may find notions and events that do not fit their explanations and challenge the themes and patterns arising from the data. It means thinking about other possibilities. Data that confirm as well as those that challenge and disconfirm have to be examined. Researchers will have to explore whether conclusions gained from them are appropriate. Indeed, even if there is just one case that does not fit or fits a rival explanation, researchers should try to revise their interpretations so they can become confident that the explanations or interpretations derived from the data are the most valid and plausible and can also account for the alternative case.

Negative or deviant case analysis involves addressing and considering alternative explanations or interpretations of the data', especially those which may be contrary to their own view of reality. Working hypotheses or propositions and search for alternative explanations can then be revised. Single or few 'dissenting voices' included in the final report demonstrate the complexity of the research. Negative case analysis always presents challenges: It is not easy to become aware of discrepant data and negative or alternative cases, but at some stage researchers must stop searching when they feel they have exhausted the alternative possibilities and can account for all the cases including those that are 'deviant'.

Peer review

It is also useful to employ the strategy of peer review or 'peer debriefing' as Lincoln and Guba (1985) called it. This means that colleagues who are competent in qualitative research procedures re-analyse the raw data, listen to the researcher's concerns and discuss them. Peers can be given the draft copy at the end of the research. They might detect bias or inappropriate subjectivity and try alternative explanations to the researcher's own working propositions and warn them against the attempt to 'fit' interpretations and explanations that cannot be substantiated by the data.

> **Example of peer debriefing**
>
> Holloway, Sofaer and Walker carried out research with people who had chronic back pain. After the collection of the data, they analysed them individually and then decided together to use those categories that in their collective view best described the experience of the participants.
>
> Holloway *et al.*, (2007)

The example cited above shows that peer review is not problematic when colleagues who review have been involved in the research. Morse (1994) states, that it can become more difficult if peers have not had any direct connection with the study, as they are less able to judge from the outside. However, peer review can be a useful tool to confirm some of the main ideas emerging from the research and to ensure coherence and plausibility.

Triangulation

Another important strategy to establish validity is to adopt triangulation procedures. Triangulation is the process by which the phenomenon or topic under study is examined from different perspectives. Triangulation in research means that the findings of one type of method (or data, researcher, theory) can be checked out by reference to another. This will provide a way of establishing whether there is generalisability in the research although researchers do not necessarily aim for this. Denzin (1989) differentiates between several types of triangulation as listed below.

- *Data triangulation*, where researchers use multiple data sources and obtain their data from different groups, settings or at different times (multiple sources of data). Data triangulation is the most common way of triangulating.
- *Investigator triangulation*, when more than one expert researcher is involved in the study. This is common in larger studies but rarely happens in student projects or theses.
- *Theoretical triangulation*, when the researcher employs several possible theoretical interpretations in the study. Competing explanations or interpretations are developed and tested against each other to find the one which is most likely to describe or explain the phenomenon.

- *Methodological triangulation*, when researchers use two or more methods in one study to answer a similar question (observations, interviews, documents, questionnaires). These are either between-method or within-method triangulation (see below).

The last method in the list is most often used in a small-scale dissertation. Researchers might consider confirming findings using one method with the findings of another. It is not always necessary, though occasionally desirable, to use quantitative methods to confirm qualitative findings, that is, using 'between-method' triangulation. Morse (2001: 210) gives a number of possibilities for triangulation, each of which has different emphases. Studies using quantitative and qualitative methods can be used simultaneously or sequentially depending on the main direction of the research and its underlying assumptions. Morse claims (p. 209) that they may generate 'a more complete understanding'.

Example of between-method triangulation

Not only does Williamson (2005) discuss the concept of triangulation but he also tries to illustrate its use in nursing research, in a mixed method action research study. In his study on the work roles of lecturer practitioners in a university and a healthcare setting, he employed a number of strategies. The between-method strategies included questionnaire surveys as the quantitative element, while he also used focus group interviews, diaries and other techniques.

However, it is more common to check observations with answers from qualitative interviews or documents and thus stay within the same methodology; this is called 'within-method' triangulation. It can include interviews and observations, diaries or other data sources. Indeed some researchers might argue that this has better 'fit' with the research view of qualitative researchers.

Example of within-method triangulation

Cloherty *et al.* (2004) developed an ethnographic study which aimed to explore mothers' and healthcare professionals' expectations, beliefs and actions concerning the supplementation of breast feeding of babies in a postnatal ward and new baby unit. The strategies adopted were both interviewing and observation of mothers and professionals. Observed behaviour was analysed and interviews took place with mothers and health professionals.

Triangulation takes place when the same phenomenon has been examined in different ways or from different perspectives. Triangulation does not, of course, automatically demonstrate the trustworthiness of the study. It is used to give more depth to the analysis and enhance its validity, although it cannot guarantee it.

The audit or decision trail

All research should have an audit trail by which others are able to judge, to some extent at least, its validity. Halpern (1983) initially discussed the inquiry audit in qualitative research, and Lincoln and Guba (1985) developed the concept of the audit trail. The audit trail is the detailed record of the decisions made before and during the research and a description of the research process. Rodgers and Cowles (1993) suggest four types of documentation:

1. Contextual
2. Methodological
3. Analytic
4. Personal response

   The *contextual* documents should contain excerpts from fieldnotes of observation and interviewing, the description of the setting, people and location. The political and social context must also be described. Rodgers and Cowles suggest that *methodological* documents include methodological decisionmaking and the rationale for these decisions. *Analytic* documents consist of reflections on the analysis of data and the theoretical insights gained. *Personal response* documents describe the thought processes and demonstrate the self-awareness of the researcher. This self-examination is part of 'reflexivity' discussed later in this chapter. An account of the decisions that were made throughout should be incorporated into the research account to point. Cutcliffe and McKenna (2004) do point out, however, that an audit trail is not always necessary though advisable for novice researchers.

Thick description

Thick description too, helps to establish the truth value of the research and is linked to the audit trail. The term was coined originally by the philosopher Ryle but developed by Geertz (1973); it means a detailed description of the process, context and people in the research, inclusive of the meaning and intentions of the participants and the researcher's conceptual developments. Thick description provides a basis for the reader's evaluation of quality.

   Thick description is an account of the complex processes in a specific context and a rich and 'holistic' and even 'artistic' portrayal of the phenomenon under study. Readers of the research report should be able to follow the research trail, empathise with the participants and draw similar conclusions to the researcher. There is a chance, however, that the research is not seen as useful if the reader cannot transfer the insight gained from the research to other settings, particularly in the healthcare arena. If the contextual description is rich and the analytical language comprehensive enough to enable readers to understand the processes and interactions involved in the context, it might be possible to generalise to the extent of stating that people in other settings have a similar way of understanding. Thick description necessitates immersion and prolonged engagement in the setting (see also Chapters 7 and 10).

Reflexivity

Reflexivity means that researchers critically reflect on their own preconceptions and monitor their relationships with the participants and their own reactions to participants' accounts and actions. As the main tool of the research, researchers are part of the phenomenon to be studied and must reflect on their own actions, feelings and conflicts experienced during the research. If they adopt a self-critical stance to the research and their own role, relationships and assumptions, the study will become more credible and dependable. A self-critical stance throughout the inquiry process and location in political and social context enhances the quality of the research. Reflexivity is ongoing through data collection, analysis, interpretation and writing up (see also Chapter 1).

Quality and creativity

There is an essential tension between the focus on method and creativity, which is sometimes neglected by those who endlessly grapple with validity and its equivalents. There is no complete consensus about the quality of qualitative research and the criteria adopted. Whittemore et al. (2001) add secondary criteria to those outlined by some of the writers mentioned before.

The obsession of qualitative researchers with validity and related issues is due to a defensive stance in relation to the critics of qualitative research by positivist writers. Sparkes (2001) claims that the topic of validity will remain unresolved and different perspectives on it can coexist because of the variety of epistemological and ontological stances. However, we suggest that as long as qualitative inquiry is seen as 'not really' valid by quantitative researchers, those who undertake qualitative studies will have to explain why their work is credible, and that the quality criteria by which to judge it are useful devices to demonstrate this.

Cho and Trent (2006) maintain, however, that just because certain techniques and strategies have been used to establish validity or trustworthiness, there are still no guarantees that the knowledge obtained is valid, especially as the researcher has transformed the data and interpreted the findings.

Whatever labels health professionals apply, they have to demonstrate that their research has truth value, and they should be consistent in the language, concepts and methods used to demonstrate this.

Summary

There are several distinct schools of thought about criteria for judging qualitative inquiry.

- Qualitative researchers use either the conventional criteria of validity and reliability or alternatives such as trustworthiness and authenticity. There are a few writers who do not see the need to make it explicit but there is no shared understanding of the concepts.
- Strategies to ensure the quality of the research include member checking, the search for alternative cases, peer debriefing, triangulation, disclosing an audit trail, thick description and reflexivity.
- It is important for researchers to spend time in the setting and immerse themselves in this.

References

Bradbury-Jones, C. (2007) Enhancing rigour in qualitative research: exploring subjectivity through Peshkin's I's. *Journal of Advanced Nursing*, **59** (3), 290–8.

Bryman, A. (2008) *Social Research Methods*, 3rd rev. edn. Oxford, Oxford University Press.

Carr, W. & Kemmis, S. (1986) *Becoming Critical: Education, Knowledge and Action Research*. London, The Falmer Press.

Cho, J. & Trent, A. (2006) Validity in qualitative research revisited. *Qualitative Research*, **6** (3), 319–40.

Cloherty, M., Alexander, J. & Holloway, I. (2004) Supplementing breast-fed babies in the UK to protect their mothers from tiredness or distress. *Midwifery*, **20** (2) 194–204.

Cutcliffe, J.R. & McKenna, H.P. (2004) Expert qualitative researchers and the use of audit trails. *Journal of Advanced Nursing*, **45** (2), 126–35.

Dahlberg, K., Drew, N. & Nyström, M. (2001) *Reflective Lifeworld Research*. Lund, SWE, Studentlitteratur.

Denzin, N.K. (1989) *The Research Act: A Theoretical Introduction to Sociological Methods*, 3rd edn. Englewood Cliffs, NJ, Prentice-Hall.

Geertz, C. (1973) *The Interpretation of Cultures*. New York, NY, Basic Books.

Guba, E.G. & Lincoln, Y.S. (1989) *Fourth Generation Evaluation*. New York, NY, Sage.

Halpern, E.S. (1983) *Auditing Naturalistic Inquiries: The Development and Application of a Model*. Unpublished doctoral dissertation. Indiana University (cited by Rodgers and Cowles (1993) qv).

Hammersley, M. (1998) *Reading Ethnographic Research: A Critical Guide*, 2nd edn. London, Longman.

Holloway, I., Sofaer-Bennett, B. & Walker, J. (2007) The stigmatisation of people with chronic pain. *Disability and Rehabilitation*, **29** (18), 1456–64.

Hope, K.W. & Waterman, H.A. (2003) Praiseworthy pragmatism? Validity and action research. *Journal of Advanced Nursing*, **44** (2), 120–7.

Lincoln, Y.S. & Guba, E.G. (1985) *Naturalistic Inquiry*. Beverly Hills, CA, Sage.

Lomberg, K. & Kirkevold, M. (2003) Truth and validity in grounded theory – a reconsidered realist interpretation of the criteria: fit, relevance and modifiability. *Nursing Philosophy*, **4** (3), 169–200.

Maxwell, J.A. (2005) *Qualitative Research Design: An Interactive Approach*, 2nd edn. Thousand Oaks, CA, Sage.

Morse, J.M. (1994) Designing funded qualitative research. In *Handbook of Qualitative Research* (eds N.K. Denzin & Y.S. Lincoln), pp. 220–35. Thousand Oaks, CA, Sage.

Morse, J.M. (2001) Qualitative verification: building evidence by extending basic findings. In *The Nature of Qualitative Evidence* (eds J.M. Morse, J.M. Swanson & A.J. Kuzel), pp. 203–20. Thousand Oaks, CA, Sage.

Moustakas, C. (1994) *Phenomenological Research Methods*. Thousand Oaks, CA, Sage.

Murphy, E., Dingwall, R., Greatbatch, D., Parker, S. & Watson, P. (1998) Qualitative research methods in health technology assessment. *Health Technology Assessment*, **2**, 16.

Onwuegbuzie, A.J. & Leech, N.L. (2007) Validity and qualitative research: an oxymoron? *Quality and Quantity*, **41** (2), 233–45.

Porter, S. (2007) Quality, trustworthiness and rigour: reasserting realism in qualitative research. *Journal of Advanced Nursing*, **60** (1), 79–86.

Reason, P. & Heron, J. (1995) Co-operative inquiry. In *Rethinking Methods in Psychology* (eds J.A. Smith, R. Harré & L. Van Langenhove), pp. 122–42. London, Sage.

Rodgers, B.L. & Cowles, V. (1993) The qualitative audit trail: a complex collection of documentation. *Research in Nursing and Health*, **16** (3), 219–26.

Sandelowski, M. (1986) The problem of rigour in qualitative research. *Advances in Nursing Science*, **8** (3), 27–37.

Sandelowski, M. (1993) Rigor or rigor mortis: the problem of rigour in qualitative research revisited. *Advances in Nursing Science*, **16** (2), 1–8.

Seale, C. (1999) *The Quality of Qualitative Research*. London, Sage.

Silverman, D. (2006) *Interpreting Qualitative Data*, 3rd edn. London, Sage.

Sparkes, A. (2001) Myth 94: qualitative health researchers will agree about validity. *Qualitative Health Research*, **11** (4), 538–52.

Strauss, A. & Corbin, J. (1998) *Basics of Qualitative Research: Techniques and Procedures for Developing Grounded Theory*, 2nd edn. Thousand Oaks, CA, Sage.

Whittemore, R., Chase, S.K. & Mandle, C.L. (2001) Validity in qualitative research. *Qualitative Health Research*, **11** (4), 522–37.

Williamson, G. (2005) Illustrating triangulation in mixed-methods nursing research. *Nurse Researcher*, **12** (4), 7–18.

Further reading

Payne, G. & Williams, M. (2005) Generalization in qualitative research. *Sociology*, **39** (2), 295–314.

Rolfe, G. (2006) Validity, trustworthiness and rigour: quality and the idea of qualitative research. *Journal of Advanced Nursing*, **53** (3), 304–10.

CHAPTER 19

Writing up Qualitative Research

The research account

Writing the report of the research is an important task for the researcher; the presentation is in the public domain and can be reviewed by others. Researchers submit the results of their work to external examiners, commissioning or funding agencies, or to a journal for peer review either in the academic or professional arena. If the study is a thesis or dissertation, the candidate will have guidelines for presentation and these should be followed. Although conventions for writing up exist, the format may vary from one institution to another. The research report mirrors the proposal though the latter is more detailed and, of course, includes the findings and discussion. There are alternative forms of presenting findings which will be discussed later.

Writers must take into account the potential readership; there is a clear difference between reports that are written for practitioners in the clinical setting, those for funding bodies, and a research dissertation or thesis. Employers and practitioners are more interested in the results and implications of the research for practice and less concerned with philosophical and theoretical issues, while academics see the latter as important and value the process of learning how to research. Occasionally health professionals or academic writers feel it is more appropriate to write two separate reports on the research, one for the university in which they are taking their degree and the other for the practice setting. In all these reports, anonymity and confidentiality of the research participants are essential elements.

The format should match the research design; in a qualitative thesis, the rationale and the methodology section sets a frame for the research. Readers and reviewers must be able to follow all the procedures and processes of the study, thus ensuring that the methods and logic of the study are explicit and open to public scrutiny (see Chapter 18 for audit trail). Background and prior assumptions of the researcher must also be divulged to others. On a practical level it is useful to have a style sheet, similar to the sheet that journal editors present to article writers, where the researcher notes down all the consistent elements, such as certain spellings, the type of referencing both in the chapters and at the end of the dissertation or report, the format for headings and other aspects, so this can be used throughout the report (advice from Wolcott, 2001). Many students lack consistency in style and spelling.

Supervisors will generally ask their own students to write an outline for the research well before they attempt to write a full draft so that they have a tentative structure.

Use of the first person

When writing up introduction and methodology, it is better that researchers write in the first person to show that they are accountable for their actions. It sounds pompous and dull when they state 'the researcher has found...the author does...the writer considers...' etc., and Webb (2002), in an editorial for the *Journal of Advanced Nursing*, claims that first person writing is more reader-friendly. Qualitative research – and increasingly quantitative research – does not proceed in an objectified and neutral way. Gilgun (2005) too, advocates the use of the first person because researcher roles become integrated into the study. Researchers can use the first person when they describe what they themselves chose to do. For instance, researchers would not say when speaking about their own actions 'the author chose a sample, or the researcher used the methods...' etc. They might write 'I chose a purposive sample of...I collected the data through...'. It is important, however, that the first person is not overused, and the use of 'I think, I feel, I believe' throughout is not appropriate. Those who do not wish to use the first person might choose the passive form (although this is not considered good English); for instance 'a purposive sample was chosen...' etc. Wolcott (2001) confirms:

> 'Recognising the critical nature of the observer's role and the influence of his or her subjective assessments in qualitative research makes it all the more important to have readers remain aware of that role, that presence. Writing in the first person helps authors achieve those purposes. For reporting qualitative research, it should be the rule rather than the exception.'
>
> (Wolcott, 2001: 21)

Geertz (1988) warned two decades ago against the 'author evacuated text'; Charmaz and Mitchell (1996) speak of the 'myth of silent authorship' and encourage the inclusion and presence of the writer in the text. This means writing sometimes in the first person.

The format of the report

The structure of a qualitative report is often organised in the following sequence, though this may differ between studies:

- *Title*
- *Abstract*
- *Table of contents* (in some guidelines this appears after acknowledgements)
- *Acknowledgement and dedication*
- *Introduction*
  - Background and rationale (justification) for the study, including its aim
  - Initial literature review (or overview of the literature)
- *Entry issues and ethical considerations*
- *Methodology and research design*
  - Description and justification of methods (including type of theoretical framework such as symbolic interactionism or phenomenology)
  - The sample and the setting
  - Specific techniques and procedures (such as interviewing or observation)
  - Data analysis
  - Trustworthiness and authenticity (or validity and reliability, depending on the terms used)
- *Findings/results and discussion*
- *Conclusion and implications*
- *Reflections on the research*
- *References*
- *Appendices*

Qualitative writing may differ substantially from a quantitative report, although commonalities exist. The main distinction lies in the flexibility of the qualitative report. The findings and discussion are the most important elements of the final write-up (see Ponterotto and Grieger, 2007 for advice on communicating qualitative research).

A list of abbreviations, acronyms, and/or a glossary of terms employed and written in alphabetical order, is useful before the first chapter or at the end of the study. The first time the terms are mentioned in the writing, they have to be written in full, with the abbreviations in brackets. From then on, abbreviations can be used.

Title

The title of a study is important, especially if it is presented as a student project, dissertation or thesis because it is the first and most immediate contact the reader has with the research, and its impact on judging the work can be considerable. We would argue for a concise but informative title which sounds interesting but not facetious. It must be remembered that it is initially a working title and may change when some of the research has been done, so it can encompass emergent ideas.

Examples of titles

Impact of euthanasia on primary care physicians in the Netherlands.
                                                    (van Marwijk *et al.*, 2007).
Recovery in Anorexia Nervosa: The struggle to develop a new identity.
                                                    (Newell, 2008)
Self within a climate of contention: Experiences of chronic fatigue syndrome.
                                                    (Travers and Lawler, 2008)

Writers often use explanatory subtitles; Silverman (2005) for instance prefers two-part titles. The title gives a clear and succinct picture of the study's content. Punch (2005) advises that the title should not be long but contain all essential information. Novice researchers sometimes include redundancies in the title such as 'A Study of ...' 'Aspects of ...' or 'Inquiry', 'Analysis', 'Investigation'. These clutter up the title. Although the title should reflect the aim of the research it would be clumsy to give the whole aim in the title. Questions usually do not make good titles, although there may be some exceptions.

The title page in a dissertation or thesis contains the title, the name of the researcher, the year and the name of the educational institution at which the student was enrolled. There is generally a pro forma for the title page at most universities. They also specify other details for the finished dissertation such as word allowance or size of margins. Obviously this differs for other types of research.

Abstract

The abstract is a summary of the study and is written when the research is completed. In a dissertation or thesis it appears on the page behind the title but before the table of contents and the full report. The abstract provides the reader with a brief overview of the research question and aim, methods adopted, and the main findings of the study. It might include the implications of the study in one or two succinct sentences.

Depending on the size and type of study, the abstract should contain between 200 and 500 words, usually contained in one sheet of A4 paper in single spacing and often written in the past tense. Writers should keep to the word limit specified for them by the university or commissioning agency and be selective about the content. Journal editors too, specify the form of the abstract which may be structured.

Example of article abstract

The stigmatisation of people with chronic back pain

Abstract

Purpose

This study responded to the need for better theoretical understanding of experiences that shape the beliefs, attitudes and needs of chronic back patients attending pain clinics. The aim was to explore and conceptualise the experiences of people of working age who seek help from pain clinics for chronic back pain.

Methods

This was a qualitative study, based on an interpretative phenomenological approach (IPA). During in-depth interviews in their homes, participants were invited to 'tell their story' from the time their pain began. Participants were 12 male and 6 female patients, aged between 28 and 62 years, diagnosed as having chronic benign back pain. All had recently attended one of two pain clinics as new referrals. The interview transcripts were analysed thematically.

Findings

Stigmatisation emerged as a key theme from the narrative accounts of participants. The findings expose subtle as well as overt stigmatising responses by family, friends, health professionals and the general public which appeared to have a profound effect on the perceptions, self esteem and behaviours of those interviewed.

Conclusions

The findings suggest that patients with chronic back pain feel stigmatised by the time they attend pain clinics and this may affect their attitudes and behaviours towards those offering professional help. Theories of chronic pain need to accommodate these responses, while pain management programmes need to address the realities and practicalities of dealing with stigma in everyday life.

(Holloway *et al.*, 2007)

The abstract for a thesis or dissertation is generally a little longer than that for an article. It does not need to include the rationale of the study or an introduction. All important information is included.

Example of abstract for thesis

The lived experience of final-year student nurses of learning through reflective processes

This scientific phenomenological study aims to explore and better understand the lived experience of learning through reflective processes, the nature, meaning and purpose of reflective learning, what is learned and the triggers and processes that enable meaningful reflective activity. Ten final year nursing students who felt that they had experienced learning through reflective processes were invited to describe their lived experiences of the phenomenon during taped phenomenological interviews. The rich and contextualised data were analysed using the four steps for descriptive phenomenological analysis proposed by Giorgi (1985).

The findings essentially differentiate between authentic reflective learning which enables the emergence of 'own knowing', and the academically driven activities often perceived as 'doing reflection'. Authentic and significant personal 'own knowing' is derived from reflective activity prompted by unpredictable, arbitrary occurrences experienced in everyday encounters in the professional and personal worlds of the participants which stimulate meaningful existential questions that, in turn, demand attention and drive the commitment to ongoing reflection. Engagement with authentic reflective activity is often triggered by an insistent and personal 'felt' sense of a need to understand and know 'something more for the self', and this activity demands far more privacy than the contemporary literature acknowledges.

On the cusp of registered practice, the participants described how the maturation of reflective activity had enabled them to engage with the struggle to locate themselves personally and professionally in the context of care, to establish and refine personal and professional values and beliefs and to consider the realities of their nursing practice. Reflection enabled the participants to recognise and affirm that they had become nurses and could fulfil the role to their own and others' expectations. Their reflective knowing and understanding was active and embodied in the way they lived their nursing practice.

Analysis of the lived experience of learning through reflective processes has raised a number of issues for nurse education, in particular how student nurses may be supported in coming to know themselves and to become reflective, the importance of supportive mentorship and the significance of role modelling in professional development, the psychological safety of the 'practicum' and the need for privacy for authentic reflective learning.

(Rees, 2007).

The abstract is the 'public face' of the research as it appears on databases, websites and in abstract books, so it is of major importance in the research. Alexandrov and Hennerici (2007) maintain that the abstract determines whether the work might be chosen for presentation and communicated in a readable and appropriate way.

Acknowledgement and dedication

Traditionally all researchers, especially PhD or MPhil candidates give credit to those who supported, advised or supervised the research, and they also acknowledge the input of the participants. Often the writing is dedicated to particular individuals such as parents or spouses. Sometimes writers overwork and exaggerate 'thank you notes' or dedications, but of course, acknowledgement of others' help is important.

Contents

Academic research reports have a table of contents before its main chapters begin. It cannot be finished before the whole project is finalised and written. The content is sectioned into chapter headings and subheadings with page numbers. In an undergraduate student project, the table of contents should be concise and need not be too long and detailed.

Introduction

Background and rationale

In the introduction the writer informs the audience about the research question or topic. The introduction consists of the background and context of the research as well as the aim – the overall purpose of the project. Writers explain why they have become interested in the question, how their project relates to the general topic area, and what gap in health knowledge might be filled by the new research through linking the question to the potential implications for practice. In the introduction, the researcher explains the significance of the study for the clinical setting and how it could improve clinical practice or policy. Researchers need to justify the chosen topic, and why it is relevant for the profession and for themselves at this time. The background section sets the scene for the study. It is useful for the researcher to ask the 'so what?' question to keep the background section relevant.

Initial literature review (or overview of the literature)

This section can stand on its own, or it can become an integral part of the introduction. The literature in qualitative studies has a different place from that in quantitative research. Of course it must show some of the relevant research that has been done in the field. The researchers summarise the main ideas from these studies, their problems and contradictions, and they show how these papers relate to the project in hand. It is important in qualitative reports not to explore every piece of research in the field at the start of the study, nor to give a critical review of *all* the literature but the main foundational studies, those which are specifically relevant and up-to-date recent research. Gaps in knowledge become apparent at this point. At this stage, the research question is linked to the literature (see Chapter 3 for more detail on literature review). By the end of the introductory section, the reader should be in no doubt that qualitative research, in the form suggested by the researcher, was most appropriate to meet the research aim.

Entry issues and ethical considerations

Health researchers describe entry and ethical issues (see Chapters 3 and 4). It must be stated how the participants were approached, for instance whether researchers advertised on a notice board or approached the potential participants personally. How did researchers gain permission from gatekeepers, those in the position of power to grant access to the setting (managers at various levels and local research ethics committees)? If patients are involved, their consultants or GPs might have to be asked for their permission if they are still under treatment.

Last, but most importantly, health professionals should make explicit how the ethical principles were followed in the study, and how the participants' rights were protected. It is important that individual participants cannot be recognised in the report. To have permission from ethics committees might be essential, but it does not necessarily ensure that the researcher behaves ethically!

Methodology and research design

The methodology chapter includes several subsections: the research design and methodology; the methods, including data collection, sampling, detailed interviewing or observation procedures and a description of the data analysis. In qualitative research, the methodology is of particular interest because the researcher is the main research tool and has to make explicit the path of the research, so that the reader knows about the details of design, biases, relationships and limitations and is able to follow the decision trail. Hence the methodology section is often longer than its equivalent in a quantitative study.

Description and justification

The research design usually includes the main methods and the theoretical framework. Researchers briefly describe the methodology they adopt and the reasons and justification for it. They also explain the fit between the research question and the methodology.

The sample and setting

The sample is described in detail. Not all purposive sampling is fixed from the beginning (for instance, not in grounded theory (GT)). The writer describes the informants, who they were, how many were chosen and the reasons for the choice. Researchers tell the reader how they obtained their sample and portray the setting in which the study took place. If there is theoretical sampling, this must also be explained (see Chapter 11).

Example 1: People and setting

[For instance] Thirty mothers, seventeen midwives, four neonatal nurses, three paediatricians, three senior house officers and three healthcare assistants were interviewed in the postnatal ward and newborn-baby unit over a period of nine months.

(from Cloherty *et al.*, 2004)

Example 2: Theoretical sampling

[For instance] The sample was not predetermined but depended on the concepts relevant to the emerging theoretical ideas. It seemed that older people tended to adhere to the advice of GPs more than the young. I approached a number of young people for the study to follow this up.

Or

Fear of loss of control seemed to arise as a major element in the study through progressive focusing. I explored this with a further sample and went back to some of the original participants to examine this concept.

Specific techniques and procedures

The methodology section gives information about the data collection. The researcher describes the procedures such as interviewing, observation or other strategies that were used and any problems encountered. The outline should not be a general essay on procedures but a step-by-step description of the work in hand so that the reader can follow it closely. It is necessary that researchers give the reasons for using a particular methodology and research strategies and describe the procedures of collecting data. The reader should know how the data were collected and stored.

> **Example**
>
> The data were collected through unstructured interviews (with an aide mémoire) which took place in the informants' own homes and were tape-recorded with their permission. Interviews lasted between one and three hours. I transcribed the interviews and locked the numbered transcriptions safely away from the list of informants' names. Collection and analysis of data took place simultaneously as is usual in GT. (A dissertation or thesis needs more descriptive detail.)

Data analysis

The data analysis needs to be explained and should include the ways in which data were coded and categorised and how theoretical constructs were generated from the data. It is useful, and essential in dissertations or theses, to give examples from the study. A detailed account of the chosen type of analysis is required. The readership is entitled to know whether a computer analysis was used.

> **Example of data analysis in grounded theory research**
>
> Using guidelines based on the GT approach of . . . (here the particular type of GT would be given, i.e. Strauss and Corbin, Glaser or Charmaz for instance), data were collected (a detailed description of the data collection procedures is necessary here) and analysed simultaneously. The method of analysing data by 'constant comparison' is one of the unique features of the GT approach. The data were coded, categorised and constantly compared (detailed examples should be given) to produce concepts grounded in the data. Through theoretical sampling, I followed theoretical concepts that had relevance to the emerging theory. Comparison with the data and the sampling of ideas in the literature were continued until saturation occurred and no new data of relevance to the developed theory emerged.

If this were a dissertation or thesis, more detail and examples of each step should have been presented, so that the audit trail is clearly demonstrated.

Trustworthiness

This section will demonstrate how the researcher ensured the validity (trustworthiness) of the research (see Chapter 18 for a discussion of this topic).

Findings/results and discussion

There are several ways to present qualitative findings and discussion. The first is written in the traditional format in which findings and discussion are separated and follow one another. Findings without discussion and comments do not always make a good storyline; therefore the findings and discussion are often integrated. This gives more meaning to the report and shows the storyline more clearly (but again, no rigid rule exists about this). Some writers present a brief summary of the results in a diagram, and then discuss each major category (or construct, or theme) in a few sentences before starting the findings and discussion chapter. In each chapter the data the researcher collected are discussed first. The relevant literature is integrated into the discussion where it fits best and serves as additional evidence for the particular category or as a challenge to the findings of the researcher. A dialogue with the literature needs to be ongoing throughout the research.

Telling the tale

In a qualitative report writers tell a story which should be vivid and interesting as well as credible to the reader. This sometimes means writing and rewriting drafts until a storyline can be discerned clearly. Although there may be similarities with journalism or fiction, writers have to keep in mind that research accounts have a different purpose, namely to give an accurate and systematic analysis of the data and a discussion of the results. A good qualitative study need not be dry and mechanistic but reflects the researcher's involvement. The events, the people and their words and actions should be made explicit, so that readers can experience the situation in a similar way to the researcher, albeit with the researcher's interpretations or more abstract descriptions of the phenomenon under study. The communicative element is of special importance in the presentation of qualitative research so it can make an impact on its readers and remind them that the participants are 'real' people. Holloway (2005: 282) reminds researchers that scientific writing need not be incomprehensible but should capture the audience's attention, have immediacy and present a good story.

The use of quotes from participants

Direct and verbatim quotes from interviews or excerpts from the fieldnotes are inserted at an appropriate place to show some of the data from which the results emerged. Sandelowski (1994) lists some of the uses of quotes in qualitative studies and argues that they give insight into people's experiences and their meanings and interpretations of the situation and illustrate the arguments of the researcher. The content of the quotes helps the reader to judge how the findings were derived from the data, to help establish the credibility of the emerging categories or themes and provide the reader with a means of auditing these. The writers, of course, must take care that the quotes convey the meanings and feelings of the participant and are directly connected with the themes the research seeks to illustrate. Sandelowski gives importance to both content and style of quote. A direct quote of the participants' words in a study makes the discussion more lively and dynamic. Long rows of quotes or continuous duplication are not needed, and frequent very short quotes might make the study look fragmented. The choice of quotes should demonstrate that the data come from a wide range of participants rather than just one or two, except when the researcher explores deviant or negative cases. The quotes, according to Green and Thorogood (2004), are indeed examples of particular concepts to demonstrate to the reader that the ideas discussed are based in the data. Corden and Sainsbury (2006: 98) point out that quotes help to 'clarify the links between data, interpretation and conclusions'. They report that participants valued the inclusion of their own words as they felt their voices were heard and represented. Corden and Sainsbury advise researchers to consider carefully the ethical issues involved with using quotes such as, for instance, protection of identity and anonymity.

The use of quotations from the literature

Trying to give substance to their own arguments, inexperienced health researchers often quote the words of experts. This can interrupt the storyline of the research. Sometimes it is better to avoid a quotation when it can be paraphrased or summarised, but of course, the idea should still be credited to the originator.

When a specific phrase is critical and written by a well-known expert or author of a classic text on the field of study, a quotation can be used. Occasionally it does enhance a piece of writing and is appropriate. When using substantial quotes from books or articles, page numbers should be given.

We must warn researchers of two common mistakes. First, researchers often write in a very complex way and use incomprehensible terminology. In their fear of sounding simplistic and not academic, researchers in the field of healthcare often complicate and obscure simple and clear issues. It is important to express ideas in clear and unambiguous terms, although they should not, of course be simplistic. The second flaw is linked to a lack of analysis. It is not enough to simply give a collection of lengthy quotes and summarise their content. This is not analysis. Researchers have to develop their theoretical ideas and interpretations, build them into the study and then illustrate them with the relevant quotes from the participants.

Conclusion and implications

Generally studies end with a conclusion. The conclusion is a summary of the findings in context. It must be directly related to the results of the specific study, and no new elements (or references) should be introduced here unless they are necessary. The conclusion reviews what has been learnt in relation to the aim, the theoretical ideas and propositions that emerged from the study. Dramatic and overly assertive conclusions can be dangerous and pretentious in a small project. Novice researchers seldom generate 'formal theory' or come to significant conclusions; their research is small in scope – though extensive in depth; however, the modest scope does not mean that the piece of research has no importance or implications for the clinical area.

Woods (2005) has a list of considerations for the conclusion. He asks researchers whether their writing has answered the questions asked, whether there are weaknesses and limitations, and how these can be addressed. Of course, it is important to demonstrate that the study has added to knowledge in the field. The conclusion often provides a new light on the topic. The conclusion should be placed in the context of conclusions of other studies, the more general framework of the area under study and how it fits within the global picture of the topic. The full discussion of relevant related literature has been given however in previous chapters as is usual in qualitative research.

In health research and other projects for clinical and professional settings, the conclusion contains the implications and, if appropriate, the recommendations that could be made on the basis of the results. The implications can be integrated into the conclusion, they can be discussed towards its end or they can form a separate section following on from the conclusion. The implications must be based *directly* on the findings of the study which has just been completed; all too often they are not linked sufficiently to the findings, or based on the work of other researchers. Any significant policy implications can also be addressed here.

Some researchers tend to overestimate the importance of their research, and this can be avoided as readers are sceptical about exaggerated claims.

To check the quality of their conclusion researchers might ask the following questions:

Why have I included this here? (on reflecting about a statement)

What are the main issues arising from the data?

How has the study achieved its aim(s)?

What were the answers to the research question?

What is new and different in my research?

How has it contributed to knowledge?

How does it fit within the wider framework of the knowledge and advances in this topic area?

What are the implications for the profession or policy that derive from my study? (Not from other people's work!)

Reflections and reflexivity

Many academic researchers reflect on their project and adopt a critical stance to it, usually towards the end of their dissertation or thesis. They demonstrate how the research could be improved, extended or illuminated from another angle. At this point they might point to its limitations and their own biases, which they might not have made explicit in the main body of the study and describe some of the problems they encountered. Not all studies contain this reflective section and sometimes they are part of the conclusion. Nurses and other health professionals who take a reflective stance could discuss at this point how they have professionally and personally developed and changed through the research. The description of their own location in the research is called reflexivity (see Chapter 18).

A statement about validation of a qualitative study by a survey or other quantitative methods might suggest a lack of awareness that a qualitative study can stand on its own, has its own validation procedures and cannot be judged from the quantitative researcher's point of view, but occasionally a direction for a different type of research might have to be indicated.

Referencing

For academic studies the Harvard system of referencing is generally used, but other formal systems of referencing may be acceptable to the students' supervisors, journals or funding bodies. It is best to find out about this before the start of the study from supervisors, course leaders or handbooks and journals. Sometimes slight variations in advice are given in libraries, but the information must be correct and detailed in a research report. Sloppy references are the cause of criticism and might well generate 'a negative halo effect'.

The writer should compare the references in the text with the selected bibliography and make sure that every reference is included. We often find that student referencing is incomplete, incorrect or insufficient. Page (the singular) is shortened to p.; pages – the plural – to pp. but for journals the pp. or p. is usually left out. The title of the book or the name of the journal should be underlined or written in italics. Page numbers are stated in the references when an article in a journal is given, or a chapter in an edited book is referenced. Direct quotations from books or articles need page numbers after name and date (for instance: Smith 2008: 7 – or – Smith 2008, p. 7; Smith 2008, pp. 7–11).

Educational institutions, within certain parameters, may have their own rules about referencing. Publishers of books and articles, too, use different ways of referencing. In this book for instance we follow the guidelines of our publisher.

Appendices

A table of informants (with pseudonyms), their ages, experience or length of service is sometimes included by writers (making sure, however, that anonymity is preserved, particularly when the participants or informants might easily be recognised). An interview guide and a sample interview transcript (in a study that uses interviews) could be attached as an example for the reader to help in understanding the development of the data collection. Some fieldnotes from observations might be given to demonstrate their use. Appendices depend on the advice given to researchers and on their own common sense, but there should not be too many sections. Sometimes researchers attach the formal initial letter to participants or an example of the letter of permission. A copy of the letter of approval from the ethical committee should be attached, and where appropriate, the researcher blocks out the address and location of the research. The words in appendices do not count as part of the study.

The appendices (plural of appendix) are placed at the very end of the study after the bibliography in the order in which they appear in the chronology of the study. For instance, the example of the initial letter to participants would be placed before the exemplar of an interview transcript. Universities might have their own rules about the use of appendices or footnotes.

Critical assessment and evaluation

Researchers must be aware that the readers of a research study or report evaluate and judge the quality and credibility of the research and look for particular components and details. For these reasons a short guide to evaluating qualitative inquiry follows which is based on a number of writings by others, such as Horsburgh (2003), Ryan *et al.* (2007) and Green and Thorogood (2004). It is clear that many, though not all the criteria and issues for appraisal are different and distinct in qualitative research. The checklist below contains important factors to consider when evaluating a qualitative research study. It would be useful for researchers to examine their own study in the light of these elements.

Guide to appraisal

The research question and method:

Is the research problem or question suitable and feasible for qualitative research?
Is there a clear rationale for the study and the methodological approach?
Does the study show that the data of the researcher have priority?

The abstract:

Does it state the aim and describe the methodology and methods, (including sampling)?

Does it summarise results, conclusions and implications?

The literature:

Is there an initial overview that demonstrates the gap in knowledge?

Are there connections to existing and relevant theories?

Has the appropriate literature related to the findings been integrated into the study?

Are the references comprehensive, relevant and up-to-date, and do they include some foundational texts?

The sample:

Does the researcher use purposive sampling (including theoretical sampling if appropriate)?

Are the criteria for sampling made explicit?

Is the sampling explained adequately?

Is the type and size of sample justified?

Entry and ethical issues:

Does the researcher state how he or she gained access to the participants?

Were the rights of participants safeguarded (including their right to withdraw from the study)?

Are issues of anonymity and confidentiality discussed in relation to the study?

Are issues of power taken into account?

If vulnerable clients are included in the sample, is this inclusion justified?

Are major ethical issues discussed?

Has the study been approved by ethics committees and review boards?

Data collection and analysis:

What are the data sources, and are they appropriate for the study?

How are the data collected, transcribed and stored?

Is the method of analysis identified and described (with examples)?

Is the data analysis systematic and detailed?

(In GT: do data collection and analysis interact?)

The findings and discussion:

Is the presentation of the findings appropriate for a qualitative approach?
How have these findings been discussed in relation to the literature?
Does the researcher explain the trustworthiness (validity) of the study?
Is the 'audit trail' traced in detail?
How have these issues been managed?
Is there an element of reflexivity?

Conclusions and implications:

Has the study met its aim?
Does the conclusion clearly state what was learned from the research?
Do the conclusions come directly from the data?
Are the implications for clinical practice discussed?
Do they emerge directly from the findings of the study?

Publishing and presenting the research

If the findings are significant, the researcher has the responsibility to disseminate them to a wider group such as colleagues and other health professionals.

Books

Sometimes health professionals produce a book based on their thesis or a chapter in an edited book. Most publishers have guidelines for writing book proposals. The proposal then goes to their editorial board to decide whether the book is worth publishing, in their view, and commercially viable. If their proposal is not accepted the study might be too esoteric or not interesting for a larger market. Commercial considerations are the main concern of publishers, and these depend on the general appeal of the piece of research. Editors are, of course, also concerned about the quality of the content and the ability of the researcher to write clearly and in an accessible style.

Articles

More often, students who have carried out research publish an article in a professional or academic journal, often with their supervisor. The length and style of the article will depend on the type of journal; for instance, articles in the *Journal of Advanced Nursing* are more academic and generally longer than those in the *Nursing Times*. Articles have higher standing in research circles than chapters in books because articles in important academic journals are refereed by experts in the field and count more in the research assessment exercise.

The detailed guidelines for scripts are laid out at the front or the back of the journal. Some journal editors want a very detailed description of the methods adopted (for instance the journal *Midwifery*), others claim that a well-known and widely published methodology, such as GT – can be summarised rather than discussed in great detail (*Sociology of Health and Illness*). Writers must take into account the different styles and guidelines of these journals. As a long research study cannot be fully discussed in article format, researchers choose what to include or exclude. For example, just one chapter, one category or a methodological issue might form the basis of the article. Journal editors or academics sometimes speak of 'salami slicing' the research; this practice is appropriate for lengthy and in-depth studies which cannot be reported in a single article.

It is important to write in a lively manner in an article or a book based on qualitative research. This can be achieved through a good storyline and enhanced through vignettes or excerpts from interviews or fieldnotes, taking into account, of course, that individuals should not be recognised in the descriptions. Good diagrams might clarify some of the aspects of the work. Different journals address different audiences.

Types of article

The book by Corbin and Strauss (2008) states that three types of paper are published in journals, intended for different readership:

1. For academic colleagues
2. For practitioners
3. For lay readers

Articles for academic colleagues

There are those colleagues who have a particular interest in the theoretical and methodological framework as well as in the research topic and implications of the findings for practice. The *Journal of Advanced Nursing, Physiotherapy: Theory and Practice, Midwifery* and *Qualitative Health Research*, for instance, are examples for journals publishing this type of article and have high impact rating for the Research Assessment Exercise. Even the *British Medical Journal* has recently had articles on qualitative research. The journals *Qualitative Research* and *Qualitative Inquiry* deal mainly with methodological issues but are not nursing publications (*Qualitative Inquiry* and *Qualitative Health Research* are journals published in the United States while *Qualitative Research* is published in Britain). *Nurse Education Today* covers educational issues and research in nurse and midwifery education. The *International Journal of Nursing Studies* and the *Journal of Clinical Nursing* are also high-ranking journals from the United Kingdom, but there are many others. The academic standard of some journals is high, and their editors and reviewers demand high standards in their articles.

Articles for practitioners

Examples of journals intended to assist practitioners are *Nursing Times* or *Senior Nurse* or the *British Journal of Midwifery*. There are many others, and their language is more accessible for professionals. In these journals one can find articles which describe findings and address the implications of these findings for clinical practice. Often the writers of these articles develop ideas that assist in the understanding of patients or the work of nurses and midwives.

Articles for the lay reader

Some articles are meant for lay readers. Although most nurse and midwife researchers do not write for this readership, occasionally an article in a specialist magazine could actually help members of a group or the general population. For instance, an article on research into hormone replacement therapy in a women's journal might give information to women, though it would have to be short, clear and accessible. It is necessary that researchers write with integrity and factual accuracy.

Student articles

All students carrying out PhD or MPhil and even MA/MSc research should attempt writing articles; some universities encourage this during the process of the research, others suggest writing after completion of the research degree. There is an academic tradition that candidates publish with their supervisors who, of course, have had a major input in the research and will help in refining the article, critiquing it and possibly writing sections for it. Nevertheless, the student's, not the supervisor's, name should be first on the list of authors. In early articles it is useful to seek the help and advice of supervisors who know the different journals and their editors' styles and preferences.

It is very useful for all students to publish, if their work is acknowledged as valuable by their supervisors or managers, as they not only get used to disseminating their research, but also because it will eventually enhance their status within the profession. Burnard (2004) notes that the research project is not properly finished until the findings have been published and Evans (2008: 1) even adds that 'research that is not written up is wasted'.

Alternative forms of presenting or disseminating the research

There are a variety of ways to present or disseminate qualitative research. Keen and Todres (2007) describe some of these non-traditional forms which might include theatrical performances, dance, poetry or others. One student who is undertaking a PhD, for instance, is writing a play based on her research with old people, others have presented films which are rooted in the research with patients. Some of alternative forms of presenting the data or findings evoke strong feelings in the audience (see Chapter 15 on performative social science).

Summary

The main points to remember when writing up research are listed below.

- Qualitative research provides flexibility for writing research accounts.
- The structure of a qualitative report might be different from that of a quantitative study.
- Ethical issues and access must be addressed.
- The findings and discussion are the major part of the study in which the literature is integrated.
- Reports in qualitative health research need a strong conclusion with implications for the profession and/or clinical practice directly based on the findings.
- The research should be presented in an interesting way which communicates with the reader.
- To be of use in practical terms, the research needs to be disseminated.

References

Alexandrov, A.V. & Hennerici, M.G. (2007) Writing good abstracts. *Cerebrovascular Diseases*, **23** (4), 256–9.

Burnard, P. (2004) Writing a qualitative report. *Nurse Education Today*, **24** (3), 174–9.

Charmaz, K. & Mitchell, R.G. (1996) The myth of silent authorship: self, substance and style in ethnographic writing. *Symbolic Interaction*, **9** (4), 285–302.

Cloherty, M., Alexander, J. & Holloway, I. (2004) Supplementing breast-fed babies in the UK to protect their mothers from tiredness or distress. *Midwifery*, **20** (2), 194–204.

Corbin, J. & Strauss, A. (2008) *Basics of Qualitative Research: Techniques and Procedures for Developing Grounded Theory*, 3rd edn. Los Angeles, CA, Sage.

Corden, A. & Sainsbury, R. (2006) Exploring 'quality': research participants' perspectives on using quotes. *International Journal of Social Research Methodology*, 9 (2), 97–110.

Evans, R. (2008) Getting the message across. *Qualitative Researcher*, (8), 1.

Geertz, C. (1988) *Works and Lives: The Anthropologist as Author*. Palo Alto, CA, Stanford University Press.

Gilgun, J.F. (2005) Grab and good science: writing up the results of qualitative research. *Qualitative Health Research*, 15 (2), 256–62.

Giorgi, A. (1985) *Phenomenology and Psychological Research*. Pittsburgh, Duquesne University Press.

Green, J. & Thorogood, N. (2004) *Qualitative Methods for Health Research*. London, Sage.

Holloway, I. (ed.) (2005) Qualitative writing. *Qualitative Research in Health Care*, pp. 270–86. Maidenhead, Open University Press.

Holloway, I., Sofaer-Bennett, B. & Walker, J. (2007) The stigmatisation of people with chronic back pain. *Disability and Rehabilitation*, 29 (18), 1456–64.

Horsburgh, D. (2003) Evaluation of qualitative research. *Journal of Clinical Nursing*, 12 (2), 307–12.

Keen, S. & Todres, L. (2007) *Communicating Qualitative Research Findings: An Annotated Bibliographic Review of Non-Traditional Dissemination Strategies*. Bournemouth University.

van Marwijk, H., Haverkate, I., van Royen, P. & The, A. (2007) The impact of euthanasia on primary care physicians in the Netherlands. *Palliative Medicine*, 21 (7), 609–14.

Newell, C. (2008) *Recovery in Anorexia Nervosa: The Struggle for a New Identity*. PhD Thesis, Bournemouth University.

Ponterotto, J.G. & Grieger, I. (2007) Effectively communicating qualitative research. *Counseling Psychologist*, 35 (3), 404–30.

Punch, K.F. (2005) *Developing Effective Research Proposals*, 2nd edn. London, Sage.

Rees, K. (2007) *The Lived Experience of Final Year Student Nurses of Learning Through Reflective Processes*. PhD thesis, Bournemouth University.

Ryan, F., Coughlan, M. & Cronin, P. (2007) A step by step guide to critiquing research. Part 2: qualitative research. *British Journal of Nursing*, 16 (12), 738–44.

Sandelowski, M. (1994) The use of quotes in qualitative research. *Research in Nursing and Health*, 17 (6), 479–83.

Silverman, D. (2005) *Doing Qualitative Research: A Practical Handbook*, 2nd edn. London, Sage.

Travers, M.K. & Lawler, J. (2008) Self within a climate of contention: experiences of chronic fatigue syndrome. *Social Science and Medicine*, 66 (2), 315–26.

Webb, C. (2002) Editorial: How to make your article more readable. *Journal of Advanced Nursing*, 38 (1), 1.

Wolcott, H.F. (2001) *Writing up Qualitative Research*, 2nd edn. Thousand Oaks, CA, Sage.

Woods, P. (2005) *Successful Writing for Qualitative Researchers*, 2nd edn. London, Routledge.

Further reading

Canter, D. & Fairbairn, G. (2006) *Becoming an Author: Advice for Academics and Other Professionals*. Maidenhead, Open University Press.

Heinrich, K. (2008) *A Nurse's Guide to Presenting and Publishing: Dare to Share*. Cambridge, MA, Jones & Bartlett.

Holliday, A. (2007) *Doing and Writing Qualitative Research*, 2nd edn. London, Sage.

Lester, J.D. (2007) *Principles of Writing Research Papers*, 2nd edn. New York, NY, Penguin.

Murray, R. (2004) *Writing for Academic Journals (Study Skills)*. Maidenhead, Open University Press.

Glossary

Abstract: A concise summary or synopsis of the research stating the aim, nature and scope of the study and its implications.

Action research: A cyclical approach to research in which researchers are, or collaborate with, practitioners to effect change or use an intervention, evaluate it and modify their practice in the light of evaluation. The process goes on until the optimum situation has been achieved.

Aide mémoire: Key words or short questions that aid the memory of the researcher and focus on areas of interest or importance for the researcher during in-depth interviewing.

Analytic induction: An approach to analysis that involves inductive processes and which makes inferences from the specific to find general rules or theories.

Appendix (pl: appendices): Additional material at the end of the study. It is not included in the word limit and is located either before or after the bibliography (depending on institutional rules).

Assumption: A belief or assertion which is taken for granted by the researcher but has not been verified.

Auditability: Research is auditable if readers or other researchers are able to follow the methodological processes of the first researcher.

Audit trail (or decision trail): A detailed explanation of the decision-making processes of the researcher to demonstrate the logic and development of the research path.

Authenticity: A term used to demonstrate that the findings of a research project are representative of the participants' perspectives, that the study is fair and helps participants to understand their social world and improve it.

Autoethnography: An approach in ethnography where researchers and their own thoughts and feelings are at the centre of the research.

Bias: A distortion or error in the data collection, analysis or interpretation which has its origin in strongly held values or feelings of the researcher or an individual participant.

Bracketing (in phenomenology): Taken-for-granted assumptions and presuppositions about a phenomenon are suspended and the researcher focuses on the phenomenon itself.

Case study: Research with and on a single unit of study such as an organisation, a person or a subculture which is bounded by time and location.

Category: A group of concepts and ideas with similar characteristics that form a unit of analysis.

Causality: A link between cause and effect.

Code: A label given to specific data.

Coding (in analysis): Examining and breaking down the data. Assigning a name to a specific datum.

Concept: An abstract or generalised idea that describes a phenomenon.

Concept mapping: Linking and relating concepts and presenting the interrelationship in a diagram.

Constant comparison (in grounded theory): Qualitative data analysis where each datum is compared with every other piece.

Construct: A construct encompasses a number of concepts or categories and has a high level of abstraction. The term is often used for a major category that has evolved from the reduction of a number of smaller categories.

Constructionism: An approach in social science based on the assumption that human beings construct their social reality, and that the social world cannot exist independently of human beings. In research terms this means that participants and researcher construct meaning together.

Contextualisation: Researchers link the data and findings to their context.

Core category (in grounded theory): A concept that links with all other categories in the project and integrates the data.

Criterion (pl criteria): A standard by which something is evaluated.

Criterion-based sample: See purposive sample.

Critical incident technique: A data collection and analysis technique focusing on critical situations, events and incidents in the research setting.

Critical theory: The view that people can critically evaluate social phenomena and change society in order to become emancipated.

Data (plural): The information collected for the research.

Data analysis: Organisation, reduction and transformation of the data by exploring meanings of research participants. Researchers search the data for concepts and categories.

Deduction: The procedure of testing a general principle or hypothesis to explain specific phenomena or cases.

Delimitations: The boundaries of the research such as inclusion or exclusion.

Description: A detailed account of the significant phenomenon or phenomena in the research to generate a picture of the world as seen by the participants.

Design: The overall plan of the research, including methods and procedures for collecting, analysing and interpreting data.

Dross rate: Information obtained from participants which is irrelevant to the outcome of a particular study.

Emic perspective (anthropological term): The 'insider's' point of view (see also etic perspective).

Epiphany: A sudden revelation or turning point in a person's life.

Epistemology: The theory of knowledge concerned with the ways in which human beings know the world.

Ethnography: Research that is concerned with a description of a culture or group and its members' experiences and interpretations. It is both the research process and the completed product, that is, the research report.

Etic perspective: The outsider's view, the perspective of the researcher (see also emic perspective).

Exhaustive description (in phenomenology): Writing that aims to capture and describe the intensity and depth of the participants' experience.

External validity: Generalisability (see generalisability).

Field: The location or setting where the research takes place.

Fieldnotes: A record of observations in the field.

Fieldwork (initially a term from anthropology): The collection of data outside the laboratory, in the field.

Focused interview: An interview in which questions are focused on emerging and relevant issues (see also funnelling).

Focus group: A group of people with similar experiences or common traits who are interviewed as a group in order to obtain their thoughts and perceptions about a particular topic.

Funnelling: The process of interviewing that starts with a broad basis and becomes progressively more specific during the interview process (see also focused interview).

Gatekeepers: Those individuals who have the power to permit or restrict access to an organisation, a setting or people.

Generalisability: The extent to which the findings of the study can be applied to other events, settings or groups in the population.

Grounded theory: A research method which generates theory from the data through constant comparison.

Hermeneutics: A branch of phenomenology that focuses on the interpretation rather than the description of a phenomenon.

Heterogeneity: The extent to which units of a sample are dissimilar in characteristics important for the study.

Homogeneity: The extent to which units of a sample are similar in traits important for the research.

Hypothesis: An assumption or statement of a relationship between variables which can be tested, verified and falsified.

Idiographic methods: Methods focused on the unique and individual. These differ from nomothetic methods (qv) that seek law-like generalities subsuming individual cases.

Immersion: The process whereby researchers stay in, learn about and become completely familiar with the field.

Inclusion criteria (singular 'criterion'): Factors or conditions that are taken into account on selection of a sample and which are included in the sample.

Induction: A reasoning process in which researchers proceed from the specific and concrete to general and abstract principles.

Informant: A person as a member of the group under study participates in the research and helps the researcher to interpret the culture of the group (see also key informant).

Informed consent: A voluntary agreement made by participants after having been informed of the nature and aim of the study.

Interpretivism: An approach in social science that focuses on human beings and the way in which they interpret and make sense of their reality.

Interviewer effect (see also observer effect): The effect of the researcher's presence on the research.

Interview guide: Loosely formed questions which are used flexibly by the interviewer in in-depth interviews.

Interview schedule: Standardised questions which are used by the quantitative researcher who uses the same sequence and wording for each respondent (Qualitative researchers use an interview guide rather than a schedule).

In vivo *code* (in grounded theory): Codes in which the researcher uses the words of the participant as a label.

Iteration: Continuous movement between parts of the research text and the whole, between raw data and analysed data.

Key informant: (in ethnography): A long-standing member of a culture or group who has expert knowledge of its rules, customs and language.

Limitations: Weaknesses, restrictions and incompleteness of the research (not always used in a negative way).

Member check: Checking and verification of the data or interpretations of the researcher by participants.

Memoing: Notes of varying degrees of abstraction when carrying out fieldwork.

Method: Procedure and strategy for collecting, analysing and interpreting data.

Methodology: The framework of theories and principles on which methods and procedures are based.

Narrative: The description of experiences by the participants. The reconstruction of their lives or experiences.

Nomothetic methods: The search for law-like generalities or rule-following behaviour that subsumes individual cases (see also idiographic methods).

Objectivity: A neutral and unbiased stance.

Observer effect: See interviewer effect.

Ontology: A branch of philosophy concerning the nature of being. It is related to assumptions about the nature of reality.

Paradigm: A theoretical perspective or approach to reality recognised by a community of scholars. A position that provides the researcher with a set of beliefs to guide the research.

Participant observation: Observation in which the researcher becomes a participant in the setting or culture under study.

Phenomenon: The central concept to be researched: in phenomenology (qv), the meaning of the experiences in the life world of the participant in a study.

Phenomenology: A philosophy which explores the meaning of individuals' lived experience through their own description. The research approach adopted is based on this philosophy.

Pilot study: A small-scale trial run of a research interview or observation.

Positivism: A direction in the philosophy of social science which aims to find general laws and regularities based on observation and experiment parallel to the methods of the natural sciences.

Premature closure: Arriving too early at explanation or theoretical ideas.

Progressive focusing: See funnelling.

Proposition: A working hypothesis which consists of linked concepts. It establishes some regularities and relationships between categories.

Pseudonym: Fictitious names given to informants to protect their anonymity.

Purposive (or purposeful) sample: A judgemental sample of individuals chosen by certain pre-determined criteria relevant to the research question (also called criterion-based sample, qv).

Reactivity: Participants react to the presence of the researcher. The researcher also reacts to the responses of the participants.

Reflexivity: Reflecting on and critically examining the researcher's location research.

Reliability: The ability of a research tool to achieve consistent results.

Research aim: The intention of the researcher to uncover something about the phenomenon under study in order to answer the research question.

Research question: The problem or statement that guides a study and establishes the baseline for other questions.

Rigour: High standard in research which seeks detail, accuracy, trustworthiness and credibility.

Saturation: A state where no new data of importance to the specific study and developing theory emerge and when the elements of all categories are accounted for.

Serendipity: A chance and unexpected discovery during data collection.

Storyline: An analytic description and overview of the story told in the research.

Subjectivity: A personal view influenced by personal background and traits.

Symbolic interactionism: An interpretive approach in sociology that focuses on meaning in interaction.

Tacit knowledge: Implicit knowledge that is shared but not openly articulated.

Theoretical sampling (in grounded theory, qv): Sampling which proceeds on the basis of emerging, relevant concepts and is guided by developing theory.

Theoretical sensitivity (concept developed by Glaser): Sensitivity and awareness of the researcher to detect meaning in the data.

Theory: A set of interrelated concepts and propositions that attempts to explain social phenomena.

Thick description (concept developed by Geertz): Dense, detailed and conceptual description which gives a picture of events and actions within the social context.

Triangulation: The combination of different methods of research, data collection approaches, investigators or theoretical perspectives in the study of one phenomenon (e.g. qualitative and quantitative methods, interviews and observation, etc.).

Validity: The extent to which the researcher's findings are accurate, reflect the purpose of the study and represent reality (validity in qualitative research differs from that in quantitative research).

Verification: Empirical validation after testing a hypothesis; in qualitative research, testing a proposition or a working hypothesis.

Index